This book is due for return not later than the last
date stamped below, unless recalled sooner.

COMPUTATIONAL MODELING OF TISSUE SURGERY

WITPRESS

WIT Press publishes leading books in Science and Technology.
Visit our website for the current list of titles.
www.witpress.com

WITeLibrary

Home of the Transactions of the Wessex Institute, the WIT electronic-library provides the
international scientific community with immediate and permanent access to individual
papers presented at WIT conferences. Visit the WIT eLibrary at www.witpress.com

COMPUTATIONAL MODELING OF TISSUE SURGERY

Editors

M.E. Zeman
Katholieke Universiteit Leuven,
Belgium

M. Cerrolaza
Universidad Central de Venezuela,
Venezuela

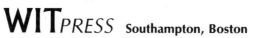

WITPRESS Southampton, Boston

Computational Modeling of Tissue Surgery

Series: Advances in Bioengineering, Vol. 1

Editors: M.E. Zeman & M. Cerrolaza

Published by

WIT Press

Ashurst Lodge, Ashurst, Southampton, SO40 7AA, UK
Tel: 44 (0) 238 029 3223; Fax: 44 (0) 238 029 2853
E-Mail: witpress@witpress.com
http://www.witpress.com

For USA, Canada and Mexico

WIT Press

25 Bridge Street, Billerica, MA 01821, USA
Tel: 978 667 5841; Fax: 978 667 7582
E-Mail: infousa@witpress.com
http://www.witpress.com

British Library Cataloguing-in-Publication Data

A Catalogue record for this book is available
from the British Library

ISBN: 1-85312-749-3
ISSN: 1464-9292

Library of Congress Catalog Card Number: 2004116355

Contents

Chapter 7
Structural analysis for pre-surgery planning: two applications in
dentistry and urology 163
C. Bignardi, E. Zanetti & G. Marino

Chapter 8
A numerical evaluation of the posterior cruciate ligament reconstruction on
the biomechanics of the knee joint 181
N.A. Ramaniraka, A. Terrier, N. Theumann & O. Siegrist

Chapter 9
Tissue modeling and visualization using virtual reality 207
O. Rodríguez, R. Carmona, E. Coto & H. Navarro

Chapter 10
Biomechanics and the cyber-infrastructure: delivering the bone and other
models to the surgeon 235
T. Impelluso and C. Negus

Preface

From an engineering perspective, biomechanics is an important and interesting discipline relating medical and natural sciences. Understanding the effects of mechanical influences on the human body is the first step towards the development of innovative models to study these effects. In recent decades, the evolution of computational modeling has been drastically determined by the increasing power and speed of data transfer, visualization and other technological tools. This positive impact has inspired a new approach to study the human body and its structures.

This book provides valuable information on the different methods to model, simulate and analyze hard and soft tissues, which is one of the many subjects concerning biomechanics. All of these techniques aim to develop tools that can offer a meaningful input in the medical practice. The book was written by very well known researchers from many disciplines, who are currently working to understand and describe the interaction of tissues and functionality.

The first chapter of the book is devoted to describing how experimental results from a bone chamber are complemented with simulations of a computational model, oriented to describe the mechanoregulation of bone tissue differentiation and adaptation around endosseous implants. Adaptation of trabecular surface is modeled and studied in Chapter 2 using real geometry microCT images for reconstruction. The methodology of 3D geometry reconstruction in order to build individualized models is another relevant topic addressed in Chapter 3. These results show the importance of accurate geometry reconstruction and material properties for medical purposes. A relevant application of this is shown in Chapter 4, when making the reconstruction of a femur with osteoporosis and modeling the effects of antiresorptive drugs. In Chapter 5 an interesting application related to femur behavior with an implant is discussed. A broad explanation about the influence of different modeling factors in numerical simulations of pre- and post-hip implant surgery situations is then presented in Chapter 6. This type of report is of extreme importance when modeling for pre-surgery planning; this topic is described in Chapter 7, showing applications in dentistry and urology.

Soft tissue is another important field where computational modeling has become a main issue in biomechanics. Knee ligaments reconstruction evaluated using numerical models is addressed in Chapter 8.

Nowadays it is mandatory to consider (and to use) the great possibilities that virtual reality offers to medical applications. The two last chapters of this book present the development of simulation platforms, which includes the numerical analyses of the models to be represented.

Although the applications of computational modeling in biomechanics are enormous and many different trends have been developed worldwide, this book attempts to show the state-of-the-art regarding some particular issues.

The editors would like to acknowledge all the authors for their great contributions to this book and encourage them to keep their enthusiasm and curiosity in order to get a better understanding of the biomechanics of the human body as well as its interaction in the presence of biomedical devices.

M.E. Zeman & M. Cerrolaza
Leuven, Belgium, May 2005

CHAPTER 1

Mechanobiology of bone regeneration and bone adaptation to achieve stable long-term fixation of endosseous implants

L. Geris[1], H. Van Oosterwyck[1], J. Duyck[2], I. Naert[2] & J. Vander Sloten[1]
[1]*Division of Biomechanics and Engineering Design, Katholieke Universiteit Leuven, Belgium.*
[2]*Department of Prosthetic Dentistry, Katholieke Universiteit Leuven, Belgium.*

Abstract

The success or failure of the clinical application of endosseous implants lies in the adequacy of the host to establish and maintain osseointegration. Although the success rate for implants is generally high, failures still occur. Mechanical loading has been identified as an important factor for both early and late biological failure. These phenomena are studied here by means of a representative member of the endosseous implants family: the oral implants. Early biological failure is a process of bone regeneration that has mostly been studied during fracture healing in long bones. Different theoretical models aim to describe these observed processes and employ different mechanical and biological parameters to drive the regeneration process. Several of these models were implemented to simulate the process of peri-implant tissue differentiation in an *in vivo* bone chamber. Qualitative agreements can be noted between the numerically predicted and experimentally observed tissue patterns in the chamber. Late biological failure has often been attributed to inappropriate implant loading. Numerous animal experiments show a distinct influence of the various types of loading on bone adaptation. Theoretical models aim to capture these observations in mathematical expressions. From an anatomical finite element model the peri-implant only part of the marginal bone loss could be related to overload. To further explore the relation between marginal bone resorption and overload one of the theoretical models was implemented. A redistribution of the peri-implant bone stresses caused by the removal of peri-implant tissue experiencing overload put a hold on the marginal bone resorption.

1 Introduction

The use of implant-supported oral prostheses for the treatment of partially and fully edentulous patients has nowadays grown into a viable alternative to removable dentures. Implants are installed into the jaw bone tissue and transfer the occlusal loads, exerted on the prosthesis to the surrounding bone. The key to a successful clinical application of oral implants lies in the establishment and maintenance of a direct connection between the implant surface and the surrounding bone tissue, without any intervening fibrous tissue layer. This is commonly termed osseointegration [1]. However, most definitions of this term remain rather vague with respect to the actual histological, physico-chemical and mechanical nature of the implant-bone interface in case of osseointegration. In most cases direct implant-bone contact is judged on a light microscopic examination of the interface, but electron microscopic studies have revealed that the implant-bone interface is much more heterogeneous at the ultrastructural level [2].

Although the clinical outcome for different commercial implant systems is in general highly successful [3], failures still occur. Failures can be divided into mechanical failure and biological failure. While a mechanical failure refers to fracture of an implant component, mostly due to fatigue, a biological failure can be defined as the inadequacy of the host to establish or to maintain osseointegration. The inability to establish osseointegration during the healing phase can be regarded as an early failure, whereas the inability to maintain the achieved osseointegration, under functional conditions, may be considered a late failure. Clinically, lack of osseointegration is generally characterized by implant mobility. A fibrous tissue layer may have developed at the interface with the mobile implant. Biological failure may also be associated with excessive marginal bone loss (i.e. bone loss around the implant neck (cf. fig. 1)), although the implant may remain clinically stable.

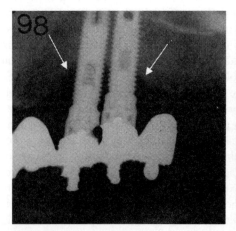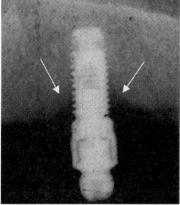

Figure 1: Röntgenograms of orals implant with excessive marginal bone loss. The crater-shaped bone defect is clearly visible (arrows).

The conservation of the marginal bone plays a crucial role in the long-term clinical success of an implant.

1.1 Early biological failure

Early implant failure can be defined as the inadequacy of the host to establish osseointegration. The bone regenerative processes at the bone implant interface are strongly influenced by the initial surface properties of the implant and the mechanical environment at the site.

Kasemo and Lausmaa [4] described the biological and chemical interactions that take place at the interface of a (bio)material, starting from the nanometer scale up to the macroscopic level. They argued that the interaction of the (bio)material surface and the biological environment is determined by the chemical composition, the (micro)structure and the topography of the surface. These are, in turn, controlled by the history (manufacturing, cleaning, environmental contamination, sterilization) of the (bio)material. Apart from its chemical composition, the implant surface can strongly vary in terms of microstructure and morphology, which are partly determined by the grain structure of the underlying metal, and partly by the oxidation conditions. When the implant is brought into the biological tissue a complex cascade of chemical and biological reactions take place at different spatial and time scales. After the initial hydration of the surface, biomolecules (like proteins) adsorb to the surface. It is likely that the nature of the biomolecule layer has an influence on the cell type that proliferates at the implant surface.

It is well accepted that mechanical factors play a role in bone regeneration, although the exact nature remains unknown. Many groups tried to qualify and quantify the exact contribution of the mechanical loading to tissue differentiation and bone regeneration, either by means of animal experiments [5–8] or numerical simulations [9–19]. One common result of these studies is that severe implant loading in the early stages of the regenerative process will lead to the establishment of a fibrous tissue layer around the implant, preventing osseointegration taking place.

Section 2 deals in greater detail with the topic of bone regeneration. It starts with an overview of the biology involved in bone regeneration. Next, a series of theoretical models describing the process of bone regeneration is presented, followed by the application of several of these models in the simulation of the peri-implant tissue differentiation in an *in vivo* bone chamber.

1.2 Late biological failure

Considering late biological failures two major etiological factors were suggested: infection and mechanical loading. Several clinical studies investigated the relation between oral hygiene (plaque accumulation) and marginal bone loss, but contradictory results were reported [20, 21]. Based on a study of Esposito *et al.* [3] it seems that plaque is not an important etiological factor for marginal bone loss in case of machined ("smooth") implant surfaces, like e.g. the Brånemark implant. However, for implants with a rougher surface, plaque-induced marginal bone loss could play a more important role, since the rough surface may promote plaque accumulation.

A number of animal experiments showed that overload can lead to excessive marginal bone resorption or even complete loss of osseointegration [22–24]. This does not however prove that the same is true in a clinical situation. A number of clinical studies hypothesized that marginal bone loss can be correlated with unfavorable prosthesis design and parafunctional habits (clenching, bruxism), both possibly leading to overload [21, 25, 26]. The risk of excessive marginal bone loading due to high bending moments was recognized by many authors. However in none of these clinical studies where excessive marginal bone loss was observed were the implant loads actually quantified.

In contrast to this overload theory, others suggested underload (disuse atrophy) to be responsible for marginal bone decrease. Pilliar *et al.* [27] reported bone loss around the smooth collar of endosseous implants that were installed in dog mandibles. They argued that due to the lack of retention, stresses cannot be transferred to the bone around the collar, resulting in disuse atrophy of the marginal bone.

Section 3 takes a closer look at the influence of mechanical loading on bone adaptation. It starts with a general description of the functional adaptation of bones based on the results from animal experiments throughout the years. This is followed by a summary of the theoretical models which have been established to describe the observations of the experiments. Finally, two case studies are discussed that aim to gain insight into the biomechanics of oral implants and to verify some of the hypotheses that relate mechanical loading to peri-implant bone responses.

2 Bone regeneration

Bone regeneration is a complex process encountered for instance in fracture healing and implant osseointegration. The course of this process is influenced by many parameters such as the size of the trauma, the mechanical nature of the regenerative site, the nature of the surrounding tissue etc. Two major types of regenerative processes can be discerned: direct and indirect healing [17]. Bone will regenerate in a direct way when there is little or no loading of the injured site (e.g. cortical defects, rigidly fixated fractures). The defect will ossify via intramembranous bone formation without any external callus formation. Indirect or secondary bone regeneration is characterized by a rapid stabilization of the trauma site. The formation of a callus ensures a rapid restoration of the mechanical integrity. After this quick initial repair, a long period of remodeling eventually returns the bone to its original shape.

The complex character of bone regeneration has mostly been studied during fracture healing of long bones. Therefore, this section starts with an overview of the biology of fracture healing. This is followed by a summary of theoretical models that aim to describe the influence of different mechanical and biological parameters on the process of fracture healing. In the case studies some of these models were implemented to simulate the process of peri-implant tissue differentiation inside an *in vivo* bone chamber.

2.1 Biology of fracture healing

Secondary fracture healing can be roughly divided in three overlapping phases: the inflammatory, reparative (including soft and hard callus formation) and remodeling phase [28, 29]. The initial stage of fracture healing is characterized by an acute inflammatory reaction. Following bone injury, the cortical bone/periosteum and surrounding soft tissues are torn, and numerous blood vessels are ruptured. This blood rapidly coagulates to form a clot enclosing the fracture area. The haematoma has inherent angiogenic and osteogenic potential [30, 31]. As a consequence of the vascular damage, the fracture site becomes hypoxic. Osteocytes at the fracture line become deprived of their nutrition and die. Severely damaged periosteum and marrow as well as injured surrounding tissues contribute necrotic tissue to the region. This necrotic material elicits an immediate inflammatory response: acute inflammatory cells and polymorpho-nuclear leukocytes are recruited to the fracture site, followed by macrophages. Concomitantly, fibroblasts, mesenchymal progenitors and endothelial cells also invade the haematoma and later replace it with connective tissue and (fibro-) cartilage. The inflammatory response is associated with pain, heat, swelling and release of several growth factors and cytokines that have important roles in subsequent healing [32, 33]. For instance, the inflammatory reaction may stimulate mesenchymal cell proliferation at the site of injury and induce angiogenesis, thus playing a key requisite role in the repair process [28].

The inflammatory stage is closely followed by the reparative phase which in its turn can be divided into two phases. During the first reparative phase, fibrous tissue forms and mesenchymal cells proliferate and differentiate, either into chondrocytes that will mature towards hypertrophy (i.e. endochondral ossification, forming mainly the internal callus), or directly into osteoblasts that deposit bone (i.e. intramembranous ossification, predominantly creating the external callus). The mechanisms that control the behavior of each individual cell at this stage are largely unknown, but are likely to derive from the cell's microenvironment. For instance, a major determinant is believed to be the extent of vascularization, with variations in oxygen tension affecting the preference to form either cartilage or bone. As such, this first reparative phase is characterized by the formation of a callus composed of (fibro-) cartilage in areas that are distant from the vasculature and of immature, woven bone predominantly in subperiosteal areas. As the immature callus envelopes the bone ends, stability of the fracture increases.

The second phase of repair is characterized by the replacement of the cartilaginous callus scaffold with bone, in a process indistinguishable from endochondral bone formation except for its lack of organization. This occurs largely concomitant with the remodeling of the already newly formed bone. Hard callus tissue, consisting of mineralized bone matrix, is produced by osteoblasts that receive enough oxygen and are subjected to the proper mechanical stimuli. The bone ends gradually become enveloped by a bone callus mass, immobilization of the fragments becomes more rigid through this internal and external hard callus formation, and eventually a clinical "union" is achieved.

In the middle of the reparative phase, the remodeling phase begins with osteoclastic resorption of unnecessary, poorly placed or inefficient parts of the callus and the formation of new haversian systems and trabecular bone. During this final phase of the healing process, the large fracture callus is replaced by secondary bone; the size of the callus is reduced to that of the pre-existing bone at the damage site, and the vascular supply reverts to a normal state. This remodeling takes place for a prolonged period of time, constantly refining the bony architecture to match the mechanical needs of the skeleton. The end result of remodeling is regenerated bone that, if it has not returned to its original form, has been altered so that it may best perform the function demanded of it.

2.2 Mathematical models

The first theoretical models to describe the mechanoregulation of skeletal tissue differentiation were introduced by Pauwels [16]. He recognized that physical factors cause stress and deformation of the mesenchymal cells and that these stimuli could determine the cell differentiation pathway. He hypothesized that deviatoric stresses, which are always accompanied by strain in some direction and thus a change in cell shape, stimulate the formation of fibrous connective tissue. Hydrostatic stresses on the other hand are a specific stimulus for the formation of cartilaginous tissue. A specific stimulus for the formation of bone, however, is not present in the theory of Pauwels. According to Pauwels, bony tissue proceeds on the basis of a rigid framework of fibrous tissue, cartilage or bone [16]. Some years later, the concept of interfragmentary strain (IFS) was developed by Perren [17] and Perren and Cordey [18]. They proposed that a tissue, with a certain failure strain, cannot be formed in a region that experiences strains higher than this level. This means that a fracture gap can only be filled with a tissue capable of sustaining the IFS without failure. The IFS concept provides a theoretical basis for evaluating fracture treatment strategies, but is not applicable for bone regeneration in general, since it disregards the structural and mechanical heterogeneity of the fracture callus. Building on the theories of Pauwels [16], Perren [17] and Perren and Cordey [18], many research groups have formulated a theoretical model relating tissue differentiation to mechanical loading. Carter and co-workers [10, 11] specifically discussed the importance of cyclic tissue loading and proposed a mechanical stimulus that takes into account the local stress or strain history. The stress acting on the regenerating tissue is described in terms of hydrostatic stress and distortional strain. Direct bone formation is permitted in regions experiencing low hydrostatic stresses and low distortional strains. Carter, however, never provided any values for stimuli that favors bone formation. Claes and Heigele [12] combined the result of their finite element analyses of the mechanical stimuli on ossifying surfaces during fracture healing with a histological analysis of a real callus geometry. From this, they derived a quantitative mechanoregulatory model relating magnitudes of hydrostatic pressure and principal strain to the bone formation process. Intramembranous bone formation occurred at the regenerating bone surface for hydrostatic pressures smaller than 0.15 MPa, while endochondral bone formation occurred when the compressive hydrostatic pressure exceeded this threshold. The above mentioned theories all considered tissues as solid elastic materials. Prendergast et al. [19] proposed a mechanoregulatory model for tissue differentiation, based on a poroelastic (biphasic) behavior of the tissues. Maximal distortional strain and relative fluid velocity constitute the stimulus that controls the differentiation process. High values of both solid strain and fluid velocity favor fibrous tissue formation, while intermediate values lead to cartilaginous tissue. Bone can only be formed if the values are sufficiently low. Huiskes et al. [13] quantified the upper and lower limits of the mechanical stimulus for the different tissue phenotypes, which yielded a mechanoregulatory diagram for tissue differentiation. The model was extended to include mesenchymal cell migration (by means of a diffusion equation), as a first step to incorporate the underlying cellular processes [34, 35]. Carter [36] defined mechanobiology as the study of how mechanical or physical conditions regulate biological processes. At the same time, it is clear that the influence of mechanical loading on tissue differentiation is mediated by other factors, like vascularization or the presence of biochemical agents. The previously described mechanoregulatory models hardly incorporate any biological parameters – apart from Lacroix and Prendergast – and treat the interaction between mechanical loading and tissue differentiation in a more phenomenological way. In contrast, Bailón-Plaza and van der Meulen [9] developed a mechanistic model for fracture healing which approaches the differentiation process from an exclusively biological point of view. In their model, they incorporate the differentiation and proliferation of the different cell types that play a role in fracture healing and the regulation of these processes by means of growth factors. In a recent study [37] they integrated the concepts of Carter et al. [11] into their model for the mechanoregulation of ossification. Such an integrated approach seems highly promising for a better understanding of mechanobiological processes and for the establishment of models that have a more quantitative predictive value.

2.3 Case studies

The predictive value of a model can only be assessed by comparison with in vivo data. Moreover, it would be interesting to compare different theoretical models by applying them to the same, well-defined problem. The following case studies discuss the simulation results of two mechanoregulatory models developed by Prendergast et al. [19] and Claes et al. [12] and of the biological model developed by Bailón-Plaza and van der Meulen [9] when implemented to simulate the peri-implant tissue differentiation in an in vivo bone chamber [38–40].

The repeated sampling bone chamber methodology was developed to investigate the exact role of the mechanical environment on the bone adaptive response around titanium implants. This is not easy because of the difficulty of isolating the implanted material and its surrounding tissues and protecting it from external

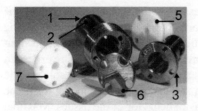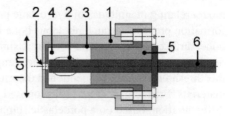

Figure 2: Picture and composition-drawing of the bone chamber. After insertion of
the outer bone chamber (1) in the rabbit's proximal tibia, there is a healing
period of six weeks during which bone ingrowth via the perforations (2)
in the wall is inhibited by a teflon inner chamber (7). After six weeks
this inner chamber is removed and replaced with an inner chamber (3), a
teflon bearing (5) and an implant (6).

influencing factors. In addition, the ruling mechanical conditions should be well-
controlled. A bone chamber which contains a central test implant, was implanted
in the proximal tibia of New Zealand white rabbits (fig. 2). Via perforations, bone
grows into the bone chamber. An actuator allows a well-controlled mechanical
stimulation of the test implant. After an experiment, the content of the bone chamber can be harvested and subjected to a variety of analyses. Consecutively, a new
inner bone chamber structure with a central test implant can be inserted in the outer
bone chamber structure and a new experiment can start. Pilot studies lead to an
acceptable surgical protocol and showed the applicability of the methodology. The
methodology offers the possibility to study tissue differentiation and bone response
around titanium implants under well-controlled mechanical conditions, protected
from external influences [41]. Repeated sampling of the bone chamber allows the
conducting of several experiments within the same animal at the same site, thereby
excluding subject- and site-dependent variability [42]. In addition, it reduces the
number of required experimental animals.

2.3.1 Mechanoregulatory models

The mechanoregulatory models developed by Prendergast *et al.* [19] and Claes *et al.*
[12] both consider mechanical factors to be the determinants of the differentiation
process. Based on the values for strain, stress or fluid flow, they predict certain
tissues (bone, cartilage, fibrous tissue) to be formed or pathways (intramembranous
vs. endochondral bone formation) to be followed.

2.3.1.1 Materials and methods   A 2D axisymmetric finite element (FE) model
of the tissue inside the chamber was created (fig. 3). For both theoretical models
the entire chamber is filled with granulation tissue at the start of the simulation.

In the model developed by Prendergast *et al.* [19] and Huiskes *et al.* [13] the
tissues are treated as biphasic (solid and fluid constituents) and the mechanical
stimulus for tissue differentiation is defined in terms of relative fluid velocity and
maximal distortional strain. Depending on the value of the stimulus, a favoured

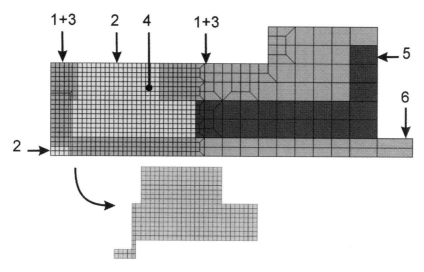

Figure 3: 2D axisymmetric finite element model of the entire bone chamber (upper – numbers cf. fig. 2) and of the tissue inside the chamber.

tissue phenotype ((im)mature bone, cartilage, fibrous tissue) is predicted. A simple diffusion law (eqn (1)) is assumed to describe the migration of mesenchymal cells throughout the chamber. D represents the diffusion coefficient, n the cell density and t represents time.

$$D\nabla^2 n = \frac{dn}{dt}.$$ (1)

Using a rule of mixtures [34] the biphasic material properties are adjusted every iteration step depending on the predicted phenotype and the local concentration of mesenchymal cells. This process is continued until a stable configuration in the chamber is obtained. Figure 4 (top) shows the flowchart of the numerical simulation, table 1 contains the material properties of the different tissues.

In the mechanoregulatory model of Claes *et al.* [12] the major principal strain and hydrostatic stress are the determinants of the differentiation process. Based on their value either soft tissue formation or endochondral or intramembranous bone formation takes place. Again, the material properties of each element are updated every iteration step until a stable configuration is reached (fig. 4, bottom).

2.3.1.2 Results and discussion There are several ways to validate a model. A comparison between the simulation outcomes and the results of an animal experiment can be performed in a qualitative way (e.g. comparison of the tissue types) or a quantitative way (e.g. comparison of measured and calculated reaction forces on the implant). The influence on the simulation outcome of the parameters that cannot be validated experimentally can be assessed by means of sensitivity analyses. The mechanoregulatory models described above are validated in all three ways.

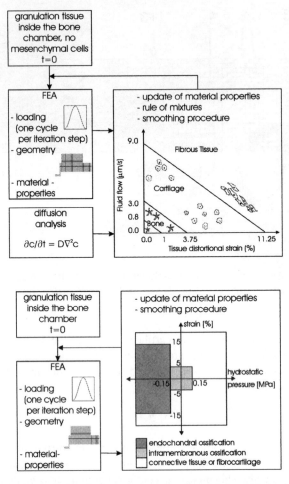

Figure 4: Flow-chart of simulation process for the mechanobiological models of Prendergast *et al.* [19] (top) and Claes *et al.* [12] (bottom).

Table 1: Material properties [43] of the tissues used in the simulations of the model developed by Prendergast *et al.* [19] and Huiskes *et al.* [13].

	Granulation tissue	Fibrous tissue	Cartilage	Immature bone	Mature bone
Young's modulus (MPa)	1	2	10	1000	6000
Poisson's ratio	0.17	0.17	0.17	0.3	0.3
Permeability $(m^4(NS)^{-1})$	10^{-14}	10^{-14}	5×10^{-15}	10^{-13}	3.7×10^{-13}

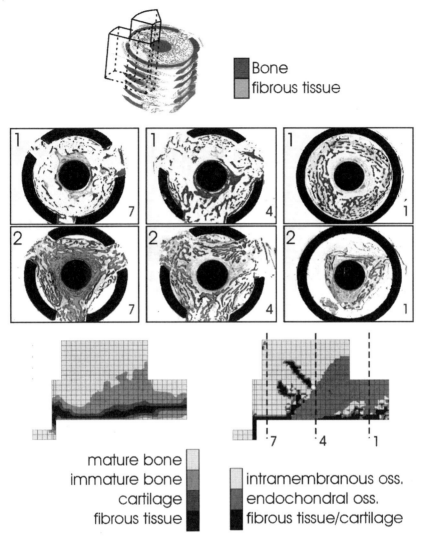

Figure 5: Top: histological sections taken from 2 animals at 3 different heights in the bone chamber (height indicated in bottom right figure). Bottom: results of the simulations with the models of Prendergast *et al.* [19] (left) and Claes *et al.* [12] (right).

Figure 5 shows the simulation result (upper left) and the histological sections taken at three different heights in the bone chamber from two rabbits. The animals were loaded twice a week for 12 weeks with an implant-displacement of $30\,\mu$m (1 Hz, 400 cycles) the first six weeks, followed by another six weeks of loading with an implant-displacement of $50\,\mu$m (1 Hz, 800 cycles).

Table 2: Numerically calculated forces needed to impose the required implant
displacements.

| | Numerically calculated forces | |
| | Model of | Model of |
Imposed displacements	Prendergast et al. [19]	Claes et al. [12]
30 μm	123 N	140 N
60 μm	30 N	14 N
90 μm	21 N	16 N

Changing the boundary values for the fluid flow stimulus (30 and 90 μm/s instead
of 3 and 9 μm/s), the simulation predicts the formation of a layer of fibrous tissue
at the implant interface, almost no cartilage formation and (im)mature bone formation in the main part of the chamber. The results from the experiments show
those same tissue types (bone and fibrous tissue) in the bone chamber. The spatial
distribution of the tissue phenotypes at the implant interface varies from animal
to animal. The forces needed to impose the required displacement of the implant
were measured during the experiments and calculated during the FE simulations.
The results in table 2 are from an experiment where all animals were loaded with
four different loading conditions (0, 30, 60 and 90 μm – 1 Hz, 800 cycles) that were
applied twice a week during six weeks. The simulation results are reasonable for the
higher displacements; they are in the same order of magnitude as the experimentally
measured forces. For the 30 μm loading condition though, the simulations predict
the entire chamber to be filled with mature bone, requiring high forces (>100 N) to
ensure the displacement of the implant, whereas the experimental measurements
indicate that only low forces (20 N) are required in reality.

The sensitivity analyses show that the fluid flow has a direct influence on the
degree of maturation of the bone in the chamber and a considerable indirect effect
(through the biphasic nature of the tissues) on the strain values and hence the differentiation patterns in the bone chamber. The number of loading cycles applied
per iteration step (e.g. one period of a sine function instead of 800 periods) has
no influence on the predicted tissue phenotypes. Variations in the diffusion rate (D
in the diffusion eqn (1)) do not influence the outcome of the simulations, only the
computational time to reach a converged situation in the bone chamber (i.e. application of additional iteration steps does not alter the tissue phenotype configuration
in the chamber).

Changing the boundary values in the model of Claes et al. [12] (3.75% and
11.25% strain and 0.75 MPa hydrostatic pressure instead of 5% and 15% and
0.15 MPa) gives rise to the simulation results represented in fig. 5 (upper right)
and table 2. Comparing to the results obtained with the model of Prendergast et al.
[19], similar trends are obtained, although quantitative differences can be noticed.
The sensitivity analyses indicate that the strain is responsible for the formation of
the layer of fibrous tissue at the implant interface and the value of the hydrostatic

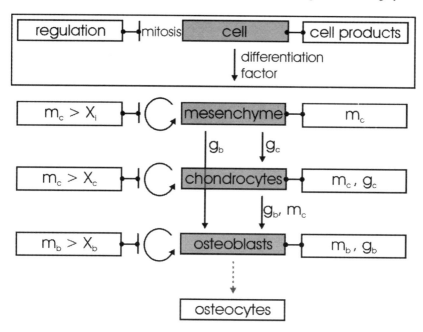

Figure 6: Schematic representation of the mathematical model of Bailón-Plaza and van der Meulen [9].

stress mainly determines the character of the ossification process (endochondral vs. intramembranous).

2.3.2 Biological model

The mathematical model of tissue differentiation by Bailón-Plaza and van der Meulen [9] is schematically represented in fig. 6. This model describes the spatiotemporal evolution of seven quantities: cell densities (mesenchymal cells, chondrocytes, osteoblasts), extracellular matrix densities (connective/cartilage and bone matrix) and growth factor concentrations (chondrogenic and osteogenic) by means of a system of seven coupled partial differential equations of the taxis-diffusion-reaction (TDR) type. This model accounts for many of the important events in fracture healing including haptokinetic and haptotactic mesenchymal cell migration depending on the matrix densities, space-limited cell proliferation as well as environment-dependent cell differentiation, growth factor and matrix production and degradation.

2.3.2.1 Materials and methods

Figure 7 shows the simplified 2D model of the tissue in the bone chamber. A time-limited inflow of mesenchymal cells and growth factors, via prescribed concentration values, through the chamber perforation in the outer wall and the bottom, (cf. the markings on the upper and left domain boundary, respectively, in fig. 7) is assumed. The bottom boundary of the domain is

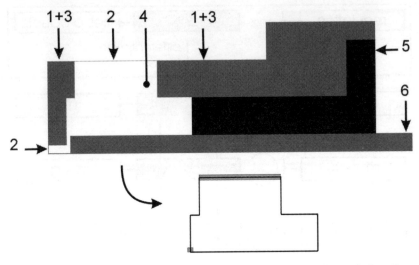

Figure 7: 2D model of the entire bone chamber (top – numbers cf. fig. 2) and simplified model of the tissue inside the chamber.

a symmetry line and there and on all remaining boundary parts no flow conditions apply. Except for a low matrix concentration, all quantities are assumed initially zero in the domain.

The seven concentrations appearing in the mathematical model are nonnegative. This qualitative property of the solution should be inherited by numerical approximations of the concentrations and hence must be obeyed by the algorithms employed. Reliable numerical methods for TDR models have been investigated extensively by Gerisch [44]. The techniques developed there are adapted to the specific system at hand. The general approach taken is the method of lines (MOL) which consists of three substeps.

- Selection of a spatial grid. With each grid cell, for each of the seven quantities a time-dependent (spatial) average concentration value is associated. The aim of the following two steps is the computation of the temporal evolution of these average concentrations.
- Spatial discretization, i.e. approximation of the spatial derivatives of the PDE system in all grid cells by using the average concentration values in neighboring grid cells (finite differences/finite volumes approach). This leads to the so called MOL-ODE, that is a system of coupled ordinary differential equations (ODEs) describing the temporal evolution of the average concentrations in the grid cells. One important characteristic of the selected spatial discretization is the requirement that the resulting ODE admits only nonnegative solutions whenever the initial data is nonnegative. The requirement leads to conditions on the discretizations employed for taxis, diffusion, and reaction terms. These are easily met for the reaction terms (point wise evaluation) and the discretization of the diffusion

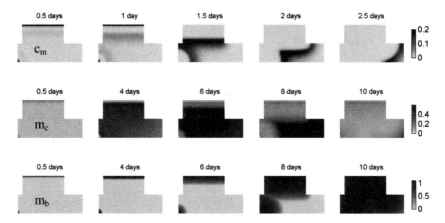

Figure 8: Simulation results for the model of Bailón-Plaza and van der Meulen [9]. Change over time of mesenchymal cell density (c_m, top), density of cartilage and fibrous tissue ECM (m_c, middle) and density of bone ECM (m_b, bottom).

term (standard second-order central differences). However, the discretization of the taxis term is not straightforward under these conditions and upwinding techniques with nonlinear limiter functions (van Leer limiter) are employed in order to satisfy them. A detailed discussion of the spatial discretization can be found in [44].

• Time integration of the MOL-ODE. Due to the enormous size of the MOL-ODE this calls for efficient numerical techniques. ODE systems arising from the discretization of PDEs involving diffusion terms are so-called stiff systems and call for implicit time integration schemes. Such a method is implemented in the efficient and reliable code ROWMAP [45] which is used in our simulations.

2.3.2.2 Results and discussion The results of the simulations with the biological model are not yet validated with specific histomorphometrical and immunohisto-chemical analyses of the tissues in the bone chambers at different stages in the experiment, therefore the values of the parameters of the model are assumed to be the same as in [9] and sensitivity analyses are performed to assess the influence of these assumptions on the final outcome.

After three days, the mesenchymal cells have spread throughout the entire chamber, describing a steep moving front (fig. 8, top). Under the influence of the chondrogenic growth factor, the cells start differentiating into chondrocytes that fill the entire chamber with a fibrous tissue/cartilage ECM by day five. Hereafter, the endochondral replacement starts. Chondrocytes are replaced by osteoblasts describing again the same steep moving fronts. A bony ECM is laid down and by day ten, the entire chamber is filled with bone. Figure 8 (middle and bottom) shows the variation of both the fibrous tissue/cartilage and the bone ECM throughout the entire simulation. Moderate changes to the values of the boundary and initial conditions have no influence on the simulation results. A too low value for the mesenchymal cells at the boundaries will lead to a bone chamber filled with cartilage ECM and a too low level of the initial ECM values will cause a delay or an arrestment in the differentiation process. Setting the initial value of the chondrogenic growth factor to zero causes intramembranous bone formation, filling the chamber with bone in four days. When the initial value of the osteogenic growth factor is set to zero, the endochondral replacement is prohibited from taking place hence no bone is formed. Not only the values of the boundary and initial conditions may determine the outcome of the process, the values of the model parameters also play an important role. Changing the values of the parameters involved in describing the cell differentiation and replacement causes a delay or an arrestment in the differentiation process. Changes in the values of the parameters that describe the formation and degradation of the ECM cause smoothening of the steep moving fronts by which all the processes run through the chamber.

3 Bone adaptation

The mechanical environment of the peri-implant tissue is not only important for the establishment of the osseointegration, but also for the maintenance thereof. Both over- and underload conditions have been shown to induce marginal bone loss and affect the osseointegration [21–27].

This sections starts with an overview of the experimental data gathered over the years that aims to provide a better understanding of the process of functional bone adaptation. This is followed by a summary of mathematical models that have been established based on these experimental data. Finally two case studies are presented that aim to gain insight into the biomechanics of oral implants and to verify some of the hypotheses that relate mechanical loading to peri-implant bone responses.

3.1 Animal experiments and observations

The observation that bone geometry and structure seem to be "optimally" adapted to its mechanical environment was already made by Galileo in 1638 [46]. It was however only in the second half of the 19th century that the first theories of bone adaptation emerged, when Karl Culmann, Hermann von Meyer and Julius Wolff compared the trabecular arrangement with the principal stress trajectories in a homogeneous bone. Especially Wolff became famous with his "Law of bone transformation" – later known as "Wolff's Law" – published in 1892 [47], in which he proposed a number of axioms related to growth and adaptation of bone tissue. Wolff stated that "every change in the form and function of bones or of their function alone is followed by certain definite changes in their internal architecture, and equally definite secondary alterations in their external conformation, in accordance to mathematical laws". Today, it is clear that Wolff's law is in fact a poorly defined law and that many of his concepts proved to be erroneous. A description of the historical context of bone adaptation can be found in [48].

Speaking about bone adaptation involves different aspects that can be described as [49]:

- The optimization of strength with respect to weight.
- The alignment of trabeculae with principal stress trajectories.
- Self-regulation of bone structure by cells responding to a mechanical stimulus.

This paragraph focuses on the last aspect. The word "adaptation" will be used here to designate modeling as well as remodeling in response to (changes in) mechanical loading. Other frequently encountered terms in literature about bone adaptation are "external remodeling" and "internal remodeling" [50]. The first refers to a change in outer bone geometry, either achieved by a movement in- or outward of the periosteum or endosteum (or both). The latter designates the change in bulk density of trabecular bone, the change in porosity of cortical bone and the change in orientation of the individual trabeculae.

The idea of self-regulation was introduced by Roux in 1881 [51], who hypothesized that organisms have the possibility to adapt to changes in their environment. Applying this to bone he stated that cells can either form or resorb bone tissue according to variations of a functional (mechanical) stimulus. The question was and still is: which mechanical stimulus? *In vitro* experiments have pointed out that cell cultures from the osteoblast lineage can respond to strain [52]. Fluid flow seems another important regulator of (osteocytic) cell activity [53]. Fluid flow may interact with the osteocytes, either by inducing shear deformation by means of electrical signals. The latter stems from the fact that the extracellular matrix in bone has a net negative electrical charge so that the extracellular fluid (which can be considered as an electrolyte) will develop a diffuse double layer of positive charges. When the solid matrix is deformed, the fluid will start to flow, thereby giving rise to streaming currents and streaming potentials, which may interact with the osteocytes [54]. The formation of micro-cracks is also suggested as another stimulus that could directly trigger a cellular response [55–57]. During *in vivo* experiments it is not possible to monitor the mechanical stimuli at the cellular level. Since osteoblasts and bone lining cells are attached to bone surfaces, it is reasonable that they will "feel" the deformation of the bone surface (although the in case of osteocytes, the relation between macroscopic bone deformation and cellular deformation seems far from straightforward). Therefore, many researchers have concentrated on the measurement of strain (by means of strain gauges) on the periosteal surface of (mostly long) bones during different levels of activity in animals [58–62].

Interestingly, for all the different animals and bones, peak strains were found between 2000 and 3000 $\mu\varepsilon$. These results sustain the hypothesis that bone adaptation takes place in order to control the level of maximum strains during function. The work of Hylander [59] is of particular interest for the field of implant dentistry, since he is the only one that performed measurements on the (macaque) mandible. He found peak strains of 2200 $\mu\varepsilon$ during biting.

Uhthoff and Jaworski studied the effect of disuse on bone tissue by immobilizing one of the forelimbs in either growing [63, 64] or older dogs [65]. In case of growing dogs they found a loss of bone mass of about 50% after 32 weeks, involving resorption at the periosteal, endosteal and intracortical envelopes. When the fore-limbs were mobilized again, 65–70% of the lost bone mass was recovered within 28 weeks. For the older dogs bone loss primarily occurred at the endosteal surface and through increased intracortical porosity. The capacity to recover the bone loss seemed lower for older dogs, recovering only 40%. Lanyon *et al.* [61] looked at the effect of increased bone loading in the radius of mature sheep, by removing the ulna (i.e. ulnar osteotomy), so that the radius must carry the entire load in the forelimb. They observed woven bone formation at the periosteal perimeter, which was most intense at the side adjacent to the osteotomised ulna. At this side, the woven bone was also secondary remodeled. However, this was not the side of the radius that experienced the largest increase in bone strains due to the ulnar osteotomy. Even more surprisingly, the strain level after adaptation had dropped below the strain level before osteotomy. These findings seem conflicting with the idea that the strain magnitude controls the adaptive response of bone. In order to try to explain their results, Lanyon *et al.* [61] argued that alterations in the "normal" strain distribution may play a role as well in the bone adaptive response. Lanyon and co-workers per-formed another series of highly interesting animal experiments with adult turkeys, in which the shaft (diaphysis) of the ulna was isolated and loaded via pins that were surgically inserted. In this way, they had much more control over the different parameters of tissue loading, since the ulna only experienced the experimentally applied loads. They performed several experiments in which they studied the effect of strain magnitude, the daily number of load cycles and the effect of static versus dynamic loading. When no loading was applied, bone loss was observed in the form of endosteal resorption and an increase in intracortical porosity. Compressive static loading up to $2000\,\mu\varepsilon$ generated the same results, but when the same compressive loading magnitude was applied dynamically (100 cycles per day, 1 Hz) an increase in cross-sectional area with 24% was observed, primarily from periosteal woven bone formation [66]. The same regime of 100 cycles per day and a frequency of 1 Hz – but now in a bending mode – was considered to study the effect of peak strain mag-nitude [67]. They found a linear relation ($R^2 = 0.69$) between peak strain magnitude and (increase in) cross-sectional area. Calculating the intercept with the x-axis (i.e. zero increase), it seemed that for the applied cyclic load a deformation of $1000\,\mu\varepsilon$ was enough to maintain bone mass. Higher strains caused bone formation, while lower strains were associated with bone resorption. In order to assess the influence of the number of daily loading cycles, a bending load was applied at a frequency of $0.5\,\mathrm{Hz}$ that produced a peak strain of $2050\,\mu\varepsilon$. The number of loading cycles was 4, 36, 360 and 1800 [62]. Only 4 cycles were sufficient to maintain bone mass. For the other regimes, similar bone increases by means of woven bone formation were observed, indicating that the adaptive response was an all-or-nothing phenomenon and not a linear response to the number of cycles. Another parameter that seems to have an effect on the bone adaptive response is the loading frequency. McLeod and Rubin [68] used the same isolated adult avian ulna model and varied the fre-quency between 1 Hz and 30 Hz for different peak strain magnitudes. For all strain magnitudes, the amount of bone formation increased with increasing frequency. At 30 Hz, the minimum strain that was necessary to maintain bone mass was $300\,\mu\varepsilon$, while in case of 1 Hz, this value increased to 1200 $\mu\varepsilon$. Moreover the sensitivity to an increase in strain magnitude was much higher for higher frequencies. A number of conclusions can be drawn from these animal experiments:

- Bone loading needs to be dynamic in order to maintain (or increase) bone mass. If only static loads are applied, resorption seems to occur.
- The bone adaptive response is not only sensitive to strain magnitude, but also to strain rate (frequency). A change in strain distribution may as well play a role.
- A limited amount of daily load cycles is sufficient to maintain or even increase bone mass. If bones are completely immobilized, disuse atrophy (resorption) takes place.
- Functional adaptation is different in mature versus growing bone.

Based on the *in vivo* measurements, different regions of strains have been defined that correspond to different adaptive responses in weight-bearing bones. Frost [69] has termed this the bone "mechanostat":

- Disuse atrophy: below a certain strain value, resorption due to disuse is initiated. Different values have been proposed by different authors, ranging between 10 $\mu\varepsilon$ [67], 50 $\mu\varepsilon$ [65] and 200 $\mu\varepsilon$ [70].
- Physiological load: comprises the range between disuse and mild overload: in this range bone tissue is in homeostatic equilibrium. Other terms that have been used to describe this region are "lazy zone" or "dead zone".
- Mild overload: the strains are between 2000 and 4000 $\mu\varepsilon$. Peak strains that are encountered in this region can trigger an increase in bone mass (bone formation). Frost [69] suggested that there is a "minimum effective strain" that has to be exceeded in order to have a net bone formation.
- Pathologic overload: above a certain strain irreversible bone damage takes place, either by fatigue or by creep (or both). A strain value of 4000 $\mu\varepsilon$ has been proposed as the lower limit of this region.

The described animal experiments were all carried out in load-bearing bones. Other bones in the skeleton, like e.g. the skull merely have a protective function and bone adaptive principles do not seem to be applicable here. In those bones the anatomy seems to be dictated by genetic and inherent physiological conditions. Moreover, the bone adaptive responses may be different in the vicinity of "special" tissues, like the periodontal ligament, that surrounds natural teeth. Orthodontic forces, which are static, are capable of translating and rotating teeth through the bone tissue by the induction of local bone resorption and formation (although even in this case a dynamic occlusal loading component is present). Bertram and Swartz [42] critically discussed the animal experiments of the 1970s and 1980s that studied bone adaptation. Based on the disuse experiments of amongst others Uhthoff and Jaworski [63–65] they argued that there are prominent differences in the response of growing versus mature bone to the removal of functional load. It seems that mature animals are less sensitive to disuse. Moreover, the amount of resorption in case of immobilization appears to be dependent on anatomical location as well: for mature dogs, Jaworski *et al.* [65] found a reduction in cross-sectional area of 40%, 10% and 3% for respectively the metacarpus, the radius and the humerus. Bertram and Swartz [42] mentioned that complete removal of loads could also interfere with other factors – like calcium regulating hormones, blood flow, oxygen and nutrient levels, pH – that are important for bone maintenance, so that mechanical load has only an indirect effect on disuse atrophy. In order to induce increased bone loading, many researchers performed an osteotomy of one of the paired limb bones (e.g. [61]). Bertram and Swartz focused attention on the fact that the surgical intervention itself can trigger an osteogenic response, even at anatomical locations that are far removed from the osteotomy. Such systemic reactions were observed by Bab *et al.* [71], who found increased bone formation at the mandibular condyle of rats, when bone marrow was removed from the tibia. As a consequence, it may not be possible in practice to distinguish the osteogenic effect of increased loading from the effect of surgical trauma. Therefore, one of the most elegant experiments that has demonstrated the bone adaptive response to dynamic loading are the experiments with the isolated adult avian ulna model, as developed by Lanyon and co-workers. In their experiments a control animal was included, that was subjected to the surgical protocol, but remained unloaded. For this animal, no possible osteogenic response to the surgery was observed, at the same time demonstrating that the bone formation encountered in the loaded animals are indeed attributed to the applied dynamic loading. To conclude this paragraph, it is important to notice that mechanical load is clearly not the only influencing factor. Nutrition (calcium deficit) and hormonal aspects are as important and can interfere with the effects of a change in loading conditions.

3.2 Mathematical models

For more than two decades researchers have tried to capture bone adaptive responses into mathematical laws. By implementing these "adaptive rules" into a feedback system that makes use of finite element modeling to calculate the local mechanical stimulus, the observed changes in bone geometry, density and/or orientation can be simulated or even – if possible – predicted. Two different approaches have emerged:

- strain-adaptive rules
- damage-based rules.

It must be noted that the existing theories concentrate on the prediction of bone resorption and formation below the range of pathologic overload. None of the theories reported in literature has incorporated pathological overload.

The founders of the strain-adaptive rules were Cowin and Hegedus [72], who developed their theory of adaptive elasticity. The adaptive rules are based on the assumption that bone tissue that is mechanically loaded, aims at an equilibrium level of strain, called the homeostatic strain level. The mechanical stimulus that drives the adaptive response is then calculated as the difference between actual and homeostatic strain. In case of external remodeling (cf. definitions previously mentioned) the equation can be written as:

$$\frac{\partial X}{\partial t} = C_{ij} \left(\varepsilon_{ij} - \varepsilon_{ij}^0 \right), \tag{2}$$

where X is the surface position of either the periosteum or endosteum, ε_{ij} is the actual strain tensor and ε_{ij}^0 is the homeostatic strain tensor. C_{ij} is a matrix of site-specific external remodeling rate constants. For internal remodeling a similar equation can be written, but now the change in (isotropic) elastic modulus E (assuming that continuum mechanics is valid) must be considered

$$\frac{\partial E}{\partial t} = C'_{ij} \left(\varepsilon_{ij} - \varepsilon_{ij}^0 \right). \tag{3}$$

Again, C'_{ij} is a matrix of internal remodeling rate constants. Instead of defining one threshold that determines the limit between bone resorption and bone formation, two threshold values can be defined as well in order to include a "lazy zone". Others, like Carter *et al.* [73] defined a different mechanical stimulus, called the daily stress stimulus ϕ, which is a magnitude-weighted summation of individual products of effective stress magnitude $\bar{\sigma}_i$ and daily count n_i for multiple activity types of similar magnitude, given by:

$$\phi = \left[\sum_{day} n_i \bar{\sigma}_i^m \right]^{1/m}. \tag{4}$$

The effective stress is defined as a fictitious stress, corresponding to a uniaxial stress and strain state that produces the same elastic strain energy density U as the real three-dimensional stress and strain state:

$$U = \frac{\bar{\sigma}^2}{2E} = \frac{1}{2} \sum \sigma_{ij} \varepsilon_{ij}, \tag{5}$$

where E is the (isotropic) elastic modulus and σ_{ij} and ε_{ij} are the stress and strain components respectively. Again, in order to simulate adaptive responses, a reference valued for ϕ must be defined. Carter and co-workers [73–75] applied the concept of the daily stress stimulus to calculate bone density distributions, starting from a homogeneous distribution. In this way, they did not distinguish between cortical and trabecular bone. One of the biggest problems in the previous equations is that a number of empirical constants must be determined. In practice, this is done by calibrating the model to animal experimental data.

Prendergast and Taylor [76] developed an alternative theory, based on damage accumulation. As was already mentioned, the formation of microcracks has been proposed to be responsible for the initiation of remodeling. Instead of assuming that bone aims at a constant level of a strain-based parameter, one could assume that the level of damage throughout the bone must remain constant. If bone is overdamaged, then new bone must be added to avoid that damage accumulation would cause fracture. Similarly, if the damage level drops below a certain level, then bone mass is removed to reach an optimal level of damage. As to the latter, one could argue that a bone is inefficiently organized when the factor of safety for fracture is too large. Indeed, in that case the metabolic cost of maintaining the bone tissue would not be optimized with respect to the risk of fracture. Therefore the damage theory could be interpreted as an optimization of strength. The damage-based theory assumes that there is an equilibrium level damage of damage ω_E. Suppose that the actual level of damage is ω, then the stimulus for bone adaptation $\Delta\omega$ is calculated as:

$$\Delta\omega = \omega - \omega_E. \tag{6}$$

In the case of external remodeling eqn (6) can be rewritten as

$$\frac{\partial X}{\partial t} = C\Delta\bar{\omega}, \tag{7}$$

where C is a rate constant that has to be determined. Equation 7 relates the apposition or resorption rate at the periosteal or endosteal envelopes to the total amount of damage in the bone. Mori and Burr [57] have observed increased remodeling in the direct vicinity of microcracks. Martin *et al.* [70] argued that one of the most important tasks of remodeling is the repair of damaged bone tissue. However, this does not prove that the presence of internal cracks can trigger a modeling response at the periosteum or endosteum.

3.3 Case studies

Although many researchers have suggested the important role of mechanical load-ing in the long-term success of oral implants, there is still a lack of quantitative data on peri-implant bone tissue loading during function. A rabbit experiment was set up to study the peri-implant bone response to cyclic loading [24, 77, 78]. At the same time, an individualized, image-based FE model was created, in order to calculate the bone stresses and strains during this cyclic loading experiment, and to relate them to the observed bone response (case study 3.3.1). The results of this finite element model only give an insight into the "initial" stress and strain distribution, i.e. before any marginal bone loss has taken place. In order to fully understand the role of mechanical loading in peri-implant bone response, it is necessary to simulate the changes in bone geometry and/or density and study their influence on stresses and strains. Therefore, a computer algorithm was programmed that simulates overload-induced bone resorption (case study 3.3.2).

3.3.1 Animal study
The aim of the study presented below was to verify whether "excessive" implant load can lead to increased (marginal) bone loss or even complete loss of implant fixation by comparing animal experimental data with data obtained from FE analyses.

3.3.1.1 Materials and methods A rabbit experiment was set up, in which a cyclic transverse force was applied to a screw-shaped titanium implant (self-tapping Brånemark implant) that was bicortically fixed in the part of the tibial diaphysis. No trabecular bone was present around the implants. Ten rabbits were included in the study and per rabbit a test (loaded) and a control (unloaded) implant were installed in the left tibia.

All implants were allowed to heal subcutaneously for 6 weeks, after which the cyclic loading experiment was started. A cyclic pulling force with amplitude of 14.7 N (1.5 kg) was manually applied perpendicular to an aluminium beam that is mounted on top of the abutment (total length of beam + abutment is 50 mm). In order to control the force amplitude in each cycle, two strain gauges were attached to the outer surface of the beam to register the either tensile or compressive bending strain. Since both strain gauges were mounted opposite to each other at the same distance of the applied force, only the sign of the measured strain is different. This configuration allowed the compensation of the strain signal for possible fluctuations in temperature. The frequency of the manually applied cyclic load was approximately 1 Hz. During the first week of the loading experiment 90 cycles per day were administered. During the second week the number of daily cycles was increased to 270, so that the total duration of the animal experiment could be shortened (in order to prevent an inflammatory reaction of the skin to manipulation of the loading device).

After animal sacrifice histomorphometrical analyses of all test and control implants were performed. One ground section was prepared in the middle of each implant parallel to the load direction (sagittal plane). For one randomly selected rabbit a μCT scan (Skyscan 1072) was taken from the test implant before section preparation. This allowed the assessment of the bone response around the entire implant (and not only in the loading plane) and the creation of an individualized, μCT-based FE model of the implant and the part of the tibia that was scanned.

Solid models were created in a computer-aided design (CAD) programme (Unigraphics) for both the bone and the implant. The μCT data was used to derive the correct anatomy and the correct position of the implant relative to the tibia. The solid model of the implant was created, based on known dimensions of the self-tapping Brånemark implant (length 10 mm, diameter 3.75 mm). For the solid model of the tibia a medical image processing programme (Mimics) was used to derive contours (polylines) that describe the outer and inner surface of the cortical bone. The contours were imported in Unigraphics, where surfaces were fitted to these contours. Once the solid models were obtained, the position of the implant solid model was aligned with the correct position of the implant, as determined from the μCT data. A Boolean operation was performed to create the implant insertion hole in the tibia. Tetrahedral meshes (four-noded tetrahedral elements) were created within Unigraphics for both solids (fig. 9). Orthotropic elastic properties were applied to the cortical bone [79] (table 3). Titanium was modeled as isotropic with a Young's modulus of 110 GPa and a Poisson ratio of 0.3.

Nonlinear, static contact analyses were performed, using the MSC.Marc/Mentat FE programme. In a first series of analyses a finite interfacial tensile strength was used, resulting in relative motion between the implant and the bone when tensile stresses exceed the tensile strength. Although exact values for the tensile strength of the implant-bone interface in case of "smooth" titanium are lacking, it can be

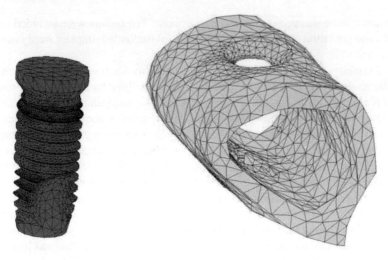

Figure 9: FE meshes for implant and bone.

Table 3: Elastic orthotropic properties of cortical bone, used in the FE model according to Ashman *et al.* [79]. The 1-direction is the radial direction of the tibia,
2-direction the circumferential direction and 3-direction the axial direction.

Young's modulus [GPa]			Shear modulus [GPa]			Poisson's ratio		
E_1	E_2	E_3	G_{12}	G_{23}	G_{31}	ν_{12}	ν_{23}	ν_{31}
12.8	15.6	20.1	4.68	6.67	5.68	0.282	0.265	0.454

estimated to be of the order of 0.5–1 MPa, based on literature values for other
biomaterials and surface roughness [80]. Additionally, an analysis was performed
with a fully-bonded interface (infinite strength), preventing any relative motion.

The nodes at the outer proximal and distal boundaries of the bone mesh were
fully constrained. Loading conditions, corresponding to the force amplitude in the
cyclic loading experiment, were applied (lateral force 14.7 N, bending moment
73.5 Ncm).

3.3.1.2 Results and discussion   The μCT scan of the test implant revealed the
occurrence of marginal bone resorption in the loading plane, but not in a direction,
perpendicular to it. As can be appreciated from fig. 10, bone craters were formed
at both the proximal ("tensile") and the distal ("compressive") side.

As to the finite element analyses, relative motion occurs at the proximal (i.e.
"tensile") side of the implant neck for all considered values of finite interfacial
tensile strength (1, 5 and 10 MPa). As a result, only large compressive forces are
developed between the implant neck and the bone at the distal side. This is reflected
in the equivalent strain distribution, shown in fig. 11: large equivalent strains (more

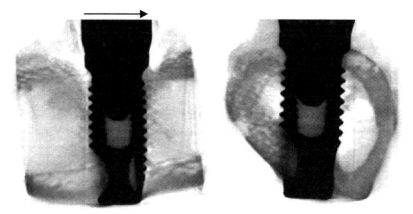

Figure 10: μCT image of a test implant in a sagittal plane (i.e. loading plane (left) and a medio-lateral plane (right)). The direction of force application is also indicated.

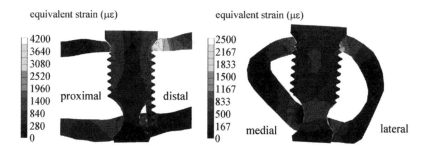

Figure 11: Equivalent strain distribution in the case of a finite interfacial tensile strength of 1 MPa: sagittal (left) and transverse (right) cross-section. Other finite strengths (5, 10 MPa) yield the same results.

than 4000 με) occur at the distal side of the implant neck, while at the proximal side much smaller strains (1100 με) exist. The equivalent (Von Mises) strains encountered around the implant neck in a medio-lateral cross-section are much lower than at the distal side (around 2000 με). They are the result of normal tensile strains in the proximo-distal direction, occurring medially and laterally from the implant neck.

For an infinite interfacial strength the maximum strains are smaller: equivalent strains proximally and distally from the implant neck amount to 2500 με. Since tensile stresses can now be transferred as well, a much more symmetric equivalent strain distribution is obtained.

Since a value of 10 MPa seems to strongly overestimate the actual interfacial tensile strength of a "smooth" machined titanium surface, it is likely that relative motion occurred during the cyclic loading experiment. Therefore, the strain distribution in fig. 11 must be regarded as more representative for the peri-implant bone tissue loading than the strain distribution in case of an infinite interfacial strength, which implies that only the distal side experienced high strains. Nevertheless, histomorphometrical analysis of all test implants did not show any statistically significant difference in crater depth, crater width or marginal bone contact between the proximal and distal sides. At both sides a continuing process of bone resorption (Howship's lacunae) was observed. For the marginal bone resorption at the distal ("compressive") side it seems reasonable that overload caused the excessive marginal bone loss, since strains were calculated that even exceeded 4000 $\mu\varepsilon$. Frost [81] considered this to be the threshold for pathologic overload, although this value might not be that absolute. Possibly, due to the high bone stresses and strains microcracks were formed at the distal side, which in turn activated osteoclasts to resorb bone tissue [57]. However, looking at the strain values at the proximal side (1100 $\mu\varepsilon$), neither overload nor underload (disuse atrophy) seem to be a plausible explanation. One could hypothesise that relative motion also plays a role in the observed bone response. Previous animal experiments have indeed shown that relative motion can interact with tissue differentiation processes around endosseous implants [7]. At the moment, it is not clear whether relative motion can also interfere with osteoclastic activity in "mature" bone. The relative displacements ("gaps") at the proximal side were in the range of 10–15 μm. This is an order of magnitude smaller than the relative motion, encountered in the experiments of Søballe *et al.* [7]. Again, it is not clear if such small relative displacements can play a significant role in bone adaptive/resorptive processes. Besides, since relative (tangential) displacement is also taking place at the medial and lateral sides of the implant neck – although to an even smaller extend – one could also expect marginal bone resorption to be present at these sides. This could not be detected in the μCT scan of the test implant.

3.3.2 Simulation of marginal bone resorption
The results of the finite element model discussed above only give insight into the "initial" stress and strain distribution, i.e. before any marginal bone loss has taken place. In order to fully understand the role of mechanical loading in peri-implant bone response, it is necessary to simulate the changes in bone geometry and/or density and study their influence on stresses and strains. Therefore, a computer algorithm was programmed that simulates overload-induced bone resorption.

3.3.2.1 Materials and methods   In order to study the interaction between a change in marginal bone level and a change in stress state a simple iterative feedback algorithm was developed that relates pathological overload to bone resorption (fig. 12). When the average effective stress in an element exceeded a pre-defined threshold value, this element was removed in order to simulate overload-induced bone resorption. This process was repeated until a new equilibrium geometry (no more overload) or until complete loss of osseointegration (no equilibrium) was obtained.

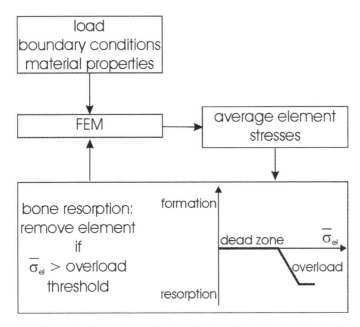

Figure 12: Schematic illustration of a simple algorithm for the simulation of bone resorption.

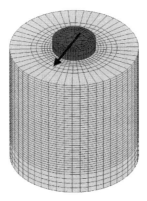

Figure 13: A simple finite element model of a cylindrical implant surrounded by a cortical bone volume. The load direction is also indicated.

The iterative feedback algorithm was applied to a finite element model of a single cylindrical implant, surrounded by a cylindrical cortical bone volume (fig. 13). Cortical bone was modeled as isotropic ($E = 15.5\,\text{GPa}$, $v = 0.31$) [82]. A fully bonded interface was assumed between bone and implant. The same load amplitude and direction as in the rabbit experiment was applied. Nodal displacements on the outer cylindrical surface were fully constrained. Eight-noded hexahedral elements were used for the mesh.

A first simulation was performed with equivalent Von Mises stress as the effective stress. It must be remarked that Von Mises stress is only physically meaningful for isotropic materials and should not be used to characterize the stress state in case of anisotropic materials – like cortical bone [83, 84]. For the purpose of this study the use of Von Mises stress is acceptable, since only qualitative results are of interest here. The simulation only considered bone resorption due to pathological overload. Other adaptive responses (resorption due to disuse, formation due to mild overload) were not yet included. Moreover no attempt was made to simulate resorption as a function of time.

3.3.2.2 Results and discussion   Overload-induced marginal bone resorption was initiated at the marginal bone edge in the loading plane. For an overload threshold of 31 MPa (in terms of Von Mises stress) resorption was arrested and a new equilibrium geometry was found, as depicted in fig. 14. Resorption (removal of elements) did not progress around the entire implant, but was limited to bone regions in or near the loading plane. The total decrease of the marginal bone level in the loading plane amounted to 1 mm. When a smaller value for the overload threshold was chosen, no equilibrium was established. Again, resorption was initiated in the loading plane, but progressed in the circumferential direction until a complete ring of elements was removed at the marginal bone edge. Subsequently, resorption advanced in the axial direction towards the implant apex along the entire implant surface until all bone at the implant surface was lost. This situation can be considered as a complete loss of osseointegration due to overload.

Due to the simplicity of the finite element model and the simulation algorithm quantitative results are of minor importance. However qualitative trends are still

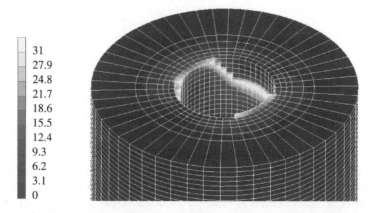

| 31 |
| 27.9 |
| 24.8 |
| 21.7 |
| 18.6 |
| 15.5 |
| 12.4 |
| 9.3 |
| 6.2 |
| 3.1 |
| 0 |

Figure 14: Marginal bone decrease for the equilibrium configuration. The Von Mises stress distribution (in MPa) is also shown.

valid. Figure 15 illustrates the change in stress distribution and stress values when marginal bone resorption takes place. It demonstrates that when overload-induced resorption is initiated in the loading plane, the maximum stresses at the marginal bone level decrease in the loading plane, while they increase in the plane perpendicular to it. These results suggest that a shift in stress transfer occurs during resorption. In the new equilibrium configuration the bone in the plane perpendicular to the loading direction carries a larger portion of the applied load than in the initial configuration. Once the stresses in the loading plane drop below the threshold, resorption is arrested. As long as the (increased) stresses in the plane perpendicular

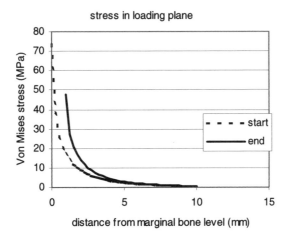

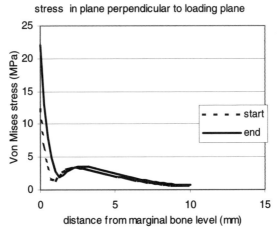

Figure 15: Bone stress distribution in the loading plane (top) and the plane perpendicular to it (bottom) for the initial bone geometry ("start") and the new equilibrium geometry ("end"). Stresses are evaluated along a straight line in the nodes at the implant-bone interface. Results were obtained for an overload threshold of 31 MPa.

to the loading plane do not exceed the threshold, resorption will not be initiated at this side. This situation was encountered for an overload threshold of 31 MPa (or larger). When resorption is initiated in the plane, perpendicular to the loading plane (either due to a lower overload threshold or due to a higher implant load), it cannot be arrested anymore. This results in a complete loss of osseointegration, as was encountered for thresholds, smaller than 31 MPa.

These results indicate that overload-induced marginal bone resorption can be arrested as long as initiation of resorption is limited to the loading plane. In reality resorption might be arrested by other mechanisms as well, e.g. densification (stiffening) of peri-implant bone. The simulation algorithm must further be elaborated to also include these adaptive responses.

4 Conclusion

This chapter described the different causes of failure that might occur in the clinical application of oral implants. A mechanical failure refers to the fracture of an implant component whereas a biological failure refers to problems with the osseointegration.

When an implant fails shortly after implantation, this is usually due to the unsuccessfulness of the osseointegration. The mechanics and the biology of the peri-implant site seem to play a major role herein. The complex process of bone regeneration is described by means of its most studied example: fracture healing in long bone. The theoretical models that aim to simulate the above described process of bone regeneration were divided into mechanoregulatory and biological models, depending on the parameters they employ to drive the differentiation process. The mechanoregulatory models predict fibrous tissue formation when the mechanical stimulus (strain, stress, fluid flow) has a high value (corresponding to a severe loading of the fracture zone or implant). The case studies presented in Section 2 described the application of different mechanoregulatory and biological models for the prediction of peri-implant tissue differentiation in an *in vivo* bone chamber. There were qualitative agreements between the numerically predicted and experimentally observed tissue phenotypes in the chamber. Additional histological analyses of samples, harvested at different phases in the regeneration process are needed however to be able to quantify these results.

Late biological failure mostly occurs due to inappropriate implant loading. Numerous animal experiments were conducted to describe the influence of the different aspects of loading (magnitude, frequency, duration) on bone adaptation. Theoretical models try to capture these phenomena into mathematical expressions. The first case study discussed in Section 3 compares the peri-implant bone stresses and strains measured during a controlled loading animal experiment with those same variables calculated from an anatomical FE-model. Marginal bone loss occurring during the experiment could only partially be related to overload. The second case study further explored the relation between marginal bone resorption and overload by implementing a theoretical model for bone adaptation. A redistribution of the peri-implant bone stresses during the adaptation process put a hold on the marginal bone resorption.

All of the theoretical models presented in Sections 2 and 3 are situated on a continuum level. The mechanical variables employed by the mechanoregulatory models are the tissue stress, strain, strain energy density or the fluid flow velocity. The biological model bases the tissue differentiation on the concentration of cells and growth factors and on ECM densities. However, the processes of bone regeneration and bone adaptation are becoming more and more understood although the exact influence of the mechanical factors and their interaction with the biochemical regulatory pathways is not yet fully unravelled. While these subcellular processes are being investigated from the biological point of view, the theoretical models also need to bring these processes into account and aim to generate mechanistic models that incorporate both mechanical and biological factors on a subcontinuum level. Only then, theoretical models really can contribute to a better understanding of the experimentally observed phenomena and help to gain insight into the mechanisms that are very hard to investigate experimentally.

Acknowledgments

This study was supported by the Research Council of the K.U.Leuven (OT/98/30 & OT/02/05). Liesbet Geris is a research assistant for the Fund for Scientific Research Flanders. Hans Van Oosterwyck and Joke Duyck are post-doctoral research fellows of the Fund for Scientific Research Flanders. The authors gratefully acknowledge A. Andreykiv and Dr. A. Gerisch for their scientific advice.

References

[1] Brånemark, P.I., Introduction to osseointegration. *Tissue-integrated Prostheses. Osseointegration in Clinical Dentistry*, eds. P.I. Brånemark, G. Zarb & T. Albrektsson, Quintessence: Chicago, pp. 1–76, 1985.

[2] Sennerby, L., Ericson, L.E., Thomsen, P., Lekholm, U. & Åstrand, P., Structure of the bone-titanium interface in retrieved clinical oral implants. *Clinical Oral Implants Research*, **2**, pp. 103–111, 1991.

[3] Esposito, M., Hirsch, J.-M., Lekholm, U. & Thomsen, P., Failure patterns of four osseointegrated oral implant systems. *Journal of Materials Science: Materials in Medicine*, **8**, pp. 843–847, 1997.

[4] Kasemo, B. & Lausmaa, J., Biomaterials and interfaces. *Osseointegration in Oral Rehabilitation*, eds. I. Naert, D. van Steenberghe & P. Worthington, Quintessence: Chicago, pp. 63–75, 1993.

[5] Moalli, M.R., Caldwell, N.J., Patil, P.V. & Goldstein, S.A., An in vivo model for investigations of mechanical signal transduction in trabecular bone. *Journal of Bone and Mineral Research*, **15**, pp. 1346–1353, 2000.

[6] Søballe, K., Rasmussen, H.B., Hansen, E.S. & Bünger, C., Hydroxyapatite coating modifies implant membrane formation (controlled micromotion in dogs). *Acta Orthopaedica Scandinavia*, **63(2)**, pp. 128–140, 1992.

[7] Søballe, K., Hansen, E.S., Rasmussen, H.B., Jorgensen, P.H. & Bünger, C., Tissue ingrowth into titanium and hydroxyapatite-coated implants during stable and unstable mechanical conditions. *Journal of Orthopaedic Research*, **10(2)**, pp. 285–299, 1992.

[8] Søballe, K., Hydroxyapatite ceramic coating for bone implant fixation. *Acta Orthopaedica Scandinavia*, **64(S255)**, pp. 1–48, 1993.

[9] Bailón-Plaza, A. & van der Meulen, M.C.H., A mathematical framework to study the effects of growth factor influences on fracture healing. *Journal of Theoretical Biology*, **212**, pp. 191–209, 2001.

[10] Carter, D.R., Mechanical loading history and skeletal biology. *Journal of Biomechanics*, **20**, pp. 1095–1109, 1987.

[11] Carter, D.R., Blenman, P.R. & Beaupré, G.S., Correlations between mechanical stress history and tissue differentiation in initial fracture healing. *Journal of Orthopaedic Research*, **6**, pp. 736–748, 1988.

[12] Claes, L.E. & Heigele, C.A., Magnitudes of local stress and strain along bony surfaces predict the course and type of fracture healing. *Journal of Biomechanics*, **32(3)**, pp. 255–266, 1999.

[13] Huiskes, R., Van Driel, W.D., Prendergast, P.J. & Søballe, K., A biomechanical regulatory model for periprosthetic fibrous-tissue differentiation. *Journal of Material Science: Materials in Medicine*, **8**, pp. 785–788, 1997.

[14] Kuiper, J.H., Ashton, B.A. & Richardson, J.B., Computer simulation of fracture callus formation and stiffness restoration. *Proc. of the 12th conference of the European Society of Biomechanics, Dublin*, eds. P.J. Prendergast, T.C. Lee & A.J. Carr, Royal Academy of Medicine in Ireland, pp. 61, 2000.

[15] Maheshwari, G. & Lauffenburger, D.A., Deconstructing (and reconstructing) cell migration. *Microscopy Research and Technique*, **43**, pp. 358–368, 1998.

[16] Pauwels, F., Eine neue Theorie über den Einfluß mechanischer Reize auf die Differenzierung der Stützgewebe. *Zeitschrift fuer Anatomie und Entwicklungsgeschichte*, **121**, pp. 478–515, 1960.

[17] Perren, S.M., Physical and biological aspects of fracture healing with special reference to internal fixation. *Clinical Orthopaedics and Related Research*, **138**, pp. 175–195, 1979.

[18] Perren, S.M. & Cordey, J., Concepts of interfragmentary strain. *Current Concepts of Internal Fixation of Fractures*, ed. H.K. Uhthoff, Springer-Verlag: New York, pp. 63–77, 1980.

[19] Prendergast, P.J., Huiskes, R. & Søballe, K., Biophysical stimuli on cells during tissue differentiation at implant interfaces. *Journal of Biomechanics*, **30(6)**, pp. 539–548, 1997.

[20] Lindquist, L.W., Carlsson, G.E. & Jemt, T., A prospective 15-year follow-up study of mandibular fixed prostheses supported by osseointegrated implants. Clinical results and marginal bone loss. *Clinical Oral Implants Research*, **7**, pp. 329–336, 1996.

[21] Quirynen, M., Naert, I. & van Steenberghe, D., Fixture design and overload influence marginal bone loss and fixture success in the Brånemark system. *Clinical Oral Implants Research*, **3**, pp. 104–111, 1992.

[22] Hoshaw, S.J., Brunski, J.B. & Cochran, G.V.B., Mechanical loading of Brånemark implants affects interfacial bone modeling and remodeling. *International Journal of Oral and Maxillofacial Implants*, **9**, pp. 345–360, 1994.

[23] Isidor, F., Histological evaluation of peri-implant bone at implants subjected to occlusal overload or plaque accumulation. *Clinical Oral Implants Research*, **8**, pp. 1–9, 1997.

[24] Duyck, J., Rønold, H.J., Van Oosterwyck, H., Naert, I., Vander Sloten, J. & Ellingsen, J.E., The influence of static and dynamic loading on the marginal bone behavior around implants: an animal experimental study. *Clinical Oral Implants Research*, **12**, pp. 207–218, 2001.

[25] Lindquist, L., Rockler, B. & Carlsson, G.E., Bone resorption around fixtures in edentulous patients treated with mandibular fixed tissue-integrated prosthesis. *Journal of Prosthetic Dentistry*, **59**, pp. 59–63, 1988.

[26] Ahlqvist, J., Borg, K., Gunne, J., Nilson, H., Olsson, M. & Åstrand, P., Osseointegrated implants in edentulous jaws: a 2-year longitudinal study. *International Journal of Oral and Maxillofacial Implants*, **5**, pp. 155–163, 1990.

[27] Pilliar, R.M., Deporter, D.A., Watson, P.A. & Valiquette, N., Dental implant design: effect on bone remodeling. *Journal of Biomedical Materials Research*, **25**, pp. 467–483, 1991.

[28] Einhorn, T.A., Enhancement of fracture-healing. *Journal of Bone and Joint Surgery America*, **77**, pp. 940–956, 1995.

[29] Einhorn, T.A., The cell and molecular biology of fracture healing. *Clinical Orthopaedics and Related Research*, **S355**, pp. S7–S21, 1998.

[30] Street, J., Winter, D., Wang, J.H., Wakai, A., McGuinness, A. & Redmond, H.P., Is human fracture heamatoma inherently angiogenic? *Clinical Othopaedics and Related Research*, **1(378)**, pp. 224–237, 2000.

[31] Street, J., Winter, D., Wang, J.H., Wakai, A., McGuinness, A. & Redmond, H.P., The angiogenic response to skeletal injury is preserved in the elderly. *Journal of Orthopaedic Research*, **19**, pp. 1057–1066, 2001.

[32] Barnes, G.L., Kostenuik, P.J., Gerstenfeld, L.C. & Einhorn, T.A., Growth factor regulation of fracture repair. *Journal of Bone and Mineral Research*, **14**, pp. 1805–1815, 1999.

[33] Hauser, C.J., Zhou, X., Joshi, P., Cuchens, M.A., Kregor, P., Devidas, M., Kennedy, R.J., Poole, G.V. & Hughes, J.L., The immune microenvironment of human fracture/soft-tissue hematomas and its relationship to systemic immunity. *Journal of Trauma*, **42**, pp. 895–903, 1997.

[34] Lacroix, D., Prendergast, P.J., Li, G. & Marsh, D., Biomechanical model to simulate tissue differentiation and bone regeneration: application to fracture healing. *Medical and Biological Engineering and Computing*, **40**, pp. 14–21, 2002.

[35] Lacroix, D. & Prendergast, P.J., A mechano-regulation model for tissue dif-
     ferentiation during fracture healing: analysis of gap size and loading. *Journal
     of Biomechanics*, **35(9)**, pp. 1163–1171, 2002.
[36] Carter, D.R., Beaupré, G.S., Giori, N.J. & Helms, J.A., Mechanobiology of
     skeletal regeneration. *Clinical Orthopaedics and Related Research*, **355S**,
     pp. 41–55, 1998.
[37] Bailón-Plaza, A. & van der Meulen, M.C.H., Beneficial effects of moderate,
     early loading and adverse effects of delayed or excessive loading on bone
     healing. *Journal of Biomechanics*, **36(8)**, pp. 1069–1077, 2003.
[38] Geris, L., Van Oosterwyck, H., Vander Sloten, J., Duyck, J. & Naert, I., Assess-
     ment of mechanobiological models for the numerical simulation of tissue
     differentiation around immediately loaded implants. *Computer Methods in
     Biomechanics and Biomedical Engineering*, **6(5–6)**, pp. 277–288, 2003.
[39] Geris, L., Andreykiv, A., Van Oosterwyck, H., Vander Sloten, J.,
     van Keulen, F., Duyck, J. & Naert, I., Numerical simulation of tissue
     differentiation around loaded titanium implants in a bone chamber. *Journal
     of Biomechanics*, **37(5)**, pp. 763–769, 2004.
[40] Geris, L., Van Oosterwyck, H., Vander Sloten, J., Duyck, J. & Naert, I.,
     Different mechanoregulatory models predict different patterns of tissue dif-
     ferentiation. *Proc. of the 6th international symposium on Computer Methods
     in Biomechanics and Biomedical Engineering, Madrid*, eds. J. Middleton,
     M.L. Jones & N. Shrive, CD–ROM, 2004.
[41] Duyck, J., De Cooman, M., Puers, R., Van Oosterwyck, H., Vander Sloten, J. &
     Naert, I., A repeated sampling bone chamber methodology for the evalua-
     tion of tissue differentiation and bone adaptation around titanium implants
     under controlled mechanical conditions. *Journal of Biomechanics*, **37(12)**,
     pp. 1819–1822, 2004.
[42] Bertram, J.E.A. & Swartz, S.M., The "Law of bone transformation": a case
     of crying Wolff? *Biological Reviews*, **66**, pp. 245–273, 1991.
[43] Lacroix, D. & Prendergast, P.J., Computational models of tissue
     differentiation-prediction of changes in mechanical stimuli (fluid flow and
     tissue microstrain) during cyclic loading. *Proc. of the 9th conference of the
     European Orthopaedic Research Society (Brussels)*, pp. 50, 1999.
[44] Gerisch, A., *Numerical Methods for the Simulation of Taxis-Diffusion-
     Reaction Systems*, PhD thesis, Martin-Luther-Universität Halle-Wittenberg,
     Germany, 2001.
[45] Weiner, R., Schmitt, B.A. & Podhaisky, H., ROWMAP – a ROW-code with
     Krylov techniques for large stiff ODEs. *Applied Numererical Mathematics*,
     25, pp. 303–319, 1987.
[46] Galileo, G., *Discorsi e dimonstrazioni matematiche, intorno a due nuove
     scienze attentanti alla meccanica ed a muovementi locali*. University of
     Wisconsin Press: Madison, 1683.
[47] Wolff, J., *The Law of Bone Remodeling*. (Translation of Wolff's *Das Gesetz der
     transformation der Knochen* by P. Maquet and R. Furlong) Springer-Verlag:
     Berlin, 1892.

[48] Vander Sloten, J., *The functional adaptation of bones in vivo and consequences for prosthesis design*. PhD thesis, K.U. Leuven, Belgium, 1990.

[49] Roesler, H., The history of some fundamental concepts in bone biomechanics. *Journal of Biomechanics*, **20**, pp. 1025–1034, 1987.

[50] Cowin, S.C., Bone remodeling of diaphyseal surfaces by torsional loads: theoretical predictions. *Journal of Biomechanics*, **20**, pp. 1111–1120, 1987.

[51] Roux, W., *Der zuchtende Kampf der Teile, oder die 'Teilauslese' im Organismus (Theorie der 'funktionellen Anpassung')*. Welhelm Engelmann: Leipzig, 1881.

[52] Jones, D.B., Nolte, H., Scholubbers, J.G., Turner, E. & Veltel, D., Biochemical signal transduction of mechanical strain in osteoblast-like cells. *Biomaterials*, **12**, pp. 101–110, 1991.

[53] Lian, J.B. & Stein, G.S., The cells of bone. *Dynamics of bone and cartilage metabolism*, Academic Press, pp. 165–185, 1999.

[54] Cowin, S.C., Bone poroelasticity. *Journal of Biomechanics*, **32**, pp. 217–238, 1999.

[55] Frost, H.M., *Bone remodeling and its relationship to metabolic bone disease*, Thomas: Springfield, 1973.

[56] Burr, D.B., Martin, R.B., Schaffler, M.B. & Radin, E.L., Bone remodeling in response to in vivo fatigue microdamage. *Journal of Biomechanics*, **18**, pp. 189–200, 1985.

[57] Mori, S. & Burr, D.B., Increased intracortical remodeling following fatigue damage. *Bone*, **14**, pp. 103–109, 1993.

[58] Goodship, A.E., Lanyon, L.E. & McFie, H., Functional adaptation of bone to increased stress. *Journal of Bone and Joint Surgery*, **61A**, pp. 539–546, 1979.

[59] Hylander, W.L., Patterns of stress and strain in the macaque mandible. *Craniofacial biology*, ed. D.S. Carlson, Center for Human Growth and Development: Ann Arbor, 1981.

[60] Rubin, C.T. & Lanyon, L.E., Limb mechanics as a function of speed and gait: a study of functional strains in the radius and tibia of horse and dog. *Journal of Experimental Biology*, **101**, pp. 187–211, 1982.

[61] Lanyon, L.E., Goodship, E.A., Pye, C.J. & McFie, H., Mechanical adaptive bone remodeling. *Journal of Biomechanics*, **15**, pp. 141–154, 1982.

[62] Rubin, C.T. & Lanyon, L.E., Regulation of bone formation by applied dynamic loads. *Journal of Bone and Joint Surgery*, **66A**, pp. 397–402, 1984.

[63] Uhthoff, H.K. & Jaworski, Z.G.F., Bone loss in response to long-term immobilization. *Journal of Bone and Joint Surgery*, **60B**, pp. 420–429, 1978.

[64] Jaworski, Z.G.F. & Uhthoff, H.K., Reversibility of nontraumatic disuse osteoporosis during its active phase. *Bone*, **7**, pp. 431–439, 1986.

[65] Jaworski, Z.G.F., Liskova-Kiar, M. & Uhthoff, H.K., Effect of long-term immobilisation on the pattern of bone loss in older dogs. *Journal of Bone and Joint Surgery*, **62B**, pp. 104–110, 1980.

[66] Lanyon, L.E. & Rubin, C.T., Static versus dynamic loads as an influence on bone remodeling. *Journal of Biomechanics*, **17**, pp. 897–905, 1984.

[67] Rubin, C.T. & Lanyon, L.E., Regulation of bone mass by mechanical strain magnitude. *Calcified Tissue International*, **37**, pp. 411–417, 1985.

[68] McLeod, K.J. & Rubin, C.T., Sensitivity of the bone remodeling response to the frequency of applied strain. *Transactions of the Orthopaedic Research Society*, **17**, pp. 533, 1992.

[69] Frost, H.M., Bone "mass" and the "mechanostat": a proposal. *The Anatomical Record*, **219**, pp. 1–9, 1987.

[70] Martin, R.B., Burr, D.B. & Sharkey, N.A., *Skeletal tissue mechanics*, Springer-Verlag: New York, 1998.

[71] Bab, I., Gazit, D., Massawara, A. & Sela, J., Removal of the tibial marrow induces increased formation of bone and cartilage in rat mandibular condyle. *Calcified Tissue International*, **37**, pp. 551–555, 1985.

[72] Cowin, S.C. & Hegedus, D.M., Bone remodeling: a theory of adaptive elasticity. *Journal of Elasticity*, **6**, pp. 313–325, 1976.

[73] Carter, D.R., Fyhrie, D.P. & Whalen, R.T., Trabecular bone density and loading history: regulation of tissue biology by mechanical energy. *Journal of Biomechanics*, **20**, pp. 785–795, 1987.

[74] Beaupré, G.S., Orr, T.E. & Carter, D.R., An approach for time-dependent bone modeling and remodeling – theoretical development. *Journal of Orthopaedic Research*, **8**, pp. 651–661, 1990.

[75] Fisher, K.J., Jacobs, C.R., Levenston, M.E. & Carter, D.R., Different loads can produce similar bone density distributions. *Bone*, **19**, pp. 127–135, 1996.

[76] Prendergast, P.J. & Taylor, D., Prediction of bone adaptation using damage accumulation. *Journal of Biomechanics*, **27**, pp. 1067–1076, 1994.

[77] Vander Sloten, J., Van Oosterwyck, H., Puers, R. & Naert, I., Finite element studies of the role of mechanical loading in bone response around oral implants. *Proc. of the 15th AIMETA Congress of Theoretical and Applied Mechanics, Taormina, Italy*, eds. G. Augusti, P.M. Mariano, V. Sepe & M. Lacagnina, CD–ROM, pp. MS-BIO-17 2001.

[78] Van Oosterwyck, H., Vander Sloten, J., Puers, R. & Naert, I., Finite element studies of the role of mechanical loading in bone response around oral implants. *Meccanica*, **37(4)**, pp. 441–451, 2002.

[79] Ashman, R.B., Cowin, S.C., Van Buskirk, W.C. & Rice, J.C., A continuous wave technique for the measurement of the elastic properties of cortical bone. *Journal of Biomechanics*, **17**, pp. 349–361, 1984.

[80] Edwards, J.T., Brunski, J.B. & Higuchi, H.W., Mechanical and morphologic investigation of the tensile strength of a bone-hydroxyapatite interface. *Journal of Biomedical Materials Research*, **36**, pp. 454–468, 1997.

[81] Frost, H.M., Some ABC's of skeletal pathophysiology. 6. The growth/modelling/remodeling distinction. *Calcified Tissue International*, **49**, pp. 301–302, 1991.

[82] Van Oosterwyck, H., Duyck, J., Vander Sloten, J., Van der Perre, G., De Cooman, M., Puers, R., Van Cleynenbreugel, J. & Naert, I., Etiology of marginal bone loss around oral implants: a finite element based approach. *Proc. of 12th Conference of the European Society of Biomechanics, Dublin,*

eds. P.J. Prendergast, T.C. Lee, & A.J. Carr, Royal Academy of Medicine in Ireland, pp. **26**, 2000.

[83] Cowin, S.C., Deviatoric and hydrostatic mode interaction in hard and soft tissue. *Journal of Biomechanics*, **23**, pp. 11–14, 1990.

[84] Natali, A.N. & Pavan, P.G., Evaluation of limit strength in implant–bone interaction with regard to dental prosthesis devices. *Proc. of 12th Conference of the European Society of Biomechanics, Dublin*, eds. P.J. Prendergast, T.C. Lee & A.J. Carr, Royal Academy of Medicine in Ireland, pp. 332, 2000.

CHAPTER 2

Computational simulation of trabecular surface remodeling using voxel finite element method

Taiji Adachi[1] and Ken-ichi Tsubota[2]

[1]Department of Mechanical Engineering, Kyoto University, Japan.
[2]Department of Bioengineering and Robotics, Tohoku University, Japan.

Abstract

Cancellous bone adapts its internal structure by trabecular surface remodeling to accomplish its mechanical function as a load bearing structure. Adaptive bone remodeling, defined as the coupled osteoblastic formation and osteoclastic resorption on the trabecular surfaces, has been investigated through both experimental and computational approaches. The computational mechanics approach allows us to test the influence of mechanical factors on adaptive bone remodeling, isolating the influence of these factors from their complex coupling with biological influences. In this study, a computational simulation method for trabecular surface remodeling using a microstructural voxel finite element modeling technique is proposed where morphological changes of trabeculae due to remodeling were directly expressed by removing/adding the elements from/to the trabecular surfaces. A rate equation of trabecular surface remodeling based on the local uniform stress hypothesis is applied. Two-dimensional simulation of trabecular surface remodeling was conducted for a human proximal femur. As a result, a distributed trabecular structure that macroscopically aligns along the principal stress directions was obtained under a multiple-loading condition. Subsequently, a cancellous bone cube was modeled using a digital image obtained by microcomputed tomography (μCT), and was uniaxially compressed. As a result of remodeling, the apparent stiffness against the applied load increased in which the trabeculae reorientated to the loading direction; and changes in the trabecular structural indices qualitatively coincided with previously published experimental observations. Through these simulation studies, it was demonstrated that the proposed voxel simulation technique enables us to simulate the trabecular surface remodeling and to compare the results with *in vivo* experimental data. In addition, this simulation method would be capable of providing insight into the hierarchical mechanism of trabecular surface remodeling at the microstructural level up to the apparent tissue level.

1 Introduction

Based on continuum mechanics, mathematical models for adaptive bone remodeling have been proposed, and have enabled us to predict the change in bone structures relating to stress/strain state at the apparent tissue level [1, 2]. However, cancellous bone remodeling is carried out by cellular activities on the trabecular surfaces in which a local mechanical stimulus plays an important role [3]. To understand the mechanism of functional adaptation in cancellous bone, it is essential to clarify the relationships between the macroscopic structural changes and the mechanical stimulus at the microstructural level.

Adding to the experimental approach taken to investigate the trabecular structural change under a controlled mechanical environment [4–8], the computational mechanics approach is indispensable to clarify the relationships between structural change and the stress/strain state at the trabecular level because the mechanical environment of trabeculae is complicated due to their complex architecture, the external shape of cortical bone, and various external-loading conditions. This approach allows us to test the influence of mechanical factors on adaptive bone remodeling, isolating the influence of these factors from their complex coupling with biological influences.

Theoretical modeling and computational simulations of bone remodeling have been developed for cortical and cancellous bone as a continuum [1, 2], and could successfully predict changes in the external shape and apparent density of bone. However, it has been recognized that anisotropic modeling and simulations are essential for evaluating local mechanical stimuli at the microstructural level, which affect the cellular activities in the bone remodeling process [3, 7]. Anisotropic continuum models have been proposed to describe the evolution of both apparent bone density and the orientation of trabecular architecture by using the fabric tensor [9], the anisotropic stiffness tensor [10], and the lattice continuum model [11]. Even though the anisotropy is not explicitly considered in the rate equation, the osteocyte-regulated bone-remodeling theory [12, 13] could predict the emergence of the anisotropic trabecular microstructure. Furthermore, the direct simulation method of trabecular surface remodeling has been proposed using a boundary element method [14, 15] and a voxel finite element method [16–20].

For the prediction of 3D trabecular structural changes caused by remodeling, detailed modeling of the complex trabecular microstructure is essential. Digital image-based voxel models of cancellous bone with high resolutions, which can be obtained by X-ray μCT scanning [21], enable modeling and stress analysis [22, 23] of the trabecular microstructure. In addition, this voxel finite element modeling technique is a useful tool for predicting microstructural changes in cancellous bone caused by remodeling; for example, structural changes in the case of osteoporosis were predicted by solving the evolution of bone relative density as a continuum [24]. However, since trabecular remodeling is due to cellular activities on the trabecular surface [25], the morphological changes due to surface movement by remodeling should be directly modeled and simulated at the trabecular level.

The purposes of this study were to propose a simulation method for trabecular surface remodeling using the microstructural voxel finite element modeling technique, and to demonstrate its applicability through case studies. A rate equation for trabecular surface remodeling [16] based on the local uniform stress hypothesis [26] was applied to voxel finite element models of cancellous bone. To investigate a characteristic of the hypothesis under a heterogeneously distributed mechanical environment, 2D simulation of trabecular surface remodeling was conducted for a proximal femur [18]. Subsequently, a remodeling simulation was carried out for a cancellous bone cube [17] that was directly modeled based on X-ray μCT digital image data using a large number of voxel finite elements, and compared with an *in vivo* experiment [7].

2 Method of voxel finite element simulation for trabecular surface remodeling

2.1 Model of trabecular surface remodeling toward uniform stress state

Trabecular structural change due to remodeling is caused by coupled bone resorption and formation by successive cellular activities on the trabecular surface [25], as shown in fig. 1(a). The relative difference between resorption and formation brings apparent movement of the trabecular surface, which leads to morphological changes of the trabeculae, as shown in fig. 1(b). In the model of trabecular surface remodeling proposed by Adachi *et al.* [16], trabecular structural change is assumed

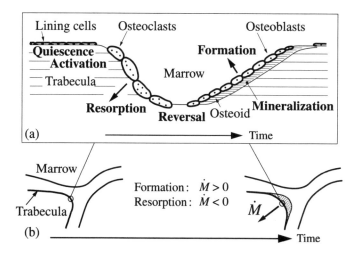

Figure 1: Trabecular surface remodeling by cellular activities leading to morphological changes in trabecular architecture of cancellous bone [18]: (a) Osteoclastic resorption and osteoblastic formation on trabecular surface and (b) Surface movement by trabecular surface remodeling.

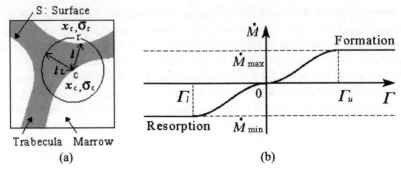

Figure 2: Model of trabecular surface remodeling driven by nonuniformity of the mechanical stimulus σ on the trabecular surface [18]: (a) Driving force of remodeling Γ is defined as the relative difference between stress σ_c at x_c and σ_d determined by integrating stress σ_r at x_r at the neighboring point $(l < l_L)$ with weight function $w(l)$ and (b) Remodeling rate equation $\dot{M} = \dot{M}(\Gamma)$ as a function of the remodeling driving force Γ representing nonuniformity in mechanical stimulus σ at x_c on the trabecular surface.

driven by a local nonuniformity of mechanical stimulus to seek a uniform state of the mechanical stimulus. The nonuniformity of the mechanical stimulus can be related to the stress/strain gradient that would cause fluid flow affecting cellular activities in remodeling [27–30].

First, using a scalar function of the stress σ, driving force for the remodeling at point x_c on the trabecular surface S is evaluated as local stress non-uniformity Γ:

$$\Gamma = \ln(\sigma_c/\sigma_d), \tag{1}$$

where σ_c denotes the stress at point x_c, and σ_d denotes the representative stress in the area around the point x_c, as shown in fig. 2(a). The stress σ_d is defined by

$$\sigma_d = \frac{\int_s w(l)\sigma_r dS}{\int_s w(l)dS}, \tag{2}$$

where σ_r denotes the stress at the point x_r on the trabecular surface S, and l denotes the distance between the points x_c and x_r. The weighting function $w(l)[w(l) > 0$ $(0 \leq l < l_L)]$ is assumed to depend on the distance l. Sensing distance l_L in fig. 2(a) is a model parameter representing the area where cells can sense a mechanical stimulus, regulating spatial distribution of apparent bone density [31].

Second, the driving force Γ determines the rate of trabecular surface movement $\dot{M}$ to seek uniform mechanical stimulus, as $\dot{M} < 0$ for $\Gamma < 0$ and $\dot{M} > 0$ for $\Gamma > 0$, by using a continuous function as shown in fig. 2(b). Model parameters Γ_u and Γ_l in fig. 2(b) are threshold values of the lazy zone [32, 33] around the remodeling equilibrium point. The parameters express the sensitivity of the cells to a mechanical stimulus in time, regulating the rate of trabecular structural change [31].

2.2 Voxel simulation method for trabecular surface remodeling

A voxel finite element model of trabeculae [22, 23, 34, 35] can be reconstructed from digital images such as those obtained by μCT scanning [21, 36], and used to represent the trabecular architecture in detail. This technique enabled direct estimation of stress and strain at the trabecular level that regulate cellular activities in bone remodeling. In this study, a model of trabecular surface remodeling [16], which was proposed to express morphological changes in the trabeculae as a local stress regulation process, is applied to the 3D microstructural voxel finite element models of cancellous bone.

Using this voxel-based modeling technique, trabecular surface remodeling is simulated by following procedures.

1. Stress in the trabecular element was analyzed under a given boundary condition using a large-scale finite element method with the element-by-element preconditioned conjugate gradients (EBE/PCG) approach [37] in which diagonal scaling was used as a preconditioner [23].
2. For all trabecular surface elements, the driving force of remodeling Γ at x_c in eqn (1) is calculated to express nonuniformity of the scalar function of the mechanical stimulus σ in space. In eqn (2), S denotes the trabecular surface and $l = |x_r - x_c|$, as shown in fig. 2(a). The weight function $w(l)$ takes a nonzero positive value at the neighbor point within the sensing distance l_L. As a simple case, the following function was used.

$$w(l) = \begin{cases} 1 - l/l_L & (0 \le l \le l_L) \\ 0 & (l_L \le l). \end{cases} \qquad (3)$$

3. The rate of surface movement $\dot{M}$ is determined by substituting the evaluated value of Γ into the function shown in fig. 2(b), in which the parameters Γ_l and Γ_u are the threshold values of remodeling. With the progress of remodeling, the nonuniformity of the surface stress becomes small, that is, $|\Gamma|$ approaches zero. As a result, the probability of remodeling also approaches zero, which represents the lazy zone of remodeling around the equilibrium state [32, 33].
4. Morphological changes are accomplished by the removal/addition of the voxel elements from/to the trabecular surfaces.
5. If a remodeling equilibrium is not attained, return to the procedure (1), in which equilibrium is attained when the number of voxel elements under resorption/formation and the change in bone volume fraction become sufficiently small.

Procedures (1) to (5) are one step of the simulation. In this paper, the von Mises equivalent stress is used as the scalar function σ of the stress as the mechanical stimulus. Other positive scalar functions that act as mechanical stimuli, such as the strain energy density, are also applicable in this theory, and similar results in bone structure at the equilibrium state can be expected [16, 26].

3 Functional adaptation of cancellous bone in proximal femur predicted by trabecular surface remodeling simulation

3.1 Finite element model of human proximal femur

A computational model of a human proximal femur was created using approximately 0.67 million voxel-based finite elements, as shown in fig. 3(a). Assuming an isotropic trabecular structure at the initial stage, the cancellous bone part was filled with a random pattern of circular trabeculae, as shown in fig. 3(b). The external and internal diameters of each trabecula were $1680\,\mu\text{m}$ and $1120\,\mu\text{m}$, respectively. The principal values of the fabric ellipse of the trabecular structure [38], $H_i(i = 1, 2, H_1 > H_2)$, were $H_1 = 714\,\mu\text{m}$ and $H_2 = 713\,\mu\text{m}$, that is, the degree of structural anisotropy H_1/H_2 was nearly equal to unity. The bone part was assumed to be a homogeneous and isotropic material with Young's modulus $E = 20$ GPa and Poisson's ratio $\nu = 0.3$. The marrow part was regarded as a cavity, and neglected in finite element analysis.

Stress for the loading case $L_i(i = 1, 2, 3)$ was analyzed by the finite element method under the plane strain condition with a 10 mm thickness. Using equivalent stress as a scalar function of the stress σ, remodeling driving force Γ_i for the loading case L_i was calculated for all the elements on a trabecular surface. Under the multiple-loading condition, the averaged value Γ_{mlt} with weighting depending

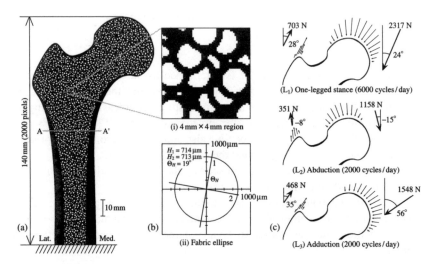

Figure 3: Computational simulation model for trabecular surface remodeling in human proximal femur using large-scale voxel-based finite elements [18]: (a) Overview of the finite element model; (b) Initial trabecular structure and its fabric ellipse; and (c) Boundary condition considering daily loading history [39].

on the loading frequency n_i:

$$\Gamma_{mlt} = \sum_{i=1}^{3} w_i \Gamma_i, \quad \text{where } w_i = \frac{n_i}{n_1 + n_2 + n_3}, \tag{4}$$

was used as a remodeling driving force.

As a representative daily loading condition, three loading cases of one-legged stance (L_1), extreme ranges of motion of abduction (L_2), and adduction (L_3) were assumed [39], as shown in fig. 3(c). These external loadings were applied as distributed forces generated by using a sine function to the joint surface and the greater trochanter. The lower boundary that corresponded to the diaphysis was fixed. Simulation results were discussed only for the proximal region of the finite element model, above the line A-A' shown in fig. 3(a), to neglect an artificial influence of the fixed boundary condition.

The model parameters in the remodeling model need to be determined from the experimental observations. However, quantitative experimental data for determining these parameters were not available because of the difficulty of *in vivo* observation of the change in trabecular architecture under a controlled mechanical environment. In this study, the parameters were set constant as the threshold values $\Gamma_u = 1.0$ and $\Gamma_l = -2.0$, and the sensing distance $l_L = 0.1$ mm to give reasonable trabecular structure, based on the previous computational study in which the effects of the model parameters on trabecular structural changes were investigated [31]. Therefore, the simulation conducted in this study was one of the case studies for discussing the basic and qualitative characteristics of the remodeling model.

The calculation was repeated for 16 simulation steps. Remodeling equilibrium was attained at 16th simulation step for all the simulation results for a proximal femur, judged by the number of voxel elements under resorption/formation becoming less than 2% of the cancellous bone area.

3.2 Trabecular structural change under single-loading condition

Remodeling simulations were conducted under both single-loading and multiple-loading conditions. Trabecular structural change under single loading at the 16th step was obtained depending on the loading case, as shown in fig. 4, due to the formation and resorption induced by the remodeling toward a local uniform stress state. In the loading case of one-legged stance (L_1), as shown in fig. 4(a), trabeculae were aligned with the compressive joint reaction force in the femoral head, represented by region 1, and with the tensile abductor force in the greater trochanter, represented by region 2. On the other hand, an orthogonal trabecular pattern emerged in the lateral side of the femoral neck, represented by region 3. This orthogonal pattern consisted of compressive trabeculae from the medial side to the lateral side near the greater trochanter, and tensile trabeculae from the lateral side to the neck of the femoral head.

In the loading case of abduction (L_2), the joint reaction force caused bending loads at the femoral neck, resulting in arcuate trabecular structure from the lateral

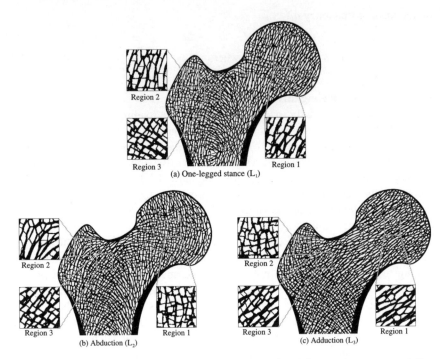

Figure 4: Trabecular structural change in the proximal femur due to remodeling under single loading at the 16th step [18]: (a) One-legged stance (L_1); (b) Abduction (L_2); and (c) Adduction (L_3).

cortical diaphysis to the femoral head, as shown in fig. 4(b). These arcuate trabeculae configured orthogonal trabecular patterns in the femoral head, represented by region 1, combined with compressive trabeculae along the joint reaction force. An orthogonal trabecular pattern also emerged in the lateral side of the femoral neck, represented by region 3. In the greater trochanter, represented by region 2, trabeculae were aligned with the tensile abductor force. The structural changes in regions 2 and 3 were similar to those obtained in the case L_1.

In the loading case of adduction (L_3), as shown in fig. 4(c), unidirectional trabeculae were distinguished in the femoral head, represented by region 1, because the compressive joint reaction force did not cause bending loads at the femoral neck. This compressive trabecular pattern spreads to the lateral side of the femoral neck, represented by region 3, and to the greater trochanter, represented by region 2. An orthogonal trabecular pattern appeared in region 2 because the trabeculae were also formed along the tensile abductor force.

The distribution of apparent bone density was obtained over the entire cancellous region. In the loading cases L_1 and L_2, the higher density emerged in the center of the femoral head, represented by region 1, and in the lateral side of the femoral neck, represented by region 3. The regions with lower density were the greater

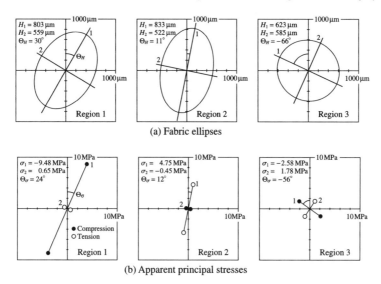

(a) Fabric ellipses

(b) Apparent principal stresses

Figure 5: Correspondence between structural property and mechanical environment at the apparent tissue level in regions $1 \sim 3$ at the 16th step under
the single-loading condition of one-legged stance (L_1) [18]: (a) Fabric
ellipses and (b) Apparent principal stresses.

trochanter, represented by region 2, and the femoral neck. Compared to these two
loading cases, the density distribution was not distinguished in the loading case L_3.

A structural property at the apparent tissue level, quantified by fabric ellipses, corresponded to the apparent stress state, as shown in fig. 5. In the loading case L_1 at the
16th step, the degree of structural anisotropy was $H_1/H_2 = 1.44$ and the principal
direction of the fabric ellipse was $\Theta_H = 30°$ in region 1, $H_1/H_2 = 1.60$ and $\Theta_H =
11°$ in region 2, and $H_1/H_2 = 1.06$ and $\Theta_H = 60°$ in region 3, as shown in fig. 5(a).

Calculating the apparent principal stresses $|\sigma_1|$ and $|\sigma_2|$ ($|\sigma_1| > |\sigma_2|$) by averag-
ing the stress components over the cancellous area, the ratio of magnitude of two
principal stresses was $|\sigma_1|/|\sigma_2| = 14.6$ and the principal direction of the stresses
was $\Theta_\sigma = 24°$ in region 1, $|\sigma_1|/|\sigma_2| = 10.6$ and $\Theta_\sigma = 12°$ in region 2, and
$|\sigma_1|/|\sigma_2| = 1.4$ and $\Theta_\sigma = -56°$ in region 3, as shown in fig. 5(b). Comparing the
fabric ellipses to the apparent principal stresses, it was shown that a unidirectional
trabecular pattern emerged in the regions of a uniaxial compressive stress state
(region 1) or tensile stress state (region 2), and that an orthogonal trabecular pattern
emerged in the regions of a biaxial compressive-tensile stress state (region 3). In
addition to the fabric ellipses obtained in the loading case L_1, the fabric ellipses
obtained in the cases L_2 and L_3 also corresponded to the apparent principal stresses.

3.3 Trabecular structural change under multiple-loading condition

Anisotropic trabecular architecture was obtained under multiple loadings at the
16th step, as shown in fig. 6. Because the one-legged stance loading (L_1) was the

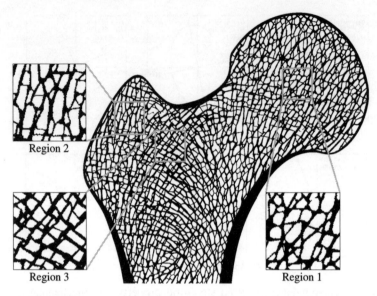

Figure 6: Trabecular structural change in the proximal femur due to remodeling under multiple loadings at the 16th step [18].

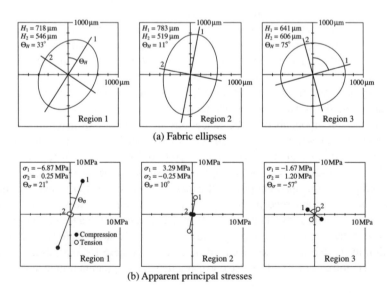

Figure 7: Correspondence between structural property and mechanical environment at the apparent tissue level in regions $1 \sim 3$ at the 16th step under the multiple loading condition [18]: (a) Fabric ellipses and (b) Apparent principal stresses.

most frequent (60%) in the three loading cases, the apparent trabecular orientation and density distribution were similar to those obtained under the single-loading condition of the case L_1, as shown in fig. 4(a).

Functional adaptation at the apparent tissue level was also exhibited, the same as in the case of single-loading condition. That is, the fabric ellipses, as shown in fig. 7(a), corresponded to the apparent principal stress state, as shown in fig. 7(b). The degree of structural anisotropy was $H_1/H_2 = 1.32$ and the principal direction of the fabric ellipse was $\Theta_H = 33°$ in region 1, $H_1/H_2 = 1.51$ and $\Theta_H = 11°$ in region 2, and $H_1/H_2 = 1.06$ and $\Theta_H = 75°$ in region 3. In evaluating the apparent principal stresses under multiple loadings, the stresses for the three loading cases were averaged with weighting depending on the loading frequency in the same manner in calculating the driving force Γ_{mlt} in eqn (4). The ratio of the two principal stresses was $|\sigma_1|/|\sigma_2| = 27.5$ and the principal direction was $\Theta_\sigma = 21°$ in region 1, $|\sigma_1|/|\sigma_2| = 13.2$ and $\Theta_\sigma = 10°$ in region 2, and $|\sigma_1|/|\sigma_2| = 1.39$ and $\Theta_\sigma = -57°$ in region 3. These characteristic parameters for the structure and mechanical environment were similar to those obtained under the single-loading condition of the case L_1.

As a result of adaptation to the multiple external loadings, the orientation of each trabecula was more distributed than that obtained under the single-loading condition. For instance, the trabecular structure and distribution of von Mises equivalent stress are illustrated for the center of region 1 at the 16th step in fig. 8. The equivalent stress of the trabeculae ranged up to 10 MPa, and varied depending on the loading cases. Driven by the various mechanical stimuli at the trabecular level, the surface remodeling brought about the distributed trabecular orientation corresponding to each loading direction. The trabeculae mainly supporting the loadings varied according to the external-loading cases, as indicated by arrows in fig. 8. Thus, multi-directional trabeculae were formed to support the multiple loadings.

3.4 Discussion

Trabecular structural changes were simulated for a human proximal femur using finite element models to investigate the characteristics of a surface-remodeling model based on the uniform stress hypothesis. To clarify the mechanism of bone remodeling driven by a local mechanical stimulus at the microstructural level, it is necessary to consider a heterogeneously distributed trabecular structure under complicated external loadings. In investigating the functional adaptation of cancellous bone brought by trabecular structural changes under such a complicated mechanical environment, a direct simulation method with a large-scale computation is advantageous compared to the models using a unit cell of trabecular structure, as was used in the lattice continuum model proposed by Adachi et al. [11] or in the homogenization method [40, 41].

Under the single-loading condition, surface remodeling driven by local stress nonuniformity caused the structural changes of trabeculae, resulting in an anisotropic trabecular structure depending on the applied loadings. Because the structural changes at the trabecular level brought the apparent structural properties that

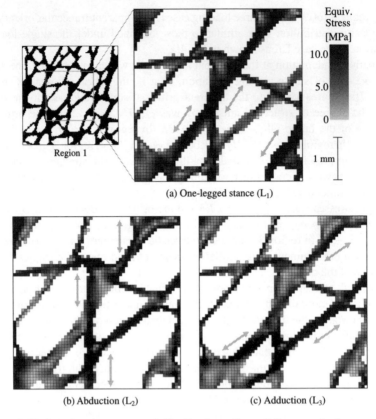

(a) One-legged stance (L₁)

(b) Abduction (L₂)   (c) Adduction (L₃)

Figure 8: Trabecular structure and distribution of von Mises equivalent stress at
the center of region 1 under multiple loadings at the 16th step [18]:
(a) One-legged stance (L_1); (b) Abduction (L_2); and (c) Adduction (L_3).

corresponded to the apparent mechanical environment, it was suggested that the
surface-remodeling model based on the uniform stress hypothesis could explain the
functional adaptation in cancellous bone under a realistic mechanical environment.
For example, the correspondence of the principal directions of fabric ellipses to
those of the apparent stresses agrees with the mathematical expression of Wolff's
law denoted by Cowin [42]. Moreover, the predicted density pattern and trabecular orientation at the apparent tissue level are consistent with those predicted by
the remodeling model that described the evolution of bone density and structural
anisotropy [10]. These results demonstrate the capability of the surface-remodeling
model investigated in this study to predict the adaptive change in cancellous bone
at both the trabecular level and the apparent tissue level.

Under the multiple-loading condition, trabeculae adapted to the various mechanical environments according to the three cases of external loadings. The obtained
trabecular structure was distributed as was predicted by the remodeling simulation
that focused on the evolution of apparent bone density under multiple loadings

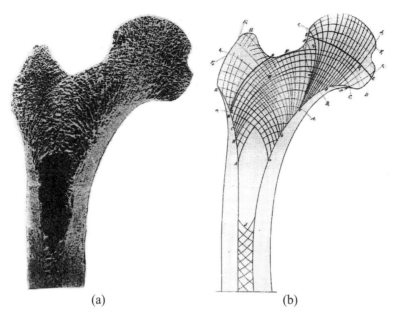

(a)   (b)

Figure 9: Trabecular architecture in proximal femur (from Wolff's monograph [44]:
(a) Section of a human proximal femur and (b) An orthogonal set of curved
lines.

[43]. One of the new things attained in this study was that the distributed structure
of each trabecula was predicted simultaneously with the apparent structural properties corresponding to the apparent principal stresses. These results successfully
predicted the trabecular structure observed in the actual bone as shown in fig. 9,
indicating the validity of the surface remodeling simulation based on the uniform
stress hypothesis using a large-scale voxel-based finite element model.

Some limitations of this study need to be addressed in order to discuss the characteristics of the surface-remodeling model. Following prior computational studies
on bone remodeling [10, 28, 33, 43], a 2D model of human proximal femur was
used in this study, considering that 2D models can represent the characteristic
mechanical environment and trabecular structure of the proximal femur. The 2D
model was sufficiently useful for investigating basic and qualitative relationships
between trabecular structural changes and their mechanical environment. However,
simulation results obtained using the 2D model do not quantitatively express the
3D structure and its mechanical environment in actual bone. The fabric ellipse and
apparent bone density predicted in this study, which are characteristic quantities
of trabecular structure, might be different from those obtained in 3D simulation,
although the trabecular structural orientation would correspond to the mechanical
environment, as was predicted in this study. In future work, 3D simulation [17]
is necessary in quantitative evaluation of trabecular structural changes driven by
local stress nonuniformity in the proximal femur, as shown in fig. 10.

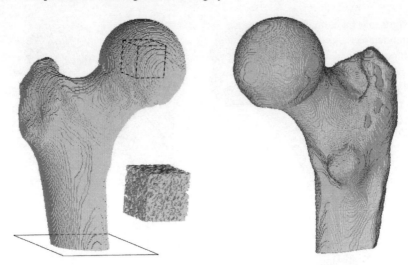

Figure 10: Three-dimensional voxel finite element model of a human proximal femur constructed based on digital images.

The obtained principal values of fabric ellipses were larger than those in the actual bone [45] due to the trabecular size used in the simulation at the initial stage. This larger size of the trabeculae was the reason why the sensing distance l_L was chosen to be 1.0 mm, which might be much larger than the physiological range of a few hundred micrometers [12, 46]. To discuss an appropriate value of the sensing distance l_L, the characteristic size of initial trabecular structure should be refined to be of the same size as that in the actual bone. In addition, quantitative comparison of the trabecular structure obtained by 3D remodeling simulation to experimental observation is necessary in determining the sensing distance l_L.

Considering that the cellular activities are influenced by local mechanical stimuli, the local stress nonuniformity, which was equivalent to the convexity and concavity of the scalar function of stress/strain, was used as a remodeling driving force, as shown in eqn (1). In terms of the uniform stress hypothesis, the difference from the reference value of stress/strain [28] or the first-order gradient could be responsible for the fluid flow that would activate bone cells. Because the distribution of apparent bone density obtained in this study did not emerge clearly compared to the remodeling models that seek a reference value of the stress/strain, the model using local stress nonuniformity as a remodeling driving force is less sensitive to the global distribution of the mechanical stimulus. A clearer density distribution is expected by choosing the larger sensing distance l_L [31]. However, if the determined parameter l_L is out of the physiological range, it might be better to explicitly introduce the sensitivity to the global distribution of the mechanical stimulus into the surface-remodeling model in addition to the local mechanical stimulus.

The time-course change in the mechanical environment was not explicitly considered in the remodeling model in which averaging of the mechanical environment in time was assumed to affect trabecular surface remodeling. For further insight into the actual remodeling phenomena, the remodeling model needs to be extended to include the effects of the time-course change in the mechanical environment on trabecular structural change by taking the stress nonuniformity in time to be the remodeling driving force in addition to the stress nonuniformity in space. An extended model will express bone formation/resorption corresponding to the increase/decrease of external loading, and more bone formation under dynamic loading than under static loading.

It was found that the external-loading condition affected the stress distribution of each trabecula, as shown in fig. 8. These figures illustrate the ability of a large-scale voxel-based finite element model to predict the micro-macro relationships in cancellous bone that has a hierarchical structure. Exploring the mechanical stimulus at the cellular level might be possible by considering the internal structure of each trabecula. Therefore, it should be noted that the large-scale computational simulation of bone remodeling would be an effective tool not only for clarifying the relationships between the functional adaptation at the apparent tissue level and the local regulation process at the trabecular level, but also for providing insight into cellular response to the mechanical stimuli *in vivo*.

4 Trabecular surface remodeling simulation for cancellous bone using microstructural voxel finite element models

4.1 Digital-image-based model of cancellous bone

Guldberg and Goldstein *et al.* [6, 7] reported experimental observation of trabecular bone adaptation adjacent to porous-coated platen implants embedded within canine distal femoral metaphyses. In the present study, adaptive changes of the trabecular bone architecture underneath the platen of 6 mm diameter were simulated and compared with the experimental results. A digital image-based model of a cancellous bone cube, $a = 5$ mm on each side, was obtained from canine distal femoral metaphyses based on 3D reconstructed μCT data, as shown in fig. 11(a). The voxel element size was 25 μm, the same as the resolution of the μCT data, and thus the total volume contained $200^3 = 8$ million voxel elements in which approximately 2.3 million elements were trabecular bone elements. The structural indices of the trabecular architecture [21] and the fabric ellipsoid of the trabecular architecture [38] could be directly calculated from the binarized 3D data.

The trabecular bone is assumed to be a homogeneous and isotropic elastic material with Young's modulus $E = 5.33$ GPa and Poisson's ratio $\nu = 0.3$ [47]; the marrow was considered to be a cavity and was excluded.

As boundary conditions, uniform displacement $U_3(< 0)$ was controlled at every simulation step on the upper plane at $X_3 = 5.0$ mm to apply the apparent stress $\sigma_3 = F_3/a^2 = -1.24$ Mpa referring to the experimental value [7], as shown in fig. 11(a), where $F_3(< 0)$ is the total force applied on the plane and $\varepsilon_3 = U_3/a$ is defined as the apparent strain in the X_3 direction. On the other five planes, shear-free boundary conditions were applied, that is, the displacements perpendicular to the plane were fixed. The sensing distance l_L in the weight function $w(l)$ was set to 500 μm, equal to the length of 20 voxel elements, and the threshold values of remodeling were set to $\Gamma_u = 4.0$ and $\Gamma_l = -5.0$. These model parameters should be determined through comparison with experimental observations [31].

4.2 Cancellous bone level

Morphological changes in the trabecular architecture of a cancellous bone cube due to remodeling under compressive loading at the 10th, 20th, and 50th steps are represented in figs 11(b)–(d), in which fabric ellipsoids of the 3D architecture and fabric ellipses of the $X_1 - X_3$ cross section show the development of trabecular anisotropy. The initial morphology shown in fig. 11(a) adapted to the applied compressive load by resorption and formation on the trabecular surface to reduce the nonuniformity of the stress. Degrees of anisotropy, defined as H_1/H_3 where

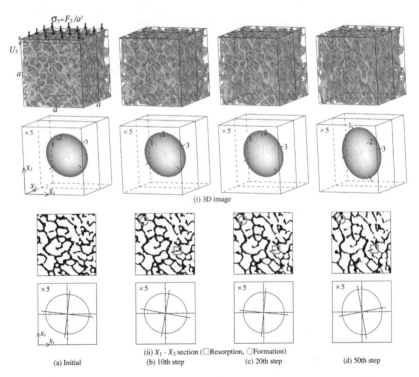

(i) 3D image

(ii) X_1 - X_3 section (□Resorption, ○Formation)

(a) Initial   (b) 10th step   (c) 20th step   (d) 50th step

Figure 11: Changes of 3D architecture of cancellous bone cube and fabric ellipsoid; $X_1 - X_3$ cross section and fabric ellipse, due to trabecular surface remodeling under compressive loading [17]: (a) Initial voxel finite element model ($200 \times 200 \times 200$ voxel elements) based on μCT digital image obtained from canine distal femur (b); 10th step; (c) 20th step; and (d) 50th step.

$H_i(H_1 \geq H_2 \geq H_3)$ are the principal values of the fabric ellipsoid, increased from 1.33 (initial) to 1.39 (50th step) upon aligning the trabecular architecture along the compressive loading axis; this can be observed in the rotation of the principal direction of the fabric ellipsoid from figs 11(a) to (d). The preferential loss of horizontal trabeculae, indicated by open rectangles in the cross-sectional image in fig. 11, and the preservation and increase in thickness of vertically oriented trabeculae directed along the compressive loading axis, indicated by open circles, contribute to the development of trabecular anisotropy.

Changes in structural indices are plotted in figs 12(a)–(d). The indices were measured using voxel finite elements at every simulation step for the center core cube of $4.0 \times 4.0 \times 4.0 \, \text{mm}^3$ from the whole volume of $5.0 \times 5.0 \times 5.0 \, \text{mm}^3$ to eliminate numerical errors adjacent to the boundary. As a result of remodeling, a decrease of 21.2% for the bone volume fraction (BV/TV), a 19.3% decrease in the trabecular thickness ($Tb.Th$), and a 2.2% decrease in the trabecular number ($Tb.N$) were found at the 50th step compared with the initial values, which resulted in a 10.0% increase in the trabecular separation ($Tb.Sp$). The increase in $Tb.Sp$ is because the resorption of horizontal trabeculae is more remarkable than the formation of vertical trabeculae. The angle Θ_{i3} between the principal directions n_i of the fabric ellipsoid and the loading axis X_3 changed upon the reorientation of the trabecular architecture, as shown in fig. 12(e). The angle Θ_{13} monotonically decreased from $7.63°$ toward zero; in contrast, Θ_{23} and Θ_{33} increased toward $90°$. These changes in

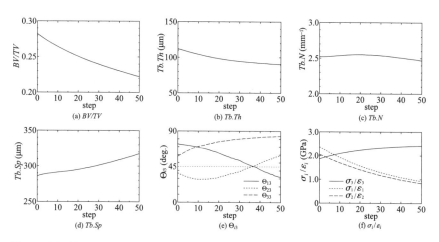

Figure 12: Changes in structural indices, principal direction of trabecular architecture and apparent stiffness of cancellous bone due to remodeling under compressive load [17]: (a) Bone volume fraction (BV/TV); (b) Trabecular bone thickness ($Tb.Th$); (c) Trabecular bone number ($Tb.N$); (d) Trabecular bone separation ($Tb.Sp$); (e) Angle Θ_{i3} between principal direction of H_i and loading axis X_3; and (f) Apparent stiffness σ_i/ε_i in X_i direction.

the structural indices and angles indicate that the trabecular orientation changes to align along the compressive axis X_3, which exhibits adaptive remodeling to support uniaxial compressive load.

In this simulation, the initial digital-image-based model was produced referring to the control trabecular bone cube from the contra-lateral side in the experiment [7], and the simulation results were compared with the experimental one within the same animal. The structural indices for the control and experimental bones for one canine and the simulation results are listed in table 1. In the simulation, the trabecular bone volume fraction (*BV/TV*) and the angle Θ_{13} of the principal axis of the trabecular architecture decreased, and the trabecular separation (*Tb.Sp*) increased by remodeling under compressive load. These results qualitatively coincide with experimental observations, in which changes in *BV/TV*, Θ_{13}, and *Tb.Sp* were statistically significant compared with the control data in the experiment. The trabecular number (*Tb.N*) slightly decreased, while that in the experiment significantly decreased. For the trabecular thickness (*Tb.Th*), the simulation result showed a decrease by remodeling; however, in the experiment, *Tb.Th* did not show significant change.

The apparent stiffness of the core cube of $4.0 \times 4.0 \times 4.0$ mm in the direction of three orthogonal axes X_1, X_2 and X_3 was numerically measured by uniaxial compression testing at each simulation step. Applied boundary conditions were similar to those in the remodeling simulation, that is, uniform displacement was applied on the upper surface and other surfaces were fixed under share-free conditions. Changes in the apparent stiffness σ_i/ε_i in the direction of coordinate axes X_i are plotted in fig. 12(f). In the compressive loading direction in the remodeling simulation, the X_3 direction, the apparent stiffness σ_3/ε_3 gradually increased by 29.4%; however, both σ_1/ε_1 and σ_2/ε_2 in the direction perpendicular to the loading axis decreased by about 60% due to remodeling. Thus, remodeling resulted in functional changes in the trabecular architecture and increases in the degree of anisotropy in the mechanical properties. Even though the average bone volume fraction decreased by remodeling, as shown in fig. 12(a), the stiffness as a structure was increased by remodeling, demonstrating the adaptive response in order to support compressive load through the reorganization of the trabecular architecture.

Table 1: Structural indices and principal direction of trabecular architecture for control, experiment, and simulation [17]: Control cancellous bone cube is from the contra-lateral side in the experiment [7], and used as the initial model in the simulation.

	BV/TV	*Tb.Th* (μm)	*Tb.N* (mm^{-1})	*Tb.Sp* (μm)	Θ_{13} (deg.)
Control	0.282	112	2.52	286	73.6
Experiment	0.230	121	1.88	421	47.9
Simulation	0.222	90	2.47	317	31.9

4.3 Discussion

As a result of remodeling, each trabecula rotated toward the compressive loading direction in order to support the load, and the apparent stiffness against load increased. In general, a reduction in bone mass is responsible for a decrease in the stiffness as a structure; however, even though the trabecular bone volume decreased, the apparent stiffness as a structure increased, through the reorganization of the trabeculae aligned along the compressive loading axis. These results, obtained under the assumption of the uniform stress hypothesis, could be understood as a functional adaptation by remodeling to the applied mechanical load.

The basic concept of introducing the weighting function $w(l)$ to express the decaying influence is from the similar approach by Mullender *et al.* [12]. The use of the integral form in eqn (2) takes into account the existence of the sensory network system [48] between multiple cells at neighboring points. The expression of eqn (2) using a weighting function $w(l)$ could be extended to consider the nonuniformity of the stress in the trabeculae by integrating over the volume element dV for the case in which the role of the osteocyte [3] is taken into account.

Driven by the nonuniformity of the stress, the adaptive reorganization of the trabecular architecture by remodeling was smoothly simulated, as shown in figs 11 and 12, and a uniform stress distribution was achieved, using digital image-based voxel finite element models. The apparent stiffness in the compressive loading axis increased with reorganizing the trabecular architecture and with increasing the degree of anisotropy, although the volume fraction decreased. This result implies that remodeling under the assumption of the uniform stress hypothesis [26] revealed the functional adaptive response of the bone as a load-bearing structure. Thus, these results demonstrate that the proposed simulation method for trabecular surface remodeling using voxel finite element models is applicable to the simulation of the functional adaptation phenomenon in cancellous bone.

Compared with a similar bone adaptation model for predicting changes in the 3D trabecular morphology using voxel-based trabecular bone models [24], in which the evolution of the bone relative density was solved as a continuum, the proposed simulation of trabecular surface remodeling has the potential to express the change in the trabecular structure directly by solving the trabecular surface movement. And, the surface movement by remodeling at the trabecular level was directly expressed by removing/adding the voxel elements from/to the trabecular surface. Quantitative comparison of the changes in the trabecular structure with the experimental observations that are obtained under a controlled mechanical environment would enable us to develop more detailed models. In addition, the reorientation of the trabeculae to correspond to the principal loading direction is a good illustration of the model developed by Cowin *et al.* [9] in which a fabric tensor is used.

The discrepancy between experiment and simulation results is because the comparison in table 1 is made for only one set of canine data, and another simulation with a different initial trabecular structure is expected to yield qualitatively the same results. To develop models that can predict the details of the remodeling phenomenon, the model parameters Γ_u, Γ_l , and l_L have to be quantitatively determined through comparison with experimental observations for multiple specimens. However, to date, because of the difficulty in observing the changes in trabecular architecture under a controlled mechanical environment *in vivo*, only a small number of remodeling experiments [6, 7, 49] have been performed to obtain quantitative results with respect to how bone remodeling is controlled by the mechanical environment.

The choice of model parameters is an important issue in the simulation. In a previous article [31], the characteristics of the model parameters, Γ_u, Γ_l, and l_L in the rate equation of trabecular surface remodeling were studied. The parameter set of Γ_u and Γ_l represents the remodeling rate sensitivity in time to the mechanical stimuli around the remodeling equilibrium, and the parameter l_L represents the area where the cells can sense the mechanical stimuli, that is, the sensitivity to the stress nonuniformity in space. From the *in vitro* experiment of observing the propagation of the calcium signaling wave to the neighboring cells [46, 50], the sensing distance l_L can be estimated to be a few hundred μm. Thus, in the simulation, l_L was set to 100 μm for a single trabecula, and 500 μm for a cancellous bone cube with rough discretization. The trabecular remodeling thresholds, Γ_u and Γ_l, need not be equal, because formation and resorption are different events. When they are set to be equal, resorption becomes more dominant, and therefore $|\Gamma_l|$ was set to be larger, in this study, to control the change in total bone volume. We believe that this set of model parameters can be extended to express an unbalanced remodeling process like that of osteoporosis-type bone resorption. From these points of view, the model parameters used in the simulation were for one of the case studies for which qualitative results could be obtained; at this stage, this is the limitation of the proposed simulation method.

One of the noteworthy features of the proposed simulation method is the capability to handle a large-scale 3D voxel model with a regular finite element mesh for complex trabecular architecture. This offers many practical advantages, such as enabling us to create voxel finite element models based on digital images such as those obtained by X-ray μCT scanning, and a variety of cancellous bone could be analyzed using images obtained from *in vivo* experiments. In addition, this simulation method could be utilized as a tool to visualize, in a computer, the morphological change of trabecular architecture by remodeling. Thus, this technique is useful for achieving further clarification of the trabecular bone-remodeling phenomenon by observing microscopic structural changes directly using the proposed simulation.

Furthermore, the application of this simulation method to bone tissue engineering would be an exciting challenge, that is, its application to the optimal design of biomaterial scaffolds for the regeneration of bone tissue [51–53]. Combined with a bone microstructure measurement system such as μCT scanning, the proposed method has the potential to be applied in designing scaffold topology and pore geometry through a process that considers bone mechanical properties, fluid diffusion through scaffold pores, deformation to control biological cellular activities, degradation of biomaterial scaffold, and new bone ingrowth/formation as a bone-scaffold system [54–56].

Acknowledgments

The support of the Japan Society for the Promotion of Science (Postdoctoral Fellowships for Research Abroad 1998) and the Computational Biomechanics Project at the Institute of Physical and Chemical Research (RIKEN, Junior Research Associate) are gratefully acknowledged. This work was supported financially in part by a Grant-in-Aid for Scientific Research from the Ministry of Education, Science, Sports and Culture, Japan and CREST from the Japan Science and Technology Agency (JST). The authors would like to thank Steve Goldstein, Scott Hollister and Nancy Caldwell at the University of Michigan and Prof. Yoshihiro Tomita at Kobe University for helpful comments.

References

[1] Cowin, S.C., Bone stress adaptation models. *Trans. ASME, J. Biomech. Eng.*, **115(4B)**, pp. 528–533, 1993.
[2] Huiskes, R. & Hollister, S.J., From structure to process, from organ to cell: Recent developments of FE-analysis in orthopaedic biomechanics. *Trans. ASME, J. Biomech. Eng.*, **115(4B)**, pp. 520–527, 1993.
[3] Cowin, S.C., Moss-Salentijn, L. & Moss, M.L., Candidates for the mechanosensory system in bone. *Trans. ASME, J. Biomech Eng.*, **113(2)**, pp. 191–197, 1991.
[4] Chambers, T.J., Evans, M., Gardner, T.N., Turner-Smith, A. & Chow, J.W.M., Induction of bone formation in rat tail vertebrae by mechanical loading. *Bone & Min.*, **20**, pp. 167–178, 1993.
[5] Cheal, E.J., Snyder, B.D., Nunamaker, D.M. & Hayes, W.C., Trabecular bone remodeling around smooth and porous implants in an equine patellar model. *J. Biomech.*, **20(11/12)**, pp. 1121–1134, 1987.
[6] Goldstein, S.A., Matthews, L.S., Kuhn, J.L. & Hollister, S.J., Trabecular bone remodeling: An experiment model. *J. Biomech.*, **24(S1)**, pp. 135–150, 1991.
[7] Guldberg, R.E., Richards, M., Caldwell, N.J., Kuelske, C.L. & Goldstein, S.A., Trabecular bone adaptation to variations in porous-coated implant topology. *J. Biomech.*, **30(2)**, pp. 147–153, 1997.
[8] Moalli, M.R., Caldwell, N.J., Patil, P.V. & Goldstein, S.A., An *in vivo* model for investigations of mechanical signal transduction in trabecular bone. *J. Bone & Min. Res.*, **15(7)**, pp. 1346–1353, 2000.
[9] Cowin, S.C., Sadegh, A.M., & Luo, G.M., An evolutionary Wolff's Law for trabecular architecture. *Trans. ASME, J. Biomech. Eng.*, **114(1)**, pp. 129–136, 1992.
[10] Jacobs, C.R., Simo, J.C., Beaupre, G.S. & Carter, D.R., Adaptive bone remodeling incorporating simultaneous density and anisotropy considerations. *J. Biomech.*, **30(6)**, pp. 603–613, 1997.
[11] Adachi, T., Tomita, Y. & Tanaka, M., Three-dimensional lattice continuum model of cancellous bone for structural and remodeling simulation. *JSME Int. J.*, **42(C-3)**, pp. 470–480, 1999.

[12] Mullender, M.G., Huiskes, R. & Weinans, H., A physiological approach to the simulation of bone remodeling as a self organization control process. *J. Biomech.*, **27(11)**, pp. 1389–1394, 1994.

[13] Huiskes, R., Ruimerman, R., Van Lenthe, G.H. & Janssen, J.D., Effects of mechanical forces on maintenance and adaptation of form in trabecular bone. *Nature*, **405**, pp. 704–706, 2000.

[14] Sadegh, A.M., Luo, G.M. & Cowin, S.C., Bone ingrowth: An application of the boundary element method to bone remodeling at the implant interface. *J. Biomech.*, **26(2)**, pp. 167–182, 1993.

[15] Luo, G., Cowin, S.C., Sadegh, A.M. & Arramon, Y.P., Implementation of strain rate as a bone remodeling stimulus. *Trans. ASME, J. Biomech. Eng.*, **117**, pp. 329–338, 1995.

[16] Adachi, T., Tomita, Y., Sakaue, H. & Tanaka, M., Simulation of trabecular surface remodeling based on local stress nonuniformity, *JSME Int. J.*, **40(C-4)**, pp. 782–792, 1997.

[17] Adachi, T., Tsubota, K., Tomita, Y. & Hollister, S.J., Trabecular surface remodeling simulation for cancellous bone using microstructural voxel finite element models. *Trans. ASME, J. Biomech. Eng.*, **123(5)**, pp. 403–409, 2001.

[18] Tsubota, K., Adachi, T. & Tomita, Y., Functional adaptation of cancellous bone in human proximal femur predicted by trabecular surface remodeling simulation toward uniform stress state. *J. Biomech.*, **35(12)**, pp. 1541–1551, 2002.

[19] Tsubota, K., Adachi, T. & Tomita, Y., Effects of a fixation screw on trabecular structural changes in a vertebral body predicted by remodeling simulation of trabecular surface remodeling. *Anna. Biomed. Eng.*, **31(6)**, pp. 733–740, 2003.

[20] Tsubota, K. & Adachi T., Changes in the fabric and compliance tensors of cancellous bone due to trabecular surface remodeling, predicted by a digital image-based model. *Comput. Methods Biomech. & Biomed. Eng.*, **7**, 2004.

[21] Feldkamp, L.A., Goldstein, S.A., Parfitt, A.M., Jesion, G. & Kleerekoper, M., The direct examination of three-dimensional bone architecture *in vitro* by computed tomography. *J. Bone Min. Res.*, **4(1)**, pp. 3–11, 1989.

[22] Hollister, S.J. & Kikuchi, N., Homogenization theory and digital imaging: A basis for studying the mechanics and design principles of bone tissue. *Biotech. & Bioeng.*, **43**, pp. 586–596, 1994.

[23] van Rietbergen, B., Weinans, H., Huiskes, R. & Odgaard, A., A new method to determine trabecular bone elastic properties and loading using micromechanical finite-element models. *J. Biomech.*, **28(1)**, pp. 69–81, 1995.

[24] Mullender, M., van Rietbergen, B., Rüegsegger, P. & Huiskes, R., Effect of mechanical set point of bone cells on mechanical control of trabecular bone architecture. *Bone*, **22(2)**, pp. 125–131, 1998.

[25] Parfitt, A.M., Osteonal and hemi-osteonal remodeling: The spatial and temporal framework for signal traffic in adult human bone. *J. Cell. Biochem.*, **55**, pp. 273–286, 1994.

[26] Adachi, T., Tanaka, M. & Tomita, Y., Uniform stress state in bone structure with residual stress. *Trans. ASME, J. Biomech. Eng.*, **120(3)**, pp. 342–347, 1998.

[27] Klein-Nulend, J., van der Plas, A., Semeins, C.M., Ajubi, N.E., Frangos, J.A., Nijweide, P.J. & Burger, E.H., Sensitivity of osteocytes to biomechanical stress *in vitro*. FASEB J., **9**, pp. 441–445, 1995.

[28] Turner, C.H., Anne, V. & Pidaparti, M.V., A uniform strain criterion for trabecular bone adaptation: Do continuum-level strain gradients drive adaptation? *J. Biomech.*, **30(6)**, pp. 555–563, 1997.

[29] Wang, L., Fritton, S.P., Cowin, S.C. & Weinbaum, S., Fluid pressure relaxation depends upon osteonal microstructure: Modeling an oscillatory bending experiment. *J. Biomech.*, **32(7)**, pp. 663–672, 1999.

[30] Weinbaum, S., Cowin, S.C. & Zeng, Y., A model for the excitation of osteocytes by mechanical loading-induced bone fluid shear stresses. *J. Biomech.*, **27(3)**, pp. 339–360, 1994.

[31] Tsubota, K., Adachi, T., Tomita, Y., Simulation study on model parameters of trabecular surface remodelling model, *Computer Methods in Biomechanics & Biomedical Engineering – 3*, eds. J. Middleton, M.L. Jones, N.G. Shrive & G.N. Pande, Gordon and Breach Science Publishers, pp. 129–134, 2001.

[32] Carter, D.R., Mechanical loading histories and cortical bone remodeling. *Calcif. Tis. Int.*, **36**, pp. S19–S24, 1984.

[33] Huiskes, R., Weinans, H., Grootenboer, H.J., Dalstra, M., Fudala, B. & Slooff, T.F., Adaptive bone-remodeling theory applied to prosthetic-design analysis. *J. Biomech.*, **20(11/12)**, pp. 1135–1150, 1987.

[34] Hollister, S.J., Brennan, J.M. & Kikuchi, N., A homogenization sampling procedure for calculating trabecular bone effective stiffness and tissue-level stress. *J. Biomech.*, **27(4)**, pp. 433–444, 1994.

[35] Ulrich, D., van Rietbergen, B., Weinans, H. & Rüegsegger, P., Finite element analysis of trabecular bone structure: A comparison of image-based meshing techniques. *J. Biomech.*, **31(12)**, pp. 1187–1192, 1998.

[36] Rüegsegger, P., Koller, B. & Muller, R., A microtomographic system for the nondestructive evaluation of bone architecture. *Calcif. Tissue Int.*, **58**, pp. 24–29, 1996.

[37] Hughes, T.J.R., Ferencz, R.M. & Hallquist, J.O., Large-scale vectorized implicit calculations in solid mechanics on a Cray X-MP/48 utilizing EBE preconditioned conjugate gradients. *Comp. Meth. Appl. Mech. Eng.*, **61**, pp. 215–248, 1987.

[38] Cowin, S.C., The relationship between the elasticity tensor and the fabric tensor. *Mech. Mat.*, **4**, pp. 137–147, 1985.

[39] Beaupré, G.S., Orr, T. E. & Carter, D.R., An approach for time-dependent bone modeling and remodeling – application: A preliminary remodeling simulation. *J. Orthop. Res.*, **8(5)**, pp. 662–670, 1990.

[40] Fernandes, P., Rodrigues, H.C. & Jacobs, C.R., A model of bone adaptation using a global optimisation criterion based on the trajectorial theory of Wolff. *Comp. Meth. Biomech. & Biomed. Eng.*, **2**, pp. 125–138, 1999.

[41] Bagge, M., A model of bone adaptation as an optimization process. *J. Biomech.*, **33(11)**, pp. 1349–57, 2000.

[42] Cowin, S.C., Wolff's law of trabecular architecture at remodeling equilibrium. *Trans. ASME, J. Biomech. Eng.*, **108**, pp. 83–88, 1986.

[43] Carter, D.R., Orr, T.E. & Fyhrie, D.P., Relationships between loading history and femoral cancellous bone architecture. *J. Biomech.*, **22(3)**, pp. 231–244, 1989.

[44] Wolff, J., The Law of Bone Remodeling, (Trans. P. Maquet and R. Furlong), Springer, (Originally published in 1892), 1986.

[45] Ciarelli, T.E., Fyhrie, D.P., Schaffler, M.B. & Goldstein, S.A., Variations in three-dimensional cancellous bone architecture of the proximal femur in female hip fractures and in controls. *J. Bone & Min. Res.*, **15(1)**, pp. 32–40, 2000.

[46] Xia, S.-L. & Ferrier, J., Propagation of a calcium pulse between osteoblastic cells. *Biochem. Biophys. Res. Commu.*, **186(3)**, pp. 1212–1219, 1992.

[47] van Rietbergen, B., Odgaard, A., Kabel, J. & Huiskes, R., Direct mechanics assessment of elastic symmetries and properties of trabecular bone architecture. *J. Biomech.*, **29(12)**, pp. 1653–1657, 1996.

[48] Donahue, H.J., McLeod, K.J., Rubin, C.T., Andersen, J., Grine, E.A., Hertzberg, E.L. & Brink, P.R., Cell-to-cell communication in osteoblastic networks: Cell line-dependent hormonal regulation of gap junction function. *J. Bone & Min. Res.*, **10(6)**, pp. 881–889, 1995.

[49] Guldberg, R.E., Caldwell, N.J., Guo, X.E., Goulet, R.W., Hollister, S.J. & Goldstein, S.A., Mechanical stimulation of tissue repair in the hydraulic bone chamber. *J. Bone & Min. Res.*, **12(8)**, pp.1295–1302, 1997.

[50] Adachi, T., Sato, K. & Tomita, Y., Directional dependence of osteoblastic calcium signaling response to mechanical stimulus. *Biomech. & Model. Mechanobiol.*, **2(2)**, pp. 73–82, 2003.

[51] Hollister, S.J., Chu, T.M., Guldberg, R.E., Zysset, P.K., Levy, R.A., Halloran, J.W. & Feinberg, S.E., Image based design and manufacture of scaffolds for bone reconstruction, *Synthesis in Bio Solid Mechanics*, eds. P. Pedersen & M.P. Bendsoe, Kluwer Academic Publishers, pp. 163–174, 1999.

[52] Taboas, J.M., Maddox, R.D., Krebsbach, P.H. & Hollister, S.J., Indirect solid free form fabrication of local and global porous, Biomimetic and composite 3D polymer-ceramic scaffolds. *Biomat.*, **24(1)**, pp. 181–94, 2003.

[53] Lin, C.Y., Kikuchi, N. & Hollister, S.J., A novel method for biomaterial scaffold internal architecture design to match bone elastic properties with desired porosity. *J. Biomech.*, **37(5)**, pp. 623–636, 2004.

[54] Adachi, T., Kawano, Y. & Tomita, Y., Computational prediction of change in stiffness of bone-scaffold structure in regeneration process. *2001 ASME Bioeng. Conf.*, ASME BED, **50**, eds. R.D. Kamm, G.W. Schmid-Schonbein, G.A. Ateshian, & M.S. Hefzy, pp. 545–546, 2001.

[55] Adachi, T., Kawano, Y., Tomita, Y. & Hollister, S.J., Design method of porous scaffold microstructure using computational simulation for bone regeneration. *Abstracts of the 4th World Cong. Biomech.*, 2002.

[56] Adachi, T., Tomita, Y. & Hollister, S.J., Three-dimensional simulation for porous scaffold degradation and new bone formation in regeneration process. *2003 ASME Sum. Bioeng. Conf.*, (CD-ROM), 2003.

CHAPTER 3

Patient specific bone and joints modeling and tissue characterization derived from medical images

M.-C. Ho Ba Tho
Laboratoire de Biomécanique et Génie Biomédical, UMR CNRS 6600
Université de Technologie de Compiègne, France.

Abstract

The objective of the paper is to address the methodology developed to model bone and joints with individualized geometric and material properties from medical image data. An atlas of mechanical properties of human bone has been investigated demonstrating individual differences. From these data, predictive relationships have been established between mechanical properties and quantitative data derived from measurements on medical images. Subsequently, geometric and numerical models of bones with individualized geometrical and mechanical properties have been developed from the same source of image data. The advantages of this modeling technique are its ability to study the 'patient' specificity. This should be of importance for quantifying bone and joint deformities and performing individualized preoperative planning surgery or orthopaedic treatment. In the same way, the efficiency of orthopaedic treatment with customised orthese or mechanical behavior of implant in bone could be evaluated. Results would suggest improvement or development of new design.

1 Introduction

Bone and joints are complex structures in their geometry and material properties. In order to assess bone deformities or understand the mechanical behavior of the implant in bone, it is necessary to model the physiological conditions of the bone and joints. The only way to obtain patient specific geometry will be to assess medical images such as magnetic resonance imaging (MRI), computed tomography (CT) and X-ray. This step has been almost achieved by most of the researchers. The other important factor to be considered is the mechanical properties of the patient. This last step is still poorly investigated as it needs basic research on the assessment of bone and joints material properties using mechanical testing and tissue characterization derived from medical images. Mechanical properties have been investigated for three decades but the data is not always of help for the modeling purpose.

This chapter will address the methodology we have developed in order to model bone and joints with appropriate geometric and mechanical properties derived from medical imaging. Medical imaging systems such as MRI, CT, X-rays are commonly used to evaluate musculo-skeletal disease. The main advantages of MRI and CT techniques are the 3D geometry assessment and the tissue characterization derived from pixels grey level density. That is why these two techniques are mainly in use.

Numerical methods are used for solving physical and mechanical engineering problems. These numerical methods are appropriate for modeling such complex systems as human bone and joints. Literature review demonstrated the extensive use of finite element modeling in biomechanics [1–3]. According to our knowledge, the first two dimensional finite element model derived from medical image were obtained by digitizing radiography [4], and a three dimensional finite element model derived from digitized CT scans [5]. Then, extensive finite element models are obtained from CT data with most often a lack of description of the method allowing to model the geometry. One should note that little attention is given to the acquisition parameters and their consequences to the accuracy of bone modeling. Some authors proposed specific protocol to optimize the reconstruction of a specific long bone (femur) from CT data [6] meanwhile others focus on the hardware and software parameters acquisition influence on the CT image assessment qualitatively and quantitatively [7]. Automatic FE generation have been developed using CT scans voxels [8, 9]. The voxels are converted directly in elements of equal size. Problems occurring with this technique are (1) their limitation in the accuracy of the model at the geometric and material boundaries and (2) the number of elements generated which would require specific algorithms of resolution. Besides these extensive numerical models, most of models are derived from CT data and a few from MRI. Few consider appropriate material properties as they are mostly issued from literature (data or relationships). When experimental data do not confirm numerical simulation, material properties data are assessed experimentally by mechanical testing. This can only be performed on cadaveric specimens.

As shown by the previous review, human bone has a non uniform geometry and a heterogeneous structure. One may expect differences from bone to bone and among individuals. In order to consider these intrinsic differences, it was necessary to develop a modeling technique describing appropriately and simultaneously the geometric and material properties. The methodology we have developed is based on a semi-automatic generation of a three dimensional geometric model of bone and joints anatomy derived from medical imaging CT or MRI data. Predictive relationships obtained from previous work demonstrated a significant correlation between the material properties and quantitative measurements derived from imaging techniques [10, 11]. Then, from the same source of medical imaging data, numerical models with individualized geometric and mechanical properties were developed.

2 Methods

The different steps of the methodology would be first to be able to decode the native medical images in order to assess the geometry and the density grey level. It is important to assess native grey level density in order to assess biological material tissue characterization.

The second step would be to determine the mechanical properties of bone or soft tissue and correlate these mechanical properties with bone and joints tissue characterization derived from medical images.

2.1 Assessment of geometry via medical imaging techniques

There are different modalities of medical imaging techniques to explore bone and joints: X-ray radiographs, CT scanner, MRI. The first two techniques are based on absorption of X-rays, and are often used to diagnose bone disease. Meanwhile the third is based on proton resonance and is more dedicated to soft tissue such as ligaments, cartilage besides bone structures are also visualised.

In order to assess the anatomical data, we have developed a pre-processing medical image CT and MRI [12].

The different steps of the image processing were (1) to decode the stack of medical image data representing the three dimensional of bone and joints structure, (2) to perform an edge detection after a threshold process and (3) to build geometric entities of the bones with creation of an output data file in a neutral format or an IGES format.

2.1.1 Medical image processing

The standard exchange format file of the medical image derived from American College of Radiology and National Electric Manufacturers Association (ACR-NEMA) specifications is Digital Imaging COmmunication in Medicine (DICOM). Once the medical images are decoded, image processing can be performed. A pixel is coded on 12 bits i.e. pixel values varies from 0 (white) to 4096 (black). The next step is to perform the threshold process. It consists in giving threshold values based on the histogram representing the distribution of pixel values. As a result only anatomical contours of interest are visualized on the binary image (only two levels 0 and 1, white and black). Then segmentation by region is used, the edge detection allowed the outlines of the anatomical structure to be obtained. The edge detection consists in Hermite parametric cubic curves interpolation. Their formulation is obtained from a parametric cubic equation (eqn (1)) and geometric constraints on two ending points.

$$P(u) = [x(u), y(u), z(u)],$$

$$P(u) = \sum_{k=0}^{3} a_k u^k, \quad u \in [0, 1]. \tag{1}$$

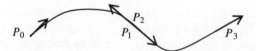

Figure 1: Hermite parametric cubic curves.

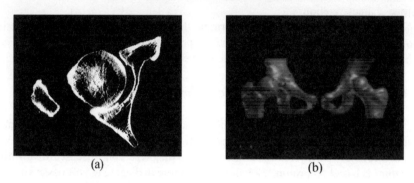

(a)   (b)

Figure 2: (a) Axial CT slice after the threshold process and (b) 3D visualization of bone contours (lines and surfaces).

Their final expression form with blending functions are expressed in eqn (2).

$$P(u) = P_0(1-3u^2+2u^3)+P_1(3u^2-2u^3)+P_0'(u-2u^2+u^3)+P_1'(-u^2+u^3) \quad (2)$$

$P(u = 0) = P_0$, $P(u = 1) = P_1$, $P_0' P_1'$: ending points and associated derivatives. The geometric continuity of two curves is obtained by defining same tangent at the ending points of the first curve and the first point of the second curve as illustrated in fig. 1.

Surfaces connecting these curves were Hermite bicubic polynomials defined by eqn (3).

$$P(u) = \sum_{i=0}^{3}\sum_{j=0}^{3} a_{ij}u^i v^j, \quad u, v \in [0, 1]. \quad (3)$$

The different steps of a 3D geometrical reconstruction *in vivo* of a human hip from CT data is illustrated in fig. 2. The pre- and post-processor Patran (MSC.Software) is used for the visualization of the geometric entities written in a neutral file.

Once the geometrical data was obtained, finite element meshing was performed via any commercial software.

In order to model realistic bone anatomy, it is necessary to associate the appropriate mechanical properties of the bone.

2.2 Mechanical properties of human bone

Mechanical properties of bone have been studied for over three decades in order to understand the mechanical behavior of bone in the process of fracture risk, repair and bone related disease. Besides, few data are available or insufficient for human bone modeling. Human bone is highly heterogeneous and anisotropic material. It can be compared to composite materials; it is made of two different tissue, spongious bone (high porosity) and cortical bone (compact bone), depending on the anatomical location. Bone was assumed to have an orthotropic behavior which stiffness matrix containing elastic constants were defined by eqn (4). By reversing the stiffness matrix, the compliance matrix allowed the elastic properties in the three axes of symmetry of the crystal to be determined eqn (5).

$$[C_{ij}] = \begin{bmatrix} C_{11} & C_{12} & C_{13} & 0 & 0 & 0 \\ C_{21} & C_{22} & C_{23} & 0 & 0 & 0 \\ C_{31} & C_{32} & C_{33} & 0 & 0 & 0 \\ 0 & 0 & 0 & C_{44} & 0 & 0 \\ 0 & 0 & 0 & 0 & C_{55} & 0 \\ 0 & 0 & 0 & 0 & 0 & C_{66} \end{bmatrix}, \tag{4}$$

$$[S_{ij}] = \begin{bmatrix} \frac{1}{E_1} & -\frac{v_{21}}{E_3} & -\frac{v_{31}}{E_3} & 0 & 0 & 0 \\ -\frac{v_{12}}{E_1} & \frac{1}{E_2} & -\frac{v_{32}}{E_3} & 0 & 0 & 0 \\ -\frac{v_{13}}{E_1} & \frac{v_{23}}{E_2} & \frac{1}{E_3} & 0 & 0 & 0 \\ 0 & 0 & 0 & \frac{1}{G_{23}} & 0 & 0 \\ 0 & 0 & 0 & 0 & \frac{1}{G_{31}} & 0 \\ 0 & 0 & 0 & 0 & 0 & \frac{1}{G_{12}} \end{bmatrix}, \tag{5}$$

where E_i is the Young's moduli in the direction i, G_{ij} is the Shear moduli in plane i-j and v_{ij} is the Poisson's ratio stress and strain respectively in directions i, j.

Experimentally, an ultrasonic transmission technique was used to assess bone material properties. Different wave propagation techniques were used for velocities measurements of bone tissue. Bulk velocities were measured for cortical bone, and then elastic constants were obtained. Cancellous bone is porous and highly heterogeneous compared to cortical bone. Homogeneous volume needed to be assumed and bar waves were used, allowing to assess directly the elastic properties Ashman et al. [13, 14]. An atlas of mechanical properties was performed in order to obtain a database of material properties of different types of bone (femur, tibia, mandible, humerus, patella, lumbar spine, scapula) Ho Ba Tho et al. [11, 15], Mansat et al. [16]. The range of values (minimum-maximum, median, average and standard deviation) of the mechanical properties of the different type of cancellous bone are summarized in table 1.

The range of values (minimum-maximum, median, average and standard deviation) of the mechanical properties of the different type of cancellous bone are summarized in table 2.

Differences of properties between bones and between subjects suggested the use of appropriate characteristic value of properties. When differences are not found to be significant, an average value of properties can be considered as the characteristic

Table 1: Minimum and maximum values, the mean and the average with standard deviation of the mechanical properties of cancellous bone.

Cancellous bone	E_1 (MPa)	E_2 (MPa)	E_3 (MPa)	ρ (kg/m^3)	σ (MPa)
Distal femur	34–2412 604 760 $\pm$ 589	39–2037 583 707 $\pm$ 555	213–4419 1536 1698 $\pm$ 993	81–883 377 395 $\pm$ 180	0.18–19 5.09 5.94 $\pm$ 4.13
Proximal humerus	82–861 392 397 $\pm$ 215	102–975 440 438 $\pm$ 245	249–1719 807 813 $\pm$ 401	117–488 245 255 $\pm$ 91	0.30–7.12 2.11 2.71 $\pm$ 2.0
Lumbar spine	75–659 264 292 $\pm$ 192	73–730 273 321 $\pm$ 218	375–1939 926 1057 $\pm$ 571	132–368 224 242 $\pm$ 96	0.66–6.23 2.76 3.14 $\pm$ 1.57
Patella	286–3553 1650 1484 $\pm$ 794	221–3183 873 1197 $\pm$ 837	569–4925 2764 2801 $\pm$ 1363	391–1210 703 731 $\pm$ 222	1.07–17.45 6.47 7.71 $\pm$ 4.56
Posimal femur	24–2492 357 713 $\pm$ 783	23–2398 530 769 $\pm$ 734	105–3669 996 1267 $\pm$ 888	73–857 285 350 $\pm$ 190	0.25–16.82 3.46 4.83 $\pm$ 3.87
Proximal tibia	27–530 171 202 $\pm$ 154	32–636 186 232 $\pm$ 180	141–1970 604 769 $\pm$ 534	55–440 181 198 $\pm$ 94	0.11–7.99 1.88 2.58 $\pm$ 2.22

value. Conversely, when differences are found to be significant, a range (minimum and maximum) would be more accurate to characterize the properties. The range of values of mechanical properties for cortical bone and cancellous bone from eight subjects are summarized in table 3.

Ultimate strength of cortical specimen was not measured, literature review gave typical values around 150 MPa. Relationships between mechanical properties of cortical and cancellous human bone is illustrated in fig. 3.

The following statements were found according to the atlas of mechanical properties measured experimentally:

- the mechanical properties of cortical bone vary around the periphery with a small variation around 10% and do not vary along the length
- the mechanical properties of cancellous bone vary around the periphery (around a factor of 2) and along the length (around a factor of 3 to 5)
- cortical and cancellous bone are orthotropic materials, however, the degree of anisotropy of cancellous bones is higher than that of cortical bones
- the mechanical properties are different from bone to bone for cortical and cancellous bones

Table 2: Minimum and maximum values, and the average with standard deviation of the mechanical properties of cortical bone.

Cortical bone	E_1 (GPa)	E_2 (GPa)	E_3 (GPa)	ρ (kg/m^3)
Femur	7.4–16.2	8–17	16.7–24.3	1581–1996
	11.8	12.2	19.8	1791
	11.7 ± 1.9	12.3 ± 2.0	19.9 ± 2.7	1821 ± 183
Humerus	6.9–14.4	7.3–16.5	13.8–25.5	1552–2075
	10.8	11.8	20.5	1790
	10.7 ± 2.0	11.6 ± 2.1	20.0 ± 2.7	1779 ± 153
Mandible	8.6–14.6	8.6–15.5	13.6–27	1731–1976
	11.7	12.1	20.5	1863
	11.6 ± 1.3	12.4 ± 2.1	20.4 ± 2.9	1858 ± 74
Tibia	8.4–15.3	8.8–15.4	15.9–24.6	1616–2063
	11.7	12.2	20.8	1859
	11.7 ± 1.3	12.2 ± 1.4	20.7 ± 1.9	1840 ± 11

Table 3: Range of values of mechanical properties obtained from eight subjects. Minimum, maximum and median values are given.

Bone	Cortical	Cancellous
E_{axial} (GPa)	14–27	0.011–3.12
	20	0.961
$E_{tangential}$ (GPa)	7–17	0.023–1.5
	12	0.341
E_{radial} (GPa)	7–16	0.024–1.5
	11	0.301
ρ (kg/m^3)	1545–2118	55–774
	1840	257
CT (HU)	1270–1835	72–512
	1560	143
σ_{ult} (MPa)	–	0.11–11
		3

- the mechanical properties of cortical and cancellous bone are not all equal between subjects but not all necessarily different
- the relationship between axial modulus and density is linear for cortical bone
- for cancellous bones, linear or power fits were found approximately equal
- powers vary from 1.3 to 1.7 for axial modulus versus density and 1.3 to 2.3 for strength versus density.

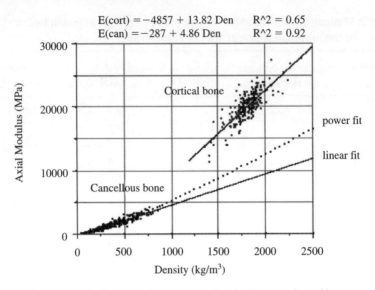

$$E(cort) = -4857 + 13.82 \, Den \qquad R^2 = 0.65$$
$$E(can) = -287 + 4.86 \, Den \qquad R^2 = 0.92$$

Figure 3: Relationships between mechanical properties of bone.

These results suggest (1) the use of appropriate characteristic values (average or range) of properties for parameterization study or finite element analysis and (2) the use of appropriate relationships of axial modulus, strength and density upon the type of bone.

Finally, these results suggest the consideration of the heterogeneity of bone material properties and the subject specificity when dealing with bone pathology. One way to consider a patient specificity is to develop numerical models with their geometric and mechanical properties.

2.3 Models with individualized geometric and material properties from CT data

In order to associate geometric and mechanical properties, we assume that measurements derived from medical imaging could predict material properties. We have investigated the relationships between CT numbers derived from CT imaging techniques and mechanical properties of bone. The CT number characterize a linear coefficient of attenuation of X-ray within the tissue. For the CT scan, the pixels values are represented by an empirical number called CT number expressed in Houndsfield units (HU) and is defined by the following empirical equation:

$$CT \, (HU) = 1000 \frac{CT - CT_{water}}{CT_{water} - CT_{air}}, \qquad (6)$$

$$CT \, (HU) = 1000 \frac{\mu - \mu_{water}}{\mu_{water} - \mu_{air}}, \qquad (7)$$

where μ is the linear coefficient of attenuation of X-ray within the tissue (cm^{-1}). CT number value is dependent on acquisitions parameters, typical values are 0 and -1000 for water and air, respectively.

Table 4 summarizes some predictive relationships between elastic properties and density and CT numbers, Rho *et al.* [10], Ho Ba Tho *et al.* [11, 15] of the proximal tibia (upper extremity of the tibia).

Until now, few investigations were performed concerning the cortical bone, as previous relationships [15] were not significant and could not be used to predict cortical bone material properties derived from CT. That is mainly due to the low range of cortical bone material properties investigated and the limitation of the CT technique at that time.

Correlation was found between mechanical properties and CT number of cortical human bone. The data are obtained from multiscale mechanical and morphological properties characterization of cortical bone, Ho Ba Tho *et al.* [17] (fig. 4). A new ultrasonic technique has been investigated to provide an acoustic image of

Table 4: Predictive relationships for the proximal tibia. Young's modulus is expressed in MPa and density in kg/m^3 and CT number in HU.

Relationships	Coefficient of determination
$E_{\text{axial}} = 0.51\rho^{1.37}$	$R^2 = 0.96$
$E_{\text{tangential}} = 0.06\rho^{1.55}$	$R^2 = 0.90$
$E_{\text{radial}} = 0.06\rho^{1.51}$	$R^2 = 0.89$
$E_{\text{axial}} = 296 + 5.2\text{CT}$	$R^2 = 0.79$
$\rho = 144 + 0.916\text{CT}$	$R^2 = 0.80$

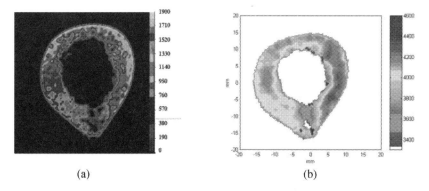

(a)   (b)

Figure 4: Cartography of CT numbers (HU) and bulk velocities (m/s) of human femur.

the cortical bone reflecting bone heterogeneity and the relation with microstructure (microporosity) has been investigated with an immersion ultrasonic technique Bensamoun *et al.* [18, 19].

2.4 Mechanical properties of soft tissue

Modeling joints are mainly obtained by MRI data. In these problems, all soft tissues have to be reconstructed such as cartilage, bone, menisci, ACL ligaments for the knee as an example. When non linear static problems are performed, the mechanical properties of the soft tissue are obtained from the literature.

Our methodology in current investigations will consist of assessing mechanical properties of soft tissue during MRI acquisition in order to correlate MRI ROI which depends mainly on different relaxation time T1, T2 with mechanical properties. The major problem would be to define appropriate MRI acquisitions to visualize and assess tissue characterization.

Mechanical properties *in vivo* can be defined as shown previously, boundary conditions can also be provided by the images (exact location of ligaments and other biological tissue). But it is still a major problem to know the *in vivo* load and muscles action of the patient. Geometry or morphological data of soft tissue can be assessed from medical image. Then, one would expect that by quantifying the morphology, the mechanical properties could be assessed. Relationships between morphological and mechanical properties of the muscle were investigated in order to provide the forces developed in relation with the muscle and fiber morphology, Bensamoun [20]. These data are of help as one may expect that forces generated are different from one patient to another.

From the same source of images data, a geometric reconstruction was performed as described previously and a finite element model was then performed via a commercial software. A custom made program matching mesh properties has been developed allowing the matching of the material properties distribution measured on the stack of CT image data and their assignment to the elements properties. The program consists in matching the measured mean CT number of a region of interest (ROI) with the characteristic geometric properties of the elements of the mesh. It should be noted that for the 3D mesh, it is necessary to match the technical acquisition parameters of the CT data with that of the protocol used to get the predictive relationships and the 3D mesh. The same methodology may be used for MRI data.

3 Applications

3.1 Modeling of bone and joints of children

The clinical application of the developed methods is to evaluate bone and joint disease in children (congenital dislocation of the hip (hip deformity) [21], clubfoot (foot deformity) [22], rotational abnormalities of the lower limbs [23, 24], scoliosis (spine deformity) [25]. Geometric model of the knee from MRI, allowed to perform

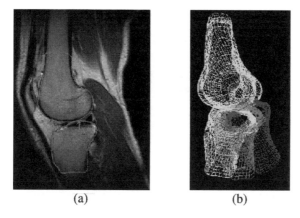

(a)   (b)

Figure 5: (a) MRI of a knee *in vivo* and (b) geometrical reconstruction.

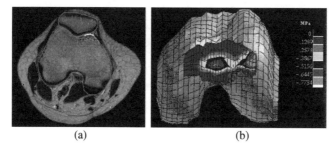

(a)   (b)

Figure 6: (a) MRI of femoro-patellar joint and (b) contact pressure visualized
on the femoral condyles.

kinematic analysis *in vivo* and quantification of contact areas using a non linear
analysis [26] (figs 5 and 6).

Geometric modeling of child foot bone *in vivo* derived from MRI [27] allowed to
distinguish the osseous nucleus and cartilage anlage (fig. 7). The length of the foot
is around 6 cm. The models allowed to quantify the bone deformity and perform
preoperative planning surgery.

Finite element models with individualized geometry and material properties
in vivo of a vertebral body of two scoliotic patients (same age and sex). They both
had a scoliotic deformity at the same level of the lumbar spine (L1). Figure 8
demonstrates clearly the individual difference in the geometry and material properties range and distribution Périé *et al.* [28].

3.2 Examples of arthroplasty

Arthroplasty consisted in changing the damaged joint (hip, knee, shoulder) by artificial joints. Figure 9 illustrates a numerical model of an acetabular implant of a
patient before and after surgery Hinrichs *et al.* [29]. In this study, significant influence of the assumptions on material properties have been demonstrated by assuming

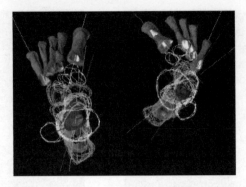

Figure 7: Geometrical model of new born clubfoot derived from MRI.

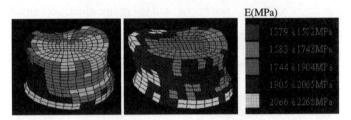

Figure 8: Finite element models with individualized geometric and mechanical properties of scoliotic patient.

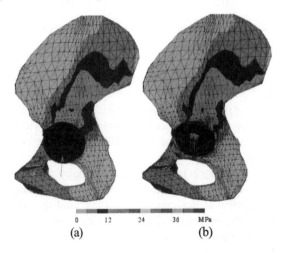

Figure 9: Von Mises Stresses for the model (a) without and (b) with implant.

the material to be isotropic or anisotropic homogeneous, isotropic or anisotropic inhomogeneous.

It should be noted that Von Mises stress is not appropriate to predict risk of failure for anisotropic elastic properties such as bone. But it is often used for these materials to simplify the interpretation and to represent the six stress components in a generalized 'stress intensity' factor Huiskes and Verdonschot [30].

The methodology has been applied to design and evaluate a customized hip implant from medical images. The protocol consists in designing a customized implant by considering the patient specific geometrical and mechanical properties. In parallel, a 3D finite element model is developed to evaluate the design and predict its mechanical behavior in the patient's femur Barré [31].

4 Discussion

4.1 Accuracy of the geometric modeling derived from medical images

Accuracy of the geometric model depends on the technical protocol acquisition of the medical images and methodology used for processing them. The geometrical errors could be introduced by the spatial resolution of the image (pixel size is equal to the field of view divided by the matrix of pixels) and algorithm of edge detection and interpolation function. A good spatial resolution allowed a better accuracy for the edge detection after the threshold process. Figure 10(a)–(b) illustrates two different spatial resolutions performed on the same image. The other source of error would be the choice of the values for the threshold process (fig. 10(b)–(c)).

For the same image with different values of thresholding may results different geometric results derived from curve interpolation.

Increasing the spatial resolution will increase the patient irradiation dose for CT image, and time examination for MRI. In general, compromise has to be taken between the quality of the images and patient welfare. An acceptable range of spatial resolution would be less than 0.5 mm (pixel value). It is clear that for each anatomical model sensitivity analysis has to be performed in order to define appropriate technical protocol of acquisition.

4.2 Models with individualized geometric and mechanical properties derived from medical images

Quantitative measurements performed on the CT images required a good 'density' resolution. In order to achieve that, the technical protocol of acquisition of the images should be optimised. Influence of these parameters on direct measurements

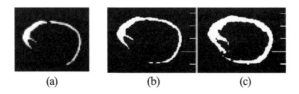

(a)   (b)   (c)

Figure 10: Geometric errors introduced by the spatial resolution (a) compared to (b) and the threshold process performed (b, c).

of CT number have been quantified and showed variation of 10% for the range of 0 to 1200 HU, Ho Ba Tho and Treutenaere [7]. This should be considered when predictive relationships are used to predict elastic properties from literature.

The methodology of bone modeling with individualized geometric and mechanical properties needed to be improved for MRI data, as tissue characterization is not reflecting significantly the material properties. In fact, the grey level of the region of interest is related to the intensity of proton density, which varies significantly with the acquisition parameters. When predictive relationships are not appropriate, the atlas database is used. When needed, this database is increased with other bones using the transmission ultrasonic technique.

4.3 Experimental validation

Before using our method in an *in vivo* case (patient case) our methodology has been validated in an *in vitro* case (cadaveric specimen) for customized hip implant Couteau *et al.* [32, 33], tibial implant Estivalèzes *et al.* [34], glenoid implants Baréa *et al.* [35]. Then *in vivo* modeling could be assessed for testing and predicting the short and long term implant behavior. The results can only be validated by clinical follow up and evaluation on the patient.

5 Conclusions and perspectives

Relevance of such techniques is their direct clinical application for modeling patient specific bone and joints. This provides an individual diagnosis and preoperative planning surgery or orthopaedic treatment.

Technical protocol of image acquisitions is of importance in the methodology; spatial and density resolution have to be achieved to reduce geometric and material properties errors.

The methodology needs to be improved by:

- the investigation of assessment of material properties of soft tissue derived from MRI
- the investigation of automatic meshing techniques dedicated to bone and joints anatomy; in order to reduce the time consumed in performing a finite element model of bone and joints.

These are challenging investigations for the next decade. From the results of *in vivo* modeling of bone and joints obtained with these techniques, one would expect objectives criterias for planning surgery or orthopaedic treatment and standardization for development of implants or orthoses.

Acknowledgments

The author would like to acknowledge Texas Scottish Rite Hospital for Children, Fondation pour la Recherche Médicale, INSERM (Institut National de la Santé et de la Recherche Médicale), CNRS (Centre National de la Recherche Scientifique) for their support. Clinicians from Orthopaedic Surgery and Radiology Departments of TSHR, CHU Purpan Toulouse and Polyclinique St Côme Compiègne are acknowledged for their scientific contribution.

References

[1] Huiskes, R. & Chao, E.Y.S., A survey of finite element analysis in orthopaedic biomechanics: the first decade. *Journal of Biomechanics*, **16**, pp. 385–409, 1983.

[2] Prendergast, P., Finite element models in tissue mechanics and orthopaedic implant design. Review paper. *Clinical Biomechanics*, **12**, pp. 343–366, 1997.

[3] Vander Sloten, J., Ho Ba Tho, M.C. & Verdonck, P., Applications of computer modeling for the design of orthopaedic, dental cardiovascular biomaterials. *Proc. Instn. Mech. Engrs.*, **212**, Part H, pp. 489–500, 1998.

[4] Carter, D.R, Vasu, R. & Harris, W.H., Stress changes in the femoral head due to porous ingrowth surface replacement arthroplasty. *Journal of Biomechanics*, **17**, pp. 737–747, 1984.

[5] Ho Ba Tho, M.C., Darmana, R., Pastor, P., Barrau, J.J., Laroze, S.& Morucci, J.P., Development of a three-dimensional finite element model of a human tibia using experimental modal analysis. *Journal of Biomechanics*, **24**, pp. 371–383, 1991.

[6] Viceconti, M., Zannoni, C., Baruffaldi, F., Pierotti, L., Toni, A. & Cappello, A., CT scan data acquisition to generate biomechanical models of bone structures. *Proc. of the 3rd Conf. on Computer Methods in Biomechanics and Biomedical Engineering*, eds. J. Middleton, M.L. Jones & G. Pande, Gordon and Breach Science Publishers, pp. 279–287, 1998.

[7] Ho Ba Tho, M.C. & Treutenaere, J.M., Influence of acquisition parameters on QCT measurements derived from CT. *Proc. of the 18th Congress of the International Society of Biomechanics*, ed. E.T.H. Zurich, pp. 102–103, 2001.

[8] Keyak, J.H., Meager, J.M., Skinner, H.B. & Mote, C.D., Automated three-dimensional finite element modeling of bone: a new method. *Journal of Biomedical Engineering*, **12**, pp. 389–397, 1990.

[9] Keyak, J.H., Fourkas, M.G., Meager, J.M. & Skinner, H.B., Validation of an automated method of three dimensional finite element modeling of bone. *Journal of Biomedical Engineering*, **15**, pp. 389–397, 1993.

[10] Rho, J.Y., Ho Ba Tho, M.C. & Ashman, R.B., Relations of mechanical properties to density and CT numbers in human bone. *Medical Engineering Physics*, **17(5)**, pp. 347–355, 1995.

[11] Ho Ba Tho, M.C., Rho, J.Y. & Ashman, R.B., Atlas of mechanical properties of human cortical and cancellous bone. *In vivo assessment of bone quality by vibration and wave propagation techniques, Part II*, eds. G. Van der Perre, G. Lowet & A. Borgwardt, ACCO publishing: Leuven, pp. 7–38, 1992.

[12] Ho Ba Tho, M.C., Logiciel SIP 305, Logiciel de prétraitement d'images médicales, Scanner, IRM. Copyright Inserm, 1993.

[13] Ashman, R.B., Cowin, S.C., Van Buskirk, W.C. & Rice, J.C., A continuous wave technique for the measurement of the elastic properties of cortical bone. *Journal of Biomechanics*, **17**, pp. 349–361, 1984.

[14] Ashman, R.B., Rho, J.Y. & Turner, C.H., Anatomical variation of orthotropic elastic moduli of the proximal human tibia. *Journal of Biomechanics*, **22**, pp. 895–900, 1989.

[15] Ho Ba Tho, M.C., Rho, J.Y. & Ashman, R.B., Anatomical variation of mechanical properties of human cancellous bone in vitro. *Bone Research in Biomechanics*, eds. G. Lowet, P. Rüegsegger, H. Weinans & A. Meunier, *IOS Press*, pp. 157–173, 1998.

[16] Mansat, P., Baréa, C., Ho Ba Tho, M.C., Darmana, R. & Mansat, M., Anatomical variation of mechanical properties of the glenoid. *Journal of Shoulder and Elbow Surgery*, **7(2)**, pp. 109–115, 1997.

[17] Ho Ba Tho, M.C., Bensamoun, S., Treutenaere, J.M. & Rey, C., Mechanical, morphological and physico-chemical multi-scale characterization of human cortical bone tissue. *Proc 14th European Society of Biomechanics*, 2004.

[18] Bensamoun, S., Ho Ba Tho, M.C., Luu, S., Gherbezza, J.M. & de Belleval, J.F., Spatial distribution of acoustic and elastic properties of human femoral cortical bone. *Journal of Biomechanics*, **37**, pp. 503–510, 2004.

[19] Bensamoun, S., Gherbezza, J.M., de Belleval, J.F. & Ho Ba Tho, M.C., Transmission scanning acoustic imaging of human cortical bone and relation with the microstructure. *Clinical Biomechanics*, **19**, pp. 639–647, 2004.

[20] Bensamoun, S., Propriétés morphologiques et mécaniques du tissu musculosquelettique. PhD Dissertation, Université de Technologie de Compiègne, 2004.

[21] Roach, J.W., Ho Ba Tho, M.C., Baker, K.J. & Ashman, R.B., Three-dimensional computer analysis of complex acetabular insufficiency. *Journal of Pediatric Orthopaedics*, **17**, pp. 158–164, 1997.

[22] Johnston, C.E., Ho Ba Tho, M.C., Baker, K.J. & Baunin, C., Three dimensional analysis of clubfoot deformity using computed tomography. *Journal of Pediatric Orthopaedics*, **4**, Part B, pp. 39–48, 1995.

[23] Limbert, G., Estivalèzes, E., Ho Ba Tho, M.C., Baunin C. & Cahuzac, J.P., In vivo determination of homogenised mechanical characteristics of human tibia. Application to the study of tibial torsion *in vivo*. *Clinical Biomechanics*, **13**, pp. 473–479, 1998.

[24] Périé, D. & Ho Ba Tho, M.C., In vivo determination of contact areas and pressure of the femorotibial joint using non linear element analysis. *Clinical Biomechanics*, **13**, pp. 394–402, 1998.

[25] Périé, D., Sales De Gauzy, J., Sévely, A. & Ho Ba Tho, M.C., In vivo geometrical evaluation of Cheneau-Toulouse-Munster brace effect on scoliotic spine using MRI method. *Clinical Biomechanics*, **16**, pp. 129–137, 2001.

[26] Ho Ba Tho, M.C., Esperet, S., Baunin, C., Darmana, R. & Cahuzac, J.P., Modélisation par la Méthode des Eléments Finis de l'articulation fémoropatellaire in vivo. *Innovation Technologie en Biologie et Médecine*, **18(5)**, pp. 327–336, 1997.

[27] Ho Ba Tho, M.C., Luu, S., Estivalèzes, E., Baunin, C. & Cahuzac, J.P., Simulation of the 3D motion of clubfoot bones using helical axes theory. *Suppl. Journal of Biomechanics*, **31**, pp. 107, 1998.

[28] Périé, D., Sales De Gauzy, J., Baunin, C. & Ho Ba Tho, M.C., Tomodensitometry measurements for in vivo quantification of mechanical properties of scoliotic vertebrae. *Clinical Biomechanics*, **16**, pp. 373–379, 2001.

[29] Hinrichs, M., Luu, S., Roux, F., Treutenaere, J.M. & Ho Ba Tho, M.C., In vivo analysis of the pelvic bone before and after acetabular reconstruction by means of a three dimensional finite element model. *Proc. of the 18th Congress of the International Society of Biomechanics*, ed. E.T.H. Zurich, pp. 102, 2001.

[30] Huiskes, R., & Verdonschot, N., Biomechanics of artificial joints: the hip. *Basic Orthopaedic Biomechanics*, eds. V.C. Mow & W. Hayes, pp. 395–460, 1997.

[31] Barré C., Mise en place d'une méthodologie pour la conception et l'évaluation d'une prothèse de hanche personnalisée. Master Sciences dissertation. Université de Technologie de Compiègne 2000.

[32] Couteau, B., Ho Ba Tho, M.C., Darmana, R., Brignola, J.C. & Arlaud, J.Y., Development of a finite element model of a human femur with individualized geometry and mechanical properties: validation by vibration analysis. *Technical Note, Journal of Biomechanics*, **31**, pp. 383–386, 1998.

[33] Couteau, B., Labey, L., Ho Ba Tho, M.C., Vander Sloten, J., Arlaud, J.Y. & Brignola, J.C., Validation of a three dimensional finite element model of a human femur with a customized hip implant. *Proc. of the 3rd Conf. on Computer Methods in Biomechanics and Biomedical Engineering*, eds. J. Middleton, M.L. Jones & G. Pande, Gordon and Breach Science Publishers, pp. 147–154, 1998.

[34] Estivalèzes, E., Limbert, G., Darmana, R. & Ho Ba Tho, M.C., Etude du comportement mécanique d'un tibia sain et prothésé, modélisation par éléments finis et validation expérimentale. *Actes du 4ème colloque national en calcul des structures*, **2**, pp. 791–796, 1999.

[35] Baréa, C., Ho Ba Tho, M.C., Darmana, R. & Mansat, M., Three dimensional finite element study of glenoid implants in total shoulder arthroplasty. *Proc. of the 3rd Conf. on Computer methods in Biomechanics and Biomedical Engineering*, eds. J. Middleton, M.L. Jones & G. Pande, Gordon and Breach Science Publishers, pp. 471–479, 1998.

CHAPTER 4

A coupled mechanical-biological computational approach to simulate antiresorbtive-drugs effects on osteoporosis

M.E. Zeman[1,2] and M. Cerrolaza[1]
[1]*Bioengineering Centre, Faculty of Engineering, Universidad Central de Venezuela.*
[2]*Division of Biomechanics and Engineering Design, Katholieke Universiteit Leuven, Belgium.*

Abstract

Most of mathematical models that describe bone adaptation deeply focus on the mechanical laws involved and less attention is paid to the biological processes. Moreover factors like drugs, hormones, genetics or nutrition also play an important role and must be considered as well. In order to have a more realistic description of the biological processes, models must be developed to incorporate biological parameters, like e.g. cellular turnover and mineralization processes. In order to achieve this we provide more insight on the coupling of biological variables to a mechanical model that handles the structural aspect. The biological model we propose is based on two elements that are changing as a consequence of an altered activation frequency of the BMUs. These affected variables are mineralization and the surface of remodeling. The model is implemented through an existent robust bone remodeling model based on damage mechanics. It considers porosity as the damage variable and the consequences of the biological changes are implemented in such a way that they affect the temporary evolution law of the damage as well as the mechanical properties of bone. The coupling of the models is applied to the study of the effects of biphosphonates in the treatment of osteoporosis. Our simulations are based on histological data reported from patients treated with alendronate, a drug used in the treatment of osteoporosis. Preliminary results show a good qualitative correlation compared to clinical data.

1 Introduction

Bone as a living tissue has the capacity to adapt to mechanical loads by modifying its external and internal structure. This process is known as adaptative bone remodeling and can occur in any bone of the skeleton during our life. Bone adaptation is associated with the evolution of apparent density and many theoretical models have been presented to study this phenomenon [1–4]. Most of these models were designed specifically to simulate changes in the bone architecture due to mechanical influences. However this is only one of the stimulus to which the bone responds during its adaptation process. Metabolic factors, such as an illness, nutrition and medication treatments also influence the bone's response to mechanical loads. In the same way, the mechanical properties of the bone are not only sensitive to the porosity and density as considered in some of these models, but to the bone's degree of mineralization [5]. This variable is included into the approach proposed in this chapter.

In order to predict the effects of these metabolic or medication induced changes, a more detailed description of the biological processes related to the remodeling is required. A model that represents the changes in the bone biology by means of histomorphometric parameters of the bone tissue is proposed in this chapter. Several authors have worked on this biological aspect, covering from cellular models in which the main variable is the probability that a new remodeling cycle would begin [6], to computer models that simulate individual time dependent remodeling zones (entities) on a bone sample [7–10]. However, these proposals do not cover rigorously the mechanical aspect and some are not implemented through numerical techniques to study the mechanical effects.

Regardless of the type of bone – cancellous or cortical – the remodeling process is a continuous sequence of bone removal by osteoclasts cells, followed by new bone formation by osteoblasts cells. Osteoclasts and osteoblasts act together and coordinated in so-called Bone Multicellular Units (BMUs), which are considered to be the main biological entity in remodeling. The mentioned sequence of events can further be divided into six phases [11]: activation: when a group of osteoclasts are recruited on the bone surface, indicating that a new BMU cycle has started; resorption: when the osteoclasts begin to resorb bone, thereby creating a cutting cone that will give rise to a new osteon (in case of cortical bone); reversal: the transition from the osteoclastic to the osteoblastic activity, which results in a spatial and temporal interval between the resorptive region and the refilling region; formation: the osteoblasts start filling the cavity with new non-mineralized bone named osteoid; mineralization: after a few days mineral starts to be deposited that will mineralize the osteoid to form mature bone and finally quiescence: is reached after osteoblasts have refilled the resorption cavity and become either osteocytes or lining cells. Two different types of mineralization are defined. On the one hand we have the primary mineralization period, which starts briefly after the apposition of new osteoid and which take place over a few days. This mineralization occurs very fast (5 days in this model) and it considers the period of time that the recently formed bone needs to reach up to 65%–75% of the maximum value of the mineralization [12]. Then a secondary mineralization starts that can take several months from the end of the primary, during this period the bone tissue continues accumulating mineral material at a decreasing exponential rate until the bone gets mature and reaches 95% of its theoretical maximum (in this model 0.7 is considered according to table 2).

The number of remodeling cycles starting in a given volume of bone in a given time can be estimated from a histological cross-section of a bone sample, and is defined as the "activation frequency" of the BMUs [13]. The intensity of the remodeling process can then be derived from the activation frequency of the BMUs. Activation frequency is the major indicator of biochemical indices of whole body resorption and formation of bone, which is very useful to analyze drug effects and pathological behavior, among others.

The "remodeling space" is another measurable variable in bone histology defined to further quantify bone remodeling. During the reversal phase there is a finite time when the resorption cavity created by the osteoclasts remains empty, while it is prepared for bone formation [14]. The number of cavities waiting to be refilled is termed the "remodeling space" and its size (and therefore the deficit of bone) depends largely on the rate of bone remodeling.

The model's applicability in this chapter focuses on the alterations and effects that the biphosphonate based medications have on the bone remodeling and specifically on the bone's mechanical properties. The alendronate_sodium or alendronate is a biphosphonate which is broadly used nowadays to increase the amount of bone mineral in patients that suffer osteoporosis. One of the consequences of osteoporosis is the negative balance that occurs during the coupling of the bone re-absorption and bone formation, which results in a loss of bone tissue, see fig. 1. This loss is accelerated due to the increase in the new BMU's activation frequency; this process is induced during menopause and persists throughout life.

The study and simulation of the alendronate is relevant, since when studying the remodeling alterations due to joint replacements, we must consider that a great part of the population that have implants are seniors with an osteopenic state or with osteoporosis.

The model we present here considers aspects of the BMU (bone multicellular units) activities and defines, in a particular way, the changes in the bone tissue's degree of mineralization and the BMU's activation frequency. The model uses measurements taken from histomorphometric studies of the human bone to represent

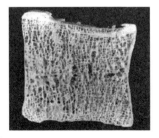 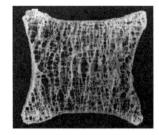

Figure 1: Details of the quality of the trabeculae in a healthy vertebra (left) and a vertebra with osteoporosis (right).

the BMU's rate of appearance, progress and life period, as well as the time periods in which the bone is reabsorbed and deposited in each individual remodeling entity. Once developed, the model is implemented and coupled to the García and Doblaré model [4], which is based on damage mechanics and will be briefly described.

2 Bone histomorphometrical values

The bone dynamic histomorphometry is a quantitative analysis of a bone sample which has been tracked with chemical markers in order to quantify the formation of bone tissue and the cellular activity.

A histomorphometric study uses a histological slice as a photograph of the cellular activity occurring immediately before the extraction of an individual's bone sample. By illustrating the activity of certain groups of cells, this photograph provides direct information about the cellular activity and its repercussion on the form and density of bone. The bone histomorphometry is especially important in bone remodeling computer models since it describes the bone's cellular activity in a quantitative way. Towards the end of the 1950's, doses of *tetracycline* were used as an innocuous and effective marker to label and identify recently formed bone (osteoid). This allowed the first studies on bone formation in humans. A series of techniques for the histomorphometric measurements were rapidly developed, many of which were created by Frost and his colleagues during the 1960's [15], likewise the inclusion of new chemical markers have evolved with these techniques. Since then, the bone histology has contributed to the understanding of the bone adaptation and the metabolic processes affected by diseases altering the bone functions.

The most common techniques that are used to measure parameters in a histological section are the perimeter and area measurements. The perimeter based measurements are achieved by superimposing a grid over the surface of the slice and counting the number of contacts or intersections between the grid and the surface being studied. The area measurements are achieved by superimposing a point grid and counting those that fall in the area being studied [16], as shown in fig. 2. The area measurements tend to be associated to volumes in the bone sample.

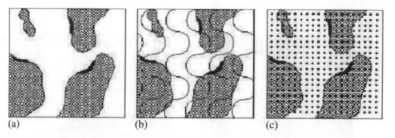

(a)   (b)   (c)

Figure 2: Some techniques to make histological measurements (a) Spongy bone slice; osteoid is shown in black and mineralized tissue in shadowed areas. (b) Perimeter measurements with Merz type grid. (c) Area measurements with point's grid.

Table 1: Some histomorphometric parameters relevant in this model.

Calculated parameter	Description	Symbol or equation
Formation period	Time over which bone formation occurs at a remodeling site (days)	FP
Eroded period	Time during which bone surface is eroded during remodeling (days)	EP
Quiescent period	Average time during which there is no active remodeling at a site (days)	QP
Total period	Time between two remodeling cycles at a site on the bone surface (days)	$Tt.P = FP + EP + QP$
Activation frequency	The rate of appearance of a BMU on the bone surface (1/days)	$Ac.f = 1/Tt.P$

From a histological slice, parameters can be either measured or calculated. Histomorphometric parameters that are directly measured are: the eroded surface, the bone surface not undergoing remodeling, the surface covered by osteoid, the total bone surface, the erosion depth and the osteon wall thickness. Some parameters that are normally calculated from the chemical marker measurements and from the value's parameter mentioned above are presented in table 1. These calculations are done by assuming that all of the bone sample's cellular activity is that of a BMU and that the activity of remodeling observed in the slice is representative of the system in equilibrium.

3 Biphosphonates: Alendronate

The biphosphonates have been known for more than 100 years, but they have only been used in the treatment of osteoporosis for 30 years. They have a characteristic structure that allows it to adhere to the hidroxiapatita crystals in the bone. They act over the precursor cells of the osteoclasts by inhibiting the resorption and modulating the bone formation. The first biphosphonates used in the treatment of osteoporosis (specifically the etidronate) had negative consequences in the mineralization process [17]. Although this problem is associated with the appropriate dosage of new biphosphonates, it is still under discussion by pharmacology field researchers. Amongst the new biphosphonates, the alendronate has received lots of attention due to its capacity to increase the bone mass with little collateral effects. Despite the therapeutic benefits of the alendronate, there still exist many effects on the bone metabolism that are not fully understood.

Nowadays alendronate is indicated in doses of 10 mg/day or 70 mg once a week. It is prescribed as an oral drug both for prevention and treatment of the post-menopausal osteoporosis, for cortico-steroids induced osteoporosis and for the treatment of the Paget's disease. To mention an example, women with post-menopausal osteoporosis under the treatment of alendronate have shown an increase in the bone mineral density (BMD) and a reduction in the tendency to fractures, including hip fractures [18, 19]. The BMD can be related directly to the mechanical properties of the bone, since the same quantity of bone showing a high or low degree of mineralization will correspond to a high or low BMD. This permits to make a follow up of the treatments with this drug through bone densimetry or Dual energy X-ray Absorbtiometry (DXA).

Studies show that after giving the doses of alendronate, the action mechanism of this medication is located in areas of the bone where there is great physiological activity [20]. This medication, as mentioned before, acts on the bone remodeling and among the results associated to the treatment is the reduction on the bone remodeling surface and the increase in the mineralization of the bone.

3.1 Characteristics of the medication to be simulated: pharmaco-kinetics and pharmaco-dynamics

To simulate the doses of the medication, the distribution of it in the body (pharmaco-kinetics), as well as the relation between the concentration of the medication and its effects (pharmaco-dynamics) should be properly understood. The pharmaco-kinetics of the alendronate is relatively simple, because the tissue response to the alendronate is related directly to the concentration of the alendronate that is present in the bone [20]. Due to this, the more relevant aspect in administrating the alendronate is the pharmaco-kinetics that describes the amount of medication that is absorbed by the bone and the rate at which it is removed or eliminated from the bone.

The rate of absortion of the alendronate by the bone is fast (less than an hour) and the fraction of the doses that is actually absorbed by the body is not influenced by the amount of the doses, this means that large doses are absorbed by the bone as well as small doses [20]. These properties of the alendronate suggest that if the medication were not eliminated by the body, no cellular response of the bone would be observed if it were to be a large dose or a number of small doses that add up to be equivalent to the large doses.

The alendronate is eliminated by the body in a natural way. Studies of the elimination of the alendronate have shown that it is captured by the bone and removed in a decreasing exponential rate in which 66% remains even after six months of taking the last doses [21]. In relation to the concentration of the alendronate that remains in the bone once the treatment has finished, it can be predicted by a logarithmic function expressed in eqn (1) [22], that represents (R_f) the physiological response to the concentration of the doses or the fraction of the medication that continues during "t" days after the take has stopped, where "m" represents a constant obtained from information on the elimination, this is, the 66% of the response that remains in the body during the next 6 months.

$$R_f = 1 - m * \ln(t + 1). \tag{1}$$

In Hernandez *et al.* [7] proposal the response of the BMUs is supposed to adopt its original level as in the pre-treatment condition in the same proportion in which the alendronate is eliminated from the mineralized tissue.

3.2 Effects of the drug on the biological parameters of the bone

Based on histomorphometric studies [18], it has been observed that the frequency of activation of the BMUs is reduced in an average of 87% per alendronate doses of 10 mg/day.

A fundamental relation of our statement is the one expressed by the Parfitt group who explained that the activation frequency, seen as a measurement of the birth rate of cross-sectional new remodeling cycles is also a valuable measure of the magnitude of the remodeling space [13]. This variable is represented in our model by the remodeling surface and the effect of the alendronate is simulated by a factor that reduces this variable in the same proportion as the one observed in the activation frequency of clinical data.

Another aspect to be considered to simulate the alendronate's effect is the degree of mineralization of the bone. In adults this variable depends on the rate of remodeling, in other words, the biological determinant of mineralization is the rate of turnover or related activation frequency of the new BMUs.

As explained in the Introduction section, there are two different types of mineralization processes happening after the deposition of osteoid, as it is represented in fig. 3.

This represents an important input in our model since the increased activation frequency that osteoporosis generates leads to a shorter lifespan of the BMUs. Consequently, the new formed bone will not have enough time to reach its total mineralization before it is prematurely reabsorbed by osteoclast of the new BMU starting a new remodeling sequence. Data obtained from patients with osteoporosis before the treatment, indicate that the average value for ash fraction (ash mass/ bone mass) was random; however, high values of this variable observed after the treatment with alendronate have been attributed to long periods in the secondary mineralization [5]. This data reinforce the hypothesis used in this chapter in which the reduction in the activation frequency, caused by the antireabsortive effect of the alendronate, is followed by a long process of secondary mineralization that increases the lifetime of the BMUs and this allows the bone to mature reaching at least normal levels of mineralization [19]. This result associated to treatments with alendronate is simulated in our model, calculating the variations of the degree of mineralization and increasing this parameter based on daily calculations. According to the proposal of these authors, the bone mass and the bone mineral density represent different entities, and it is important to observe the therapeutic implications in this difference, especially when analyzing the effects of the medication that acts on bone resorption.

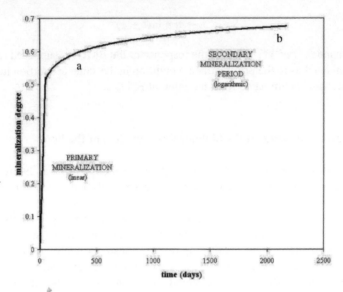

Figure 3: Graphical representation of the two mineralization periods. Point "a" represents 70% of the maximum *ash* value, point "b" represents 95% of the maximum *ash* value.

4 Proposed model

4.1 The mechanical model: overview

To establish the biological model and combine it with a mechanical approach, a model based on damage mechanics was used. This model developed by Doblaré & García [4] considers the porosity of a bone sample as the damage variable which is defined through a tensor for the two possible cases in bone adaptation:

Damage ⇔ Bone resorption,
Repair ⇔ Bone formation.

Since there is a relation between porosity and apparent density (eqn (2)),

$$p = 1 - \left(\frac{\rho_a}{\hat{\rho}} \right). \tag{2}$$

They proposed a damage tensor directly related to this concept of porosity with two possible values:

$D = 0$ corresponding to a intact state or no damage (no local porosity)
$0 < D \leq 1$ corresponding to local damage.

The changes within this range of damage are reflected as well in the mechanical properties of the bone through the eqn (3) which is an experimental relation proposed by Beaupré *et al.* [23] and Jaocbs *et al.* [24] where the differences between

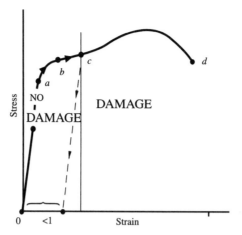

Figure 4: Representation of the limits in an elastoplatic law in order to define one or the other criteria.

the mechanical properties of cortical and trabecular bone can be expressed as (Young modulus is expressed in MPa):

$$E = \begin{cases} 2014\rho^{2.5}, & \text{if } \rho \le 1.2\,\text{g/cc} \\ 1763\rho^{3.2}, & \text{if } \rho \ge 1.2\,\text{g/cc}, \end{cases}$$

$$\nu = \begin{cases} 0.2, & \text{if } \rho \le 1.2\,\text{g/cc} \\ 0.32, & \text{if } \rho \ge 1.2\,\text{g/cc}. \end{cases} \tag{3}$$

The model of Doblaré and García defines the damage D variable through an intermediary tensor $\mathbf{H}$ directly related to the damage in resorption and in formation.

Since the model studies the evolution in time of the damage, a stimulus variable is defined to generate a change in the damage value. For this statement the formulation from the Stanford model [1, 23] defining a mechanical stimulus that involves the effective stress is used with some considerations to make it coherent regarding the differences between formation and resorption.

As a function of this stimulus they proposed the two conditions under which either formation or resorption mechanism are activated. This can be interpreted as the limits established in an elastoplastic law, depicted in fig. 4.

Then, following the formulation of a damage theory, a flow law is defined to establish the evolution in time of the damage variable, as it was done in the Stanford model for the density through eqn (4)

$$\dot{\rho} = k\dot{r}S_v\hat{\rho}, \tag{4}$$

where $\dot{r}$ is the surface remodeling rate that quantifies the volume of bone generated or eliminated by site per unit of time, S_v is the bone available surface to be under remodeling per volume unit of bone and k is the percentage of active surface that is available for remodeling.

Then, a formulation is developed for the continuous variations of the formation and resorption tensors in the damage model. The $\beta, \mathbf{J}, \hat{\omega}$ are variables related to anisotropy calculations.

$$\text{Resorption} \quad \dot{\mathbf{H}} = \frac{3\beta k\dot{r}S_v}{4\,\mathrm{tr}(\mathbf{H}_n^{-1}\mathbf{J}_n^{-3}\hat{\omega}_v)}\frac{\hat{\rho}}{\rho_n}\mathbf{J}_n^{-3}\hat{\omega}_n, \tag{5}$$

$$\text{Formation} \quad \dot{\mathbf{H}} = \frac{3\beta k\dot{r}S_v}{4\,\mathrm{tr}(\mathbf{H}_n^{-1}\mathbf{J}_n\hat{\omega}_v)}\frac{\hat{\rho}}{\rho_n}\mathbf{J}_n\hat{\omega}_n. \tag{6}$$

4.2 The biological model

As an initial condition in the model, there is a known apparent density (ρ) in each integration point. This apparent density is related to the mechanical properties of the bone through the expressions in eqn (3).

Using the definition of the ash fraction that indicates the quantity of mineral that contains a bone sample, experimental measurements relating this variable to the density [25] were used to establish a relationship as:

$$ash_0 = 0.2264 * \ln(\rho) + 0.1772. \tag{7}$$

With this relation, after the apparent density is taken from i.e CTs, the initial ash fraction is calculated.

It is known for humans that the values of the degree of mineralization range from osteoid ($ash = 0$) to completely mineralized bone ($ash = 0.70$). The dry density values for this range correspond to 1.41 g/cc and 2.31 g/cc, respectively [26, 27], see table 2. From these data Martin [27] suggests that it is possible to use these points in order to define a linear relation between density of the total mineralized sample ($\hat{\rho}$) and its degree of mineralization

$$\hat{\rho}(g/cc) \approx 1.41 + 1.29 * ash. \tag{8}$$

The mineralization periods, as already defined, are implemented in the model through a linear curve representing the primary mineralization period and a logarithmic curve to represent the secondary mineralization period. This is shown in fig. 3 and values used are in table 3. From the graph the temporary variations of the degree of mineralization are easily defined.

Table 2: Range of values for the total mineralized bone and the ash values used in our statement.

	$\hat{\rho}$ (g/cc)	ash
Osteoid	1.41	0
Cortical bone	2.31	0.70

It is possible to calculate the variations in the degree of mineralization per increment of time. The slope is then calculated for each of the two different zones (m_p for the linear zone and m_s for the logarithmic zone):

$$m(ash/t) = \frac{\Delta\alpha}{\Delta t} \tag{9}$$

and for each zone the variation of the mineralization per time interval:

$$\Delta\alpha_p = m_p * \alpha_{max} * \Delta t, \tag{10}$$

$$\Delta\alpha_s = |\alpha - \alpha_{max}| \frac{\log(0.05/0.3)}{P\_MinSec} * \Delta t. \tag{11}$$

Once the daily variation of the degree of mineralization is known, the variable "*ash*" is updated:

$$\alpha_n = \alpha_{n-1} + \Delta\alpha_n \tag{12}$$

and the total mineralized density ($\hat{\rho}$) is then recalculated (in eqn (8)) for the next increment and its implications in the mechanical properties of the bone are reflected in the mechanical model. All these parameters are loaded in arrays by integration point and then recalculated for each new increment.

In histology the remodeling space represents the volume that is occupied by a porous (hole) and only appears temporarily during the resorption and reversal periods before deposition of osteoid by the osteoclasts preceding mineralization [14].

Table 3: Some parameters used to describe bone remodeling process and the values used in our simulation.

Remodeling parameter	Description	Nominal values
Resorption period	Time during which resorption occurs at a remodeling site	60 days[a]
Reversal period	Time between osteoclast and osteoblast activity	57 days[a]
Mineralization lag time	Time between osteoid formation and the start of mineralization	22 days[a]
Primary mineralization period	Time required for bone to mineralize up to 70% of its theoretical maximum	5 days[a]
Secondary mineralization period	Time required for bone to mineralize from 70% to 95% theoretical maximum	6 years[b]

[a] Value based on healthy postmenopausal women's histology [32].
[b] Estimated value can take from 6 month [6] to many years [22].

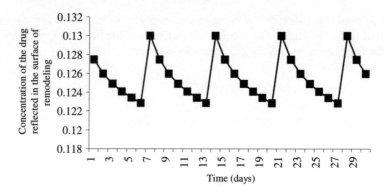

Figure 5: Curves displaying the pharmaco-kinetics and pharmaco-dynamics behaviors for weekly alendronate doses.

When the activation frequency decreases, only few of these temporary spaces are present. This implies a reduction in the remodeling space. As well, an increase in the bone mass and volume is observed. As we have seen before, the treatment with alendronate generates a significant decrease in the activation frequency of the BMUs [18]. A decrease in this parameter causes a reduction in the remodeling space [27, 28].

To reflect these changes in the remodeling surface we use in this model the eqn (1) to represent the pharmaco-kinetics and pharmaco-dynamics and their influence on these temporary spaces or surfaces. To fit the clinical data to the behavior expressed by this equation a factor "a" is added modulating the decreased percentage in the activation frequency induced by alendronate (see eqn (8)).

$$S_{vf} = a * (1 - m * \ln(t + 1)). \qquad (13)$$

Being S_{vf} the value that will multiply the existent value of the remodeling surface under healthy conditions; "a" is the value representing a decrease of 87% of the remodeling surface; "m" is a constant to fit the clinical data depending on the concentration of the doses (70 mg/week, m = 0.06); "t" represents dimensionless values for daily, weekly or monthly takes of the drug. The simulations performed in this chapter only consider weekly doses that are the ones currently prescribed to patients. A graphical detail of eqn (13) is depicted in fig. 5.

The resultant changes of the biological simulation were implemented using two dynamic feedback loops. One of the loops is established between the surface of remodeling and the flow law indicating the temporary evolution of the damage (porosity) in the mechanical model.

The second loop is implemented between the total mineralized density in the mechanical model, and the variations of the degree of mineralization calculated in the biological model. All the calculated parameters for the biological model are loaded in arrays by keeping the sampling points and updated for every new increment. A diagram of the coupling between the two models is depicted in fig. 6.

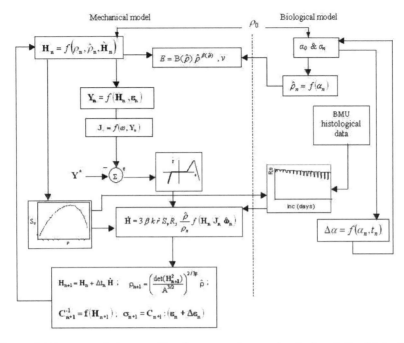

Figure 6: Diagram of the coupling between the mechanical and the biological model.

5 Results

5.1 Simple model of a cantilever beam

To obtain preliminary results a cyclic load of 40 N was applied to a beam in which control nodes were defined as shown in fig. 7. Hexahedral elements were used to build the mesh and 18 month simulations were performed.

In the control nodes an average increment of 5.6% in the density was obtained for the first 12 simulated months and an increase of 6.6% at the end of the 18th simulated month. These tendencies are depicted in fig. 8.

Regarding the degree of mineralization, simulations in which the secondary mineralization period were longer, showed a pronounced increment in the apparent density [7, 29, 30]. The simulation considering a secondary mineralization period of 6 years lead to more accurate predictions compared to clinical data.

Results from the simulations on the pharmaco-kinetics and pharmaco-dynamics of alendronate showed a periodic decrease of the activation frequency, interpreted in our model as the changes in the surface of remodeling depicted in fig. 9. Although the high non-linearity characteristics of the mechanical model, the results offer a good evaluation of the coupling between the two models, this can be observed when induced changes by the biological model bring coherent results overall.

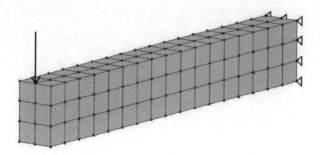

Figure 7: Schematic of the beam's example.

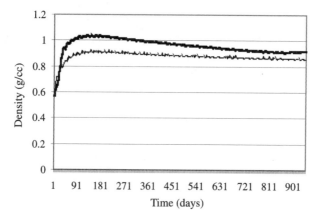

Figure 8: Results of the density variations in time. The upper line shows the predictions for the alendronate in reference with the lower line stands for the control simulation done with the mechanic model.

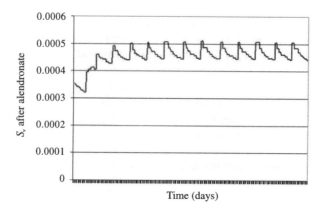

Figure 9: Detail of the variations of the surface of remodeling after introducing the weekly doses of alendronate.

We consider relevant the comprehension of which parameter is more influential with respect to others in the resultant density predictions. This point is analyzed as well when important changes in the histomorphometric indicate some metabolic disorder [31]. Due to this, a sensibility analysis was performed for the model to evaluate which of the feedback loop is more influential in the density results. The analysis showed that variations in the parameters involved in the mineralization equations induce relevant changes in the resultant density. Less correlation was found regarding changes in the remodeling surface and the density.

5.2 Female patient with osteoporosis

Once the algorithm and the coupling with the main program were tested, a simulation of data from a female osteoporotic femur was performed. Figure 10 is showing a detail of the quality of the head of the femur observed in a CT prior to surgery for a total hip replacement.

A technique developed in the Bioengineering Centre of the Central University of Venezuela [33] allows the capture of the bone quality of the patient and to have it as the initial condition of the simulation. The methodology reads the Hounsfield

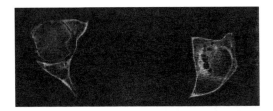

Figure 10: Detail of the tomography showing the damage in the head of the femur caused by osteoporosis.

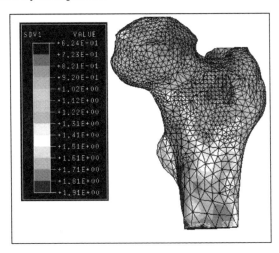

Figure 11: Initial density (g/cc) distribution in the outer surface of the model.

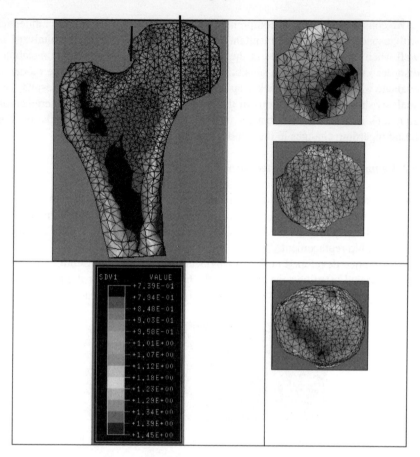

Figure 12: Left: Anterior-posterior cut showing the density distribution of the patient with osteoporosis. Right detailed cuts related to the axial lines marked in the head of the femur.

units from the CTs and then creates a voxel matrix. Once these values are converted into mechanical properties, the program enables the coupling of the data to each sampling Gauss point of the finite element model directly from the voxel model; this allows a personalized model with high heterogeneous data.

The proximal part of the femur was meshed with 50.717 linear tetrahedral finite elements and 9541 nodes. Loads and boundary conditions were applied regarding the body weight of the patient ($\approx$600 N). Since we focus on the simulation of the head of the femur only the proximal part is considered thus avoiding really huge and unwieldy models.

Different cuts of the head of the femur are showing the internal density distribution. A representation of the initial density distribution in the outer surface is depicted in fig. 11 while fig. 12 presents a longitudinal cut and different axial cuts in the zone of interest: femoral head.

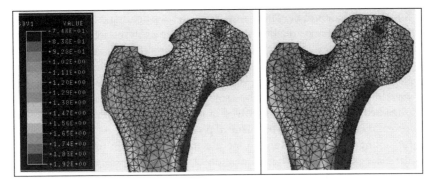

Figure 13: Density distribution in an anterior-posterior cut of the proximal femur. Left: control predictions obtained with the mechanical model. Right: result for the coupled models for the same number of increments (50). An evident change in the density values of the head and cortical layers is obtained, being the most critical areas affected by the osteoporosis (fig. 12).

The apparent density increments for the 12th month of weekly doses simulated treatment are depicted in fig. 13. The results are coherent with the preliminary ones giving increments between 5 to 6%.

Although the model generates less accurate results at the beginning of the simulation (very high density increase), the response of the coupling tends to be stable and logical for the rest of the period simulated. Further work should be done in order to correct this misfit during the first increments; meanwhile results should be read only from the first year simulated and on. Under this convention we consider that the model offers a good correlation with the expected results. Simulations considering long term treatments (10 years) should be studied as well in order to test accuracy and stability of the model.

Due to differences between the surface-volume relationships in different types of bones, the rate of cellular activity is slower in cortical bone than in cancellous bone. As a future step this behavior will be included in the model in order to improve the accuracy of the results. This represents a difficulty when modeling drugs effect; in the model a filter is preventing the alendronate effect to act on low densities representing bone marrow. This can cause that points with a low density value affected by osteoporosis are only analyzed under the mechanical model laws for adaptation but they are not considered in the biological actions we attempt to model.

6 Conclusion

A biomechanics simulation platform that couples mechanical and biological behavior of the bone under the administration of a drug used to treat osteoporosis was developed and discussed. The biological model is based on histological data that allows the evaluation of the metabolic activity of the bone tissue.

Simplified models of the femur were analyzed considering its geometry, boundary conditions and bone quality from the CTs. The analyses are done under static assumptions but they consider cyclic loads. The simplifications done to the boundary conditions of the femur i.e. the muscular forces, are not the best approach to these type of problems, more relevant muscle forces should be involved in order to have more accurate results. The same considerations should be done regarding ligaments and soft tissues involved in the articulation, but this implies a large deformation approach of the mechanical problem.

Regarding the changes done to the mechanical model in order to integrate it to the biological one, we should mention that it was necessary to redefine some variables that where originally either constant values ($\hat{\rho}$) or dependent only on one variable (S_v). These changes imply some instability and were done taking care of the coherence of the results as well as the high non linearity of the mechanical model based on damage mechanics. The coupling of the two models affects the numerical convergence of the analysis since introducing more variables brought more iterations for every increment. Nevertheless this increased calculation time is not dramatic and the convergence of the problem remains stable.

It should be remarked herein that this type of simulation represents a powerful predicting tool for medical doctors but the manipulation of all the parameters involved to create and analyze the model is no longer straightforward. A future goal after quantitative validations of the model should be to develop a friendly interface to make this model more useful for the health sector.

Acknowledgments

The authors wish to thanks Jose Manuel García for all his support understanding the mechanical model and pertinent comments. This work was partially supported by a doctoral scholarship of the Fonacit (Ministry of Science and Technology, Venezuela).

References

[1] Carter, D.R., Fyhrie, D.P. & Whalen, R.T., Trabecular bone density and loading history: regulation of tissue biology by mechanical energy. *Journal of Biomechanics*, **20(8)**, pp. 785–795, 1987.

[2] Prendergast, P.J. & Taylor, D., Prediction of bone adaptation using damage accumulation. *Journal of Biomechanics*, **27**, pp. 1067–1076, 1994.

[3] Kuiper J.H. & Huiskes R., The predective valve of stress shielding for quantification of adaptive bone resorption around hip replacements. *Journal of Biomechanical Engineering*, **119**, 228–231, 1997.

[4] Doblaré, M. & García, J.M., Anisotropic bone remodelling model based on a continuum damage-repair theory. *Journal of Biomechanics*, **35**, 1–17, 2002.

[5] Meunier P. & Boivin G., Bone mineral density reflects bone mass but also the degree of mineralization of bone: therapeutic implications. *Bone*, **21**, 373–377, 1997.

[6] Parfitt, A.M., Bone age, mineral density, and fatigue damage. *Calcified Tissue Int.*, **53(Suppl 1)**, S82–S86, 1993.

[7] Hernandez, C.J., Beaupre, G.S., Marcus, R. & Carter, D.R., A theoretical analysis of contributions of remodeling space, mineralization and bone balance to change in bone mineral density during alendronate treatment. *Bone*, **29(6)**, 511–516, 2001.

[8] Hazelwood, S.J. & Martin, R.B., Simulated effects of menopause on femoral remodeling rate, bone loss and microdamage. *Proc. Bioengineering Conference* (ASME), BED-42, ASME, 1999.

[9] Lacy, M.E., Bevan J.A., Boyce R.W. & Geddes A.D., Antiresorptive drugs and trabecular bone turnover: validation and testing of a computer model. *Calcified Tissue Int.*, **54(3)**, 179–185, 1994.

[10] Thomsen, J.S., Mosekilde, L., Boyce, R.W. & Mosekilde E., Stochastic simulation of vertebral trabecular bone remodeling. *Bone*, **15(6)**, 655–666, 1994.

[11] Parfitt, A.M, Osteonal and hemi-osteonal remodeling: The spatial and temporal framework for signal traffic in adult human bone. *Journal of Cellular Biochemistry*, **55**, 273–286, 1994.

[12] Roberts, E., Bone tissue interface. *Journal of Dental Ed.*, **52**, 804–809, 1988.

[13] Parfitt, A.M., Mundy G.R., Roodman G.D., Hughes D.E. & Boyce B.F. A new model for the regulation of bone resorption, with particular reference to the effects of bisphosphonates. *Journal of Bone and Mineral Research*, **11(2)**, 150–157, 1996.

[14] Jee, W. S., Integrated bone tissue physiology: anatomy and physiology. *Bone Mechanics Handbook*, ed. S.C. Cowin, CRC, 2nd edition: 1/1-1/68, 2001.

[15] Frost, H.M., Tetracycline-based histological analysis of bone remodeling. *Calc. Tiss. Res.*, **3**, 211–237, 1969.

[16] Parfitt, A.M., Stereologic basis of bone histomorphometry: Theory of quantitative microscopy and reconstruction of the third dimension. *Bone Histomorphometry: Techniques and Interpretation*, ed. R. Recker. Boca Raton, FL, CRC Press: 53–88, 1983.

[17] McCloskey, E.V., Yates, A.J. & Beneton M.N., Comparative effects of intravenous diphosphonates on calcium and skeletal metabolism in man. *Bone*, **8(Suppl 1)**, S35–S41, 1987.

[18] Chavassieux, P.M., Arlot, M.E., Reda, C., Wei, L., Yates, A.J. & Meunier, P.J., Histomorphometric assessment of the long-term effects of alendronate on bone quality and remodeling in patients with osteoporosis. *J. Clin. Invest.*, **100(6)**, 1475–1480, 1997.

[19] Boivin, G.Y., Chavassieux, P.M., Santora A.C., Yates J. & Meunier, P.J., Alendronate increases bone strength by increasing the mean degree of mineralization of bone tissue in osteoporotic women. *Bone*, **27(5)**, 687–694, 2000.

[20] Porras, A., Holland, S. & Gertz, B., Pharmacokinetics of alendronate. *Clin. Pharmacokinet.*, **36**, 315–328, 1999.

[21] Khan, S.A., Kanis, J.A., Vasikaran, S., Kline, W.F., Matuszewski, B.K., McCloskey, E.V., Beneton, M.N., Gertz, B.J., Sciberras, D.G., Holland, S.D.,

Orgee, J., Coombes, G.M., Rogers, S.R. & Porras, A.G., Elimination and bio-chemical responses to intravenous alendronate in postmenopausal osteoporo-sis. *J. Bone Miner. Res.*, **12(10)**, 1700–1707, 1997.

[22] Hernandez, C.J., Beaupre, G.S., Marcus, R. & Carter, D.R. Long term predic-tions of the therapeutic equivalence of daily and less than daily alendronate dosing. *J. Bone Min. Res.*, **17(9)**, 1662–1666, 2002.

[23] Beaupré, G.S., Orr, T.E. & Carter, D.R., An approach for time-dependent bone modeling and remodeling – theoretical development. *Journal of Orthopaedic Research*, **8**, pp. 651–670, 1990.

[24] Jacobs, C.R., Levenston, M.C., Beaupré, G.S., Simo J.C. & Carter D.R. Numerical instabilities in bone remodeling simulations: The advantages of a node-based finite element approach. *Journal of Biomechanics*, **28(4)**, pp. 449–459, 1995.

[25] Keller, T. Predicting the compressive mechanical behavior of bone. *Journal of Biomechanics*, **27**, 1159–1168, 1994.

[26] Robinson, R.A. Physiocochemical structure of bone. *Clin. Orthop.*, **208(112)**, 263–315, 1975.

[27] Martin, R.B., Porosity and specific surface of bone. *Crit. Rev. Biomed. Eng.*, **10(3)**, 179–222, 1984.

[28] Martin, R.B., Burr D.B. & Sharkey N.A., *Skeletal Tissue Mechanics*, Springer; New York, 1998.

[29] Bone, H., Greenspan, S., McKeever, C., Bell, N., Davidson, M., Downs, R.W., Emkey, R., Meunier, P.J., Miller, S.S., Mulloy, A.L., Recker, R.R., Weiss, S.R., Heyden, N., Musliner, T., Suryawanshi, S., Yates, A.J. & Lombardi, A., Alendronate and estrogen effects in postmenopausal women with low bone mineral density. Alendronate/Estrogen Study Group. *J. Clin. Endocrinol. Metab.*, **85(2)**, 727–733, 2000.

[30] Tonino, R.P., Meunier, P.J., Emkey, R., Rodriguez-Portales, J.A., Menkes, C., Wasnich, R.D., Bone, H.G., Santora, A.C., Wu, M., Desai, R. & Ross, P.D. Skeletal benefits of alendronate: 7-year treatment of postmenopausal osteo-porotic women. *J. Clin. Endocrinol. Metab.*, **85(9)**, 3109–3115, 2000.

[31] Eriksen, E.F., Normal and pathological remodeling of human trabecular bone: three dimensional reconstruction of the remodeling sequence in normals and in metabolic bone disease. *Endocr. Rev.*, **7(4)**, 379–408, 1986.

[32] Eriksen E.F., Hodgson S.F., Eastell R., Cedel S.L., O'Fallon, W.M. & Riggs, B.L. Cancellous bone remodeling in type I (postmenopausal) osteo-porosis: quantitative assessment of rates of formation, resorption, and bone loss at tissue and cellular levels. *J. Bone Miner. Res.*, **5(4)**, 311–319, 1990.

[33] Müller-Karger C.M. & Zeman M.E., Cerrolaza M. Highly heterogeneous finite element model using computerized tomographies. *International Symposium on Computer Methods in Biomechanics & Biomedical Engineering*, Roma, Italy, CD ROM: 7_7C.pdf, Nov. 2001.

CHAPTER 5

A computational model to analyze the bone behavior after a Total Hip Arthroplasty

P.R. Fernandes and J. Folgado
IDMEC – Instituto Superior Técnico, Technical University of Lisbon, Portugal.

Abstract

This chapter presents a computational model to analyze the bone behavior after a hip implant. The model addresses simultaneously the remodeling of bone tissue around the implant due to stress shielding effect and the bone ingrowth on implant interface. The remodeling model is obtained by the solution of a material optimization problem while the ingrowth model is based on a displacement criterion. The objective function for bone remodeling considers both the structural stiffness and the metabolic cost of bone formation. The trabecular bone is modeled as an orthotropic material with effective properties computed by the homogenization method. The model is presented in two steps. Firstly the model for bone remodeling is developed and applied to an intact femur. Then, it is extended for two bodies in contact in order to predict the bone remodeling around the stem, and an ingrowth algorithm is incorporated to a full simulation of the bone behavior after Total Hip Arthroplasty. The obtained results permit us to analyze the stability of existing stems with respect to material and shape, as well as to learn new improvements on stem design.

1 Introduction

The bone behavior after a Total Hip Arthroplasty is an important factor for the hip implants success. The bone is a natural material subject to a continuous process of apposition and resorption, corresponding to changes in density and architecture. These changes depend on diverse factors including the mechanical environment of bone. In fact, if the local mechanical conditions are adverse, resorption can outpace apposition resulting in a weaker bone, with a higher probability of fracture. A critical situation occurs when an orthopaedic implant is employed to treat disease or in fracture repair. In this case, an adverse redistribution of stresses may lead to resorption, thus to insufficient bone mass if a revision is required. Moreover it may increase the incidence of fractures and prosthesis failure. For hip implants with cementless stems, the mechanical conditions also affect the capacity of bone to attach to the stem (bone ingrowth) and consequently the long term stem stability.

Different models for bone remodeling have been developed and applied to hip prosthesis analysis [1–5]. Usually these models consider only the stress shield effect while with respect to interface condition they assume the bone and stem to be fully bonded. This approach is correct if one considers complete bone ingrowth. However, the bone remodeling after a total hip arthroplasty is an evolutionary process, i.e., in a post operative situation the bone ingrowth does not exist but, if the local mechanical conditions permit, it can appear. Even models that assume contact between stem and bone, as the one presented by Terrier *et al.* [4] does not fully address the ingrowth problem, since the bone ingrowth will change the interface condition during the prosthesis life time. The interface conditions and the bone ingrowth process have also been studied in several research works [6–9], but numerical methods that integrate ingrowth analysis and bone remodeling have not been used.

In this chapter a computational model to study concurrent bone remodeling and bone ingrowth around cementless femoral stems in total hip arthroplasty is presented. Firstly, the bone remodeling model is introduced. This model is formulated as a material optimization problem, where bone is considered a porous material with orthotropic microstructure [10]. The distribution of bone density and orientation is obtained solving the optimal conditions for a problem where the objective is a function of bone structural stiffness and the biological cost associated with metabolic maintenance of the bone tissue.

The concept behind this bone remodeling model is suitable to develop a remodeling model around hip stems since it is reported that it becomes stationary after few years [11]. Thus one can speculate that the remodeling around the stem stops when a "globally optimal" structure is achieved. However, to accommodate contact conditions on the interface between bone and stem, the model has to be adjusted. Thus, an extended model considering bone and stem in contact with friction is developed [12]. With this approach it is possible to simulate a large range of interface conditions, actuating on the friction coefficient value. An uncoated stem is simulated having zero friction while a fully coated stem has a finite value of friction on the whole surface. It is possible to simulate different coating surfaces, as well as different coating lengths, changing the friction coefficient.

For the contact approach mentioned above, the interface conditions are fixed during the remodeling process. Thus, the bone ingrowth process is not correctly simulated. In other words, if contact with friction is assumed between stem and bone, only the post-operative situation is described. On the other hand, if a fully bonded interface is considered, it corresponds to having bone ingrowth on whole coated zone, even immediately after prosthesis insertion. To overcome this problem a bone ingrowth control algorithm is introduced using a relative interface displacement criterion [13]. Besides to obtain the bone remodeling around the stem, the model predicts the zones where bone attaches to the stem, emphasizing the bone behavior on interface and addressing the problem of prosthesis stability.

The model is very useful to analyze existing stems as well as to design new ones. To show the capabilities of the computational model, changes in bone density and patterns of ingrowth are compared for different stem geometries (tapered wedge stem vs. cylindrical section stem), different stem materials (titanium vs. Co−Cr), and variable lengths of ingrowth surface coating.

2 Bone remodeling model

The dependence of bone morphology on applied loads was described by Wolff [14] at the end of nineteenth century. According with Wolff's observations, generally known as Wolff's Law, bone adaptation to mechanical environment can be described by mathematical rules [14, 15]. Since then, researchers have proposed numerous mathematical models for bone remodeling. Usually these models assume bone to be a linear elastic material and consider changes in bone density as a function of a local mechanical stimulus. This stimulus is recognized by bone cells, which regulate the coupled apposition and resorption leading to a change in bone architecture as an adaptative process. Examples of this type of model are the work of Cowin and Hegedus [16], Weinans *et al.* [17], Beaupré *et al.* [18], Mullender *et al.* [19], Jacobs *et al.* [20], Garcia *et al.* [21] and Doblaré and Garcia [22]. Additionally, there are some models, which propose structural optimization methods to compute the optimal distribution of a cellular material with a variable density. The works of Fyhrie and Carter [23], Hollister *et al.* [7] and Fernandes *et al.* [10] are examples of these methods.

The way the bone is modeled as a variable density material is an important issue, which distinguishes existing remodeling models. Some of them consider bone an isotropic material with effective properties computed by an empirical power law relationship between Young's Modulus and relative density [17–19, 23], while others assume the bone an non-isotropic material and couple material density and orientation in a single model [7, 10, 16, 20–22].

For the model developed in this chapter, such coupling is modelled assuming bone as a cellular material with an orthotropic microstructure and identifying remodeling with a material optimization process (see e.g. Fernandes *et al.* [10]). This formulation has the advantage to consider simultaneously bone density and orientation. It can be shown in general that the optimal solution is achieved when the microstructure is locally aligned with the local principal strain directions as observed by Wolff.

2.1 Material model for trabecular bone

To accomplish the purpose of coupling bone density and orientation, trabecular bone is approximated as a cellular material obtained by the periodic repetition of a unit cell with prismatic holes, as shown in fig. 1. The relative density at each

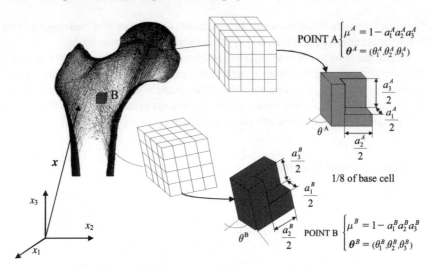

Figure 1: Material model for trabecular bone.

point depends on local hole dimensions, a_1, a_2 and a_3, i.e., $\mu = 1 - a_1, a_2, a_3$. In addition, since the selected cellular material is orthotropic, this model allows for the consideration of an optimal orientation of unit cells as shown in Pedersen [24] and, consequently, simulation of bone as an oriented material. Thus, at each point in the body, there is a microstructure characterized by the parameters $a = \{a_1, a_2, a_3\}^T$, which define the local material relative density, and by an orientation characterized by the Euler angles $\theta = \{\theta_1, \theta_2, \theta_3\}^T$. It should be noticed that the periodicity is local, thus it can change from point to point.

Assuming trabecular bone tissue has the same material properties as cortical bone, relative density values equal to one correspond to dense cortical bone while intermediate values correspond to trabecular bone. The effective (homogenized) elastic properties for this material are computed using the homogenization method and are given by,

$$E_{ijkl}^{H}(\mu) = E_{ijkl}\mu - \frac{1}{|Y|}\int_{\yen} E_{ijpm}\frac{\partial \chi_p^{kl}}{\partial y_m}dY \tag{1}$$

as a function of the relative density $\mu = 1 - a_1, a_2, a_3$, where Y is the unit cell domain and $\yen$ is the unit cell sub-domain occupied by homogeneous material (compact bone) with properties E_{ijkl}. The superscript H denotes homogenized properties. In eqn (1), the periodic functions χ^{kl} are solutions of the set of equilibrium equations,

$$\int_{\yen} E_{ijpm}\frac{\partial \chi_p^{kl}}{\partial y_m}\frac{\partial v_i\,(y)}{\partial y_j}dY = \int_{\yen} E_{ijkl}\frac{\partial v_i\,(y)}{\partial y_j}dY, \quad \forall v \; Y\text{-Periodic} \tag{2}$$

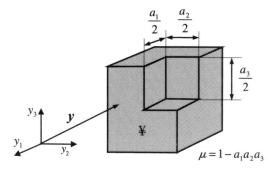

Figure 2: 1/8 of base cell.

defined on ¥ (see fig. 2). The definition of the apparent mechanical properties (eqn (1)) involves the contribution of two terms. The first is only a function of the relative density, and so, is independent of the specific geometry of the cell. The second (a correcting factor) introduces the influence of the microstructure geometry via the six displacement functions, χ^{kl}, which are the solutions of a set of equilibrium equations (eqn (2)) on the micro cell domain.

Besides the dependence on $\mu(a)$, the material properties depend also on the material orientation θ of the cells. This effect is taken into consideration by the rotation of the homogenized material properties tensor,

$$\left(E_{ijkl}^{H}\right)_{\theta} = R_{im} R_{jn} R_{kp} R_{lq} E_{mnpq}^{H}, \tag{3}$$

where R is the coordinate transformation tensor associated to cell orientation θ. The reader is referred to Sanchez-Palencia [25] for a full mathematical description of the homogenization method, and to Guedes and Kikuchi [26] for computational implementation.

2.2 The optimization problem – Law of bone remodeling

The bone remodeling model consists of the computation of relative bone density, at each point, by the solution of an optimization problem formulated in the continuum mechanics context. Assuming that bone adapts to the mechanical environment so that it can obtain the stiffest structure for the applied loads, the optimization problem is defined by the minimization of a linear combination of structural compliance and the metabolic cost to the organism maintaining bone tissue. The design variables are the hole dimensions of the microstructure defined above, and cell orientation θ. Hole dimensions have values in the interval [0, 1], where the extreme values, $a = 0$ and $a = 1$, correspond to compact bone and void, respectively, whereas intermediate values correspond to trabecular bone with a given apparent density. In that case, one assumes trabecular bone (cell walls) has the mechanical properties of compact bone. The solution to this optimization problem yields the stiffest bone structure with total mass regulated by parameters that quantifies biological factors. Thus, it reflects both mechanical advantage and metabolic cost.

Considering bone to be as a structure occupying a volume Ω_b, with boundary Γ, subject to a set of surfaces loads f^P, with the corresponding displacement fields u^P, defining the design variables $a = \{a_1, a_2, a_3\}^T$, and using a multiple load optimization criterion, the problem can be stated as,

$$\min_{a,\theta}\left[\sum_{P=1}^{NC}\alpha^P\left(\int_{\Gamma_f}f_i^P u_i^P\,d\Gamma\right) + \kappa\int_{\Omega_b}(\mu(a))^m\,d\Omega\right] \tag{4}$$

subjected to,

$$0 \leq a_i \leq 1, \tag{5}$$

$$\int_{\Omega_b}E_{ijkl}^H(a,\theta)\,e_{ij}\left(u^P\right)e_{kl}\left(v^P\right)d\Omega - \int_{\Gamma_f}f_i^P v_i^P\,d\Gamma = 0,$$

$$\forall v\ \text{admissible},\ P = 1...NC, \tag{6}$$

where E_{ijkl}^H are the homogenized material properties, e_{ij} is the strain field and v^P the set of virtual displacements. In the problem stated above, the first term of the objective function is a weighted average of the structural compliance for each load case, where α^P are the load weight factors satisfying $\sum_{P=1}^{NC}\alpha^P = 1$ and NC is the number of applied load cases. The parameters κ and m in the second term are biological factors, κ is the metabolic cost associated with a unit of bone volume and m regulates the porosity level of trabecular bone. The cost parameter κ in the second term plays an important role, since the resulting optimal bone mass will depend strongly on its value. It is known that even in the presence of identical loading conditions, the remodeling response is different for different individuals (Cowin [27]). Therefore, the parameter κ and m would include biological factors such age, hormonal status, disease, and so on.

The optimization problem formulated by eqns (4–6), is solved using a Lagrangian method (see for instance Luenberger [28]). The first variation of the associated Lagrangian functional with respect to design variables, state variables and Lagrange multipliers, permits to obtain the necessary condition for optimum. The stationarity conditions with respect to the design variables a and θ are, respectively,

$$\sum_{P=1}^{NC}\left\{\int_{\Omega_b}\left[-\alpha^P\frac{\partial E_{ijkl}^H}{\partial a}e_{kl}\left(u^P\right)e_{ij}\left(u^P\right)\right]\delta a\,d\Omega\right\}$$

$$+ \kappa\int_{\Omega_b}\left(m\mu^{m-1}\frac{\partial\mu}{\partial a}\right)\delta a\,d\Omega = 0,\quad \forall\,\delta a \tag{7}$$

and

$$\sum_{P=1}^{NC} \left\{ \int_{\Omega_b} \left[-\alpha^P \frac{\partial E_{ijkl}^H}{\partial \theta} e_{kl} \left(u^P \right) e_{ij} \left(u^P \right) \right] \delta\theta \, d\Omega \right\} = 0, \quad \forall \, \delta\theta. \tag{8}$$

In the previous equations the adjoint fields (Lagrange multipliers of the equilibrium constraints) v^P were substituted by the relation $v^P = \alpha^P u^P$, that results from the stationarity conditions with respect to u^P and v^P.

The cost function (eqn (4)) is a global criterion, and the solution of the problem gives the stiffest trabecular bone structure for the given loads, described by its relative density and orientation. The total bone mass is regulated, not only by the load values, but also by the parameter κ and m. Thus, it characterizes the law of bone remodeling in the sense that whenever they are satisfied no remodeling will occur (remodeling equilibrium). Moreover, it can be shown [10, 29] that eqn (7) under certain conditions is equivalent to local stimulus criterion models. Equations (7–8) are solved numerically using a suitable finite element discretization with the optimization algorithm based on a steepest descent method.

Since the main objective of this chapter is to analyze the bone behavior after implants, details for the optimal conditions derivation and numerical procedure will be given for the extended model with contact conditions presented below. For further details on the bone remodeling model presented in this section, including discussion on bone microstructure and material orientation for single and multiple load cases the reader is referred to [10] and [29].

2.3 Some results of bone remodeling for an intact femur

To illustrate the performance of the bone remodeling model described in the previous section, the bone density distribution on a femur is computed for different load cases and compared with a real femur. A 3D finite element model of the proximal femur was built using 5616 eight node solid elements (see fig. 3). The femur geometry is based on the *Standardized Femur* (Viceconti *et al.* [30]). The applied forces are shown in table 1 and correspond to load cases used by Kuiper [31]. The first and the second case correspond to walking and the third corresponds to stair climbing. The problem was first solved for the single load case situation applying each load case individually, and then considering the multiple load criterion, for equal load weights, i.e., $\alpha_1 = \alpha_2 = \alpha_3 = 1/3$. It was assumed that the bone tissue material has the mechanical properties of compact bone, with Young's modulus of 20 GPa [32]. This means that dense compact bone corresponds to a cellular material with relative density equal to 1 and trabecular bone has values less than 1.

The optimal material distribution obtained for the single load case (load case 2) is presented in fig. 4. These results show that the optimization model produces a material distribution that reflects certain morphological features of the femur. One obtains a hollow cylinder for the diaphyses, with high densities on the periphery corresponding to cortical bone. The epiphysis exhibits low densities, corresponding

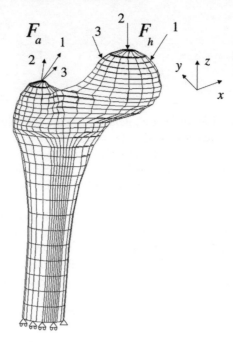

Figure 3: Three-dimensional model of an intact femur.

Table 1: Load cases.

LOAD		$F_x(N)$	$F_y(N)$	$F_z(N)$
1	F_a	768	726	1210
	F_h	−224	−972	−2246
2	F_a	166	382	957
	F_h	136	−630	−1692
3	F_a	383	669	547
	F_h	457	−796	−1707

to trabecular bone. A dense strut of trabecular bone was predicted to form from the medial cortex to the load application point. These features were also similar in the other two load cases.

The optimal orientation for this load case is presented in fig. 5. The predicted optimal orientations follow the principal strain directions. The trabecular arching system on metaphysis is particularly evident. Also, the dense strut from the medial cortex to the load application point is oriented with the direction of load application.

For one single load case, however, the tubular structure is not properly predicted in that the anterior and posterior densities are lower and the cortex is thinner than expected as compared with the medial and lateral regions. For an accurate prediction

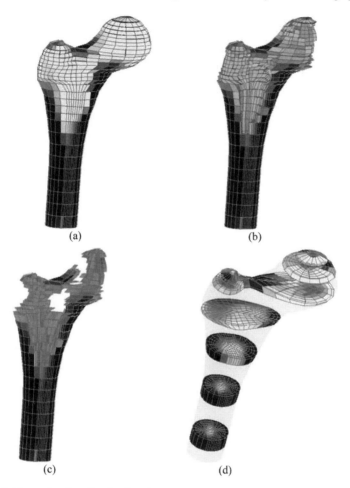

(a)

(b)

(c)

(d)

Figure 4: Bone density distribution, load case 2. (a) Whole femur, (b) elements with $\mu > 0.2$, (c) elements with $\mu > 0.4$, (d) femur cross sections.

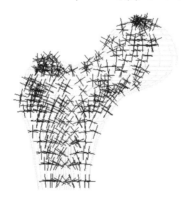

Figure 5: Trabecular bone orientation for load case 2.

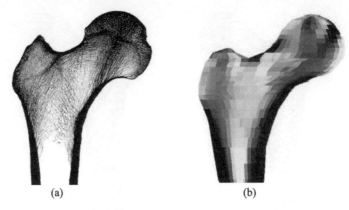

(a)   (b)

Figure 6: (a) Real femur, (b) density distribution obtained computationally.

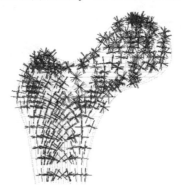

Figure 7: Orientation for multiple loads.

of bone distribution the problem was solved for multiple loads. Figure 6 shows a comparison between the obtained densities and a real femur. For the solution with multiple load, the material reorientation was not performed during the optimization procedure, but was computed for each load case individually for the final material distribution. For comparison purposes, the obtained orientations are overlaid in fig. 7. This result shows that in the region between the epiphyses and the diaphyses the orientations are roughly similar. This means that the material has a preferential orientation. Therefore, the trabecular bone in this zone can not be isotropic. In the epiphysis the three orientations are significantly different, since the trabecular bone microstructure in this region should behave as an isotropic material to support equally stresses from all directions.

3 Bone remodeling around implants

To model the bone behavior around implants the bone remodeling model briefly described above has to be extended to accommodate the interface conditions between

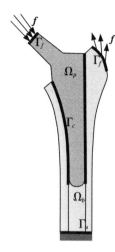

Figure 8: Generalized elastic problem with contact.

bone and stem. In fact, the bone remodeling formulated in eqns (4–6) can be applied to implants only if one considers the interface fully bonded [33]. This assumption for the interface is restrictive, since it only can simulate a situation with complete ingrowth, without relative displacement on interface. Thus, it is not possible to consider the post-operative situation and to investigate the long-term stability. Actually, the bone remodeling after a total hip arthroplasty is an evolutionary process, i.e., in a post operative situation the bone ingrowth does not exist but, if the local mechanical conditions permit, it can appear. To overcome this limitation the model is extended to include contact conditions on interface. It should be noted that, although contact formulation permits us to consider different friction coefficients, and therefore to simulate several coating types and extensions, it still does not reproduce the ingrowth process. This effect is obtained combining the remodeling process with an ingrowth control algorithm based on interface displacement.

3.1 The optimization problem

The assumption that bone adapts in order to reach the stiffest structure is also valid for the case of an implanted bone. Thus, using the material model described in Section 2.1, it is possible to define the optimization problem for two bodies in contact (bone and prosthesis) that yields the stiffest bone structure with total mass regulated by parameters that quantifies biological factors.

Let us consider the implanted femur as a structure occupying a volume $\Omega = \Omega_b \cup \Omega_p$, with boundary Γ, subject to surface loads f on Γ_f and fixed at Γ_u, where the bone/stem interface is denoted by Γ_c (fig. 8). Defining the cell parameters $a = \{a_1, a_2, a_3\}^T$, and $\theta = \{\theta_1, \theta_2, \theta_3\}^T$ as design variables, and using a multiple load optimization criterion, the problem can be stated as,

$$\min_{a,\theta} \left[\sum_{P=1}^{NC} \alpha^P \left(\int_{\Gamma_f} f_i^P u_i^P \, d\Gamma \right) + \kappa \int_{\Omega_b} (\mu(a))^m \, d\Omega \right] \tag{9}$$

subjected to,

$$0 \le a_i \le 1, \tag{10}$$

$$\int_{\Omega} E_{ijkl}\, (a, \theta)\, e_{kl} \left(u^P \right) e_{ij} \left(v^P \right) d\Omega - \int_{\Gamma_f} f_i^P v_i^P \, d\Gamma$$

$$+ \int_{\Gamma_c} \tau_n^P \left(v_n^{\mathrm{rel}} \right)^P - \tau_t^P \cdot \left(v_t^{\mathrm{rel}} \right)^P d\Gamma = 0, \quad \forall v \text{ adm.}, \ P = 1...NC, \tag{11}$$

$$\begin{cases} \left(u_n^{\mathrm{rel}} \right)^P - g \le 0, \ \tau_n^P \ge 0, \ \tau_n^P \left(\left(u_n^{\mathrm{rel}} \right)^P - g \right) = 0 \\ \left| \tau_t^P \right| \le \vartheta \left| \tau_n^P \right| \rightarrow \begin{cases} \left| \tau_t^P \right| < \vartheta \left| \tau_n^P \right| \ \Rightarrow \ u_t^{\mathrm{rel}} = 0 \quad \text{in } \Gamma_c, \ P = 1...NC \\ \left| \tau_t^P \right| = \vartheta \left| \tau_n^P \right| \ \Rightarrow \ \exists \Lambda \ge 0 : \left(u_t^{\mathrm{rel}} \right)^P = -\Lambda \tau_t^P \end{cases} \end{cases} \tag{12}$$

for *NC* load cases, with the load weight factors α^P satisfying $\sum_{P=1}^{NC} \alpha^P = 1$. In the previous problem statement, eqns (11–12) correspond to the set of equilibrium equations for two bodies in contact, in the form of a virtual displacement principle. In these equations, E_{ijkl} is the material properties tensor (homogenized properties for trabecular bone), e_{ij} is the strain field, and v_i^P is the set of virtual displacements. The last term of eqn (11) is the contribution of contact loads τ^P, the subscripts n and t denote normal and tangential directions, respectively, g is the gap between the two bodies and ϑ is the friction coefficient. In the objective function (eqn (9)) κ and m are the biological parameters as defined for the problem without contact. As previously stated, the first term of the cost function is a weighted average of the structural compliance for each load case while the second term controls the total bone mass and porosity by the action of κ and m.

3.2 Necessary conditions for optimum – Law of bone remodeling

The optimization problem with contact is solved using a Lagrangian method, and the stationarity conditions obtained following the work of Rodrigues [34] for shape optimal design.

Let us introduce the Lagrangian functional,

$$llL = \sum_{P=1}^{NC} \alpha^P \int_{\Gamma_f} f_i^P u_i^P \, d\Gamma + \kappa \int_{\Omega_b} (\mu(a))^m \, d\Omega - \int_{\Omega_b} \lambda_i^0 a_i d\Omega - \int_{\Omega_b} \lambda_i^1 (1 - a_i) d\Omega$$

$$+ \sum_{P=1}^{NC} \left[\int_{\Omega} E_{ijkl} e_{kl} \left(u^P\right) e_{ij} \left(v^P\right) d\Omega - \int_{\Gamma_f} f_i^P v_i^P \, d\Gamma \right.$$

$$+ \int_{\Gamma_c} \tau_n^P \left(v_n^{\text{rel}}\right)^P d\Gamma - \int_{\Gamma_{cs}} \boldsymbol{\tau}_t^P \cdot \left(\boldsymbol{v}_t^{\text{rel}}\right)^P d\Gamma$$

$$+ \int_{\Gamma_c} (\rho^-)^P \left(\left(u_n^{\text{rel}}\right)^P - g\right) d\Gamma - \int_{\Gamma_c} (\rho^+)^P \tau_n^P d\Gamma$$

$$+ \int_{\Gamma_c} (\rho^0)^P \left[\tau_n^P \left(\left(u_n^{\text{rel}}\right)^P - g\right)\right] d\Gamma$$

$$\left. + \int_{\Gamma_{cs}^0} (\eta^0)^P \left(|\tau_t^P| - s^P\right) d\Gamma + \int_{\Gamma_{cs}^{\pm}} (\eta^{\pm})^P \left(|\tau_t^P| - s^P\right) d\Gamma \right], \quad (13)$$

where the $\lambda^0, \lambda^1, v^P, \rho^P, \eta^P$ are Lagrange multipliers related to the constraint eqns (10–12) and Γ_{cs} is the part of Γ_c where the frictional load $\boldsymbol{\tau}_t$ is prescribed in order to obtain a well-posed mathematical problem [34], $\Gamma_{cs} = \Gamma_{cs}^0 \cup \Gamma_{cs}^{\pm}$, where Γ_{cs}^0 is the part of Γ_{cs} where $\boldsymbol{u}_t^{\text{rel}} = \boldsymbol{0}$ (non-slide region). The dependency of frictional on normal load, $s(x) = \vartheta \cdot \tau_n(\boldsymbol{u})$, is not explicit. Thus, the prescription of frictional load, i.e., $|\boldsymbol{\tau}_t| \leq s$ on Γ_{cs}, means that variations of s with respect to $\boldsymbol{u}$ vanish. Defining $V_{a0} = \{v : v = \boldsymbol{0}$ on $\Gamma_u, v_n^{\text{rel}} = 0$ on $\Gamma_{c0}, \boldsymbol{v}_t^{\text{rel}} = \boldsymbol{0}$ on $\Gamma_{cs}^0\}$, Γ_{c0} is part of Γ_c where contact actually happens, stationarity conditions of the functional with respect to the state variables $\boldsymbol{u}^P, \tau_n^P$ and τ_t^P can be written as,

$$\int_{\Omega} E_{ijkl} e_{kl}(\delta \boldsymbol{u}^P) e_{ij}(v^P) d\Omega + \alpha^P \int_{\Gamma_f} f_i^P \delta u_i^P d\Gamma = 0,$$

$$\forall \delta \boldsymbol{u}^P \in V_{a0}, \ P = 1...NC. \quad (14)$$

Thus, the stationarity of the Lagrangian with respect to $\boldsymbol{u}$ yields a linear elastic problem with additional displacement constraints on contact boundary, obtained from the solution of the state problem. Finally, the stationarity condition with respect to adjoint variables yields the state problem defined by eqns (11–12).

To sum up, the introduction of contact conditions in the optimization problem leads to a non-self-adjoint problem, i.e., the adjoint problem (eqn (14)) is different from the state problem (eqns (11–12)). Therefore, to obtain the solution, we have to solve two finite element problems for each load case instead of the one required for the original bone remodeling model given by eqns (4–6).

The stationarity conditions with respect to the design variables a and θ are,

$$
\sum_{P=1}^{NC} \left[\int_{\Omega_b} \frac{\partial E_{ijkl}}{\partial a} e_{kl} \left(u^P \right) e_{ij} \left(v^P \right) \delta a \, d\Omega \right]
$$
$$
+ \int_{\Omega_b} \left(\lambda^1 - \lambda^0 \right) \delta a \, d\Omega + \kappa \int_{\Omega_b} m \mu^{m-1} \frac{\partial \mu}{\partial a} \delta a \, d\Omega = 0, \quad \forall \, \delta a \qquad (15)
$$

and

$$
\sum_{P=1}^{NC} \int_{\Omega_b} \frac{\partial E_{ijkl}}{\partial \theta} e_{kl} \left(u^P \right) e_{ij} \left(v^P \right) \delta\theta \, d\Omega = 0, \quad \forall \, \delta\theta. \qquad (16)
$$

These two eqns (15–16) are similar to eqns (7–8), however in this case the adjoint displacement v^P is not directly related with the state field u^P, and it has to be determined at each iteration, solving the adjoint problem (eqn (14)).

The solution of this problem gives the distribution of density and orientation of trabecular bone after a total hip arthroplasty. They are now the equations that characterize the remodeling equilibrium.

4 The ingrowth control

A characteristic of cementless stems is the biological fixation by bone/metal inter-action [35]. After insertion, the bone starts to attach to the stem surface, thus sta-bilizing the prosthesis. This process is enhanced by the high coefficient of friction of a coated surface [36]. However and despite the coating, high relative displace-ments can occur in certain regions resulting in inhibition of bone ingrowth [6]. This dynamic behavior in the bone/stem interface has been poorly reproduced in exist-ing computational models. The model described in this chapter proposes a dynamic procedure to determine where ingrowth occurs.

In the immediate post-operative situation no bone ingrowth is considered. Thus, the initial contact condition to solve the problem stated above is contact with fric-tion in the coated surface and contact without friction in the smooth noncoated surface. After each time step (an iteration of the optimization algorithm) the rela-tive displacement is computed. If, at a certain point (contact node), contact actually happens and the bone/stem relative displacement is less than a threshold value, a connection between the interface bone/prosthesis is established. Initially this con-nection has low stiffness. This stiffness is increased, for favorable displacement conditions, until the interface condition is set to completely bond. Note that this condition must be verified for every load case. Consequently, on the coated sur-face, we simultaneously have regions where contact with friction occurs and bonded regions, as determined by the relative displacement at each location. Furthermore, these conditions can change at each time step depending upon the instantaneous relative displacement.

It should be noted that this process differs from the algorithm proposed in [13] only by the fact that a contact node, with favourable condition to exist ingrowth, is not immediately bonded, but the connection is progressive in order to simulate the process of bone growing into the coating pores.

A consequence of this methodology is that once a point is set to bonded, it will remain bonded until the end of the process; this condition recapitulates the observed biologic behavior *in vivo*. Another issue is the choice of the threshold displacement value. Some authors reference values between 50 and 150 μm [9, 37]. An experimental study with dogs relates occurrence of bone ingrowth for test values of 0 and 20 μm, and no ingrowth appears with 40 and 150 μm [38]. In this chapter a parametric study is done using two different values, 25 and 50 μm.

5 Numerical implementation

Computationally, eqns (15–16) are satisfied as follows: firstly the bone homogenized elastic properties are computed for an initial solution. Next, one computes the set of displacement fields u^P and the set of adjoint fields v^P using the finite element method. Based on the finite element approximation, the necessary optimality conditions are checked. If they are satisfied the process stops; if not, improved values of the design variables are computed, the interface conditions are updated and the process restarts (fig. 9).

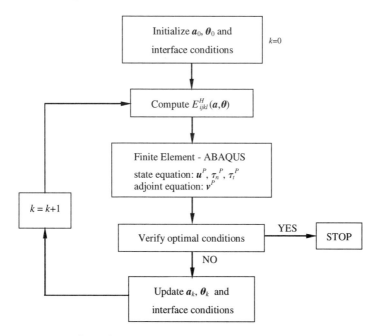

Figure 9: Computational model flow diagram.

To minimize computational cost the properties $E_{ijkl}^H(a)$ are obtained for each new optimization iteration by a polynomial interpolation on the interval $[0,1]^3$. This was accomplished with the values at the interpolation points computed using the homogenization code PREMAT [26]. The approximated solution for the set of displacement fields u^P and set of adjoint fields v^P are obtained by the finite element code ABAQUS [39]. The contact problem (to obtain u^P) is solved using standard parameters of ABAQUS with an infinitesimal-sliding formulation and Lagrange multipliers to compute the tangential force.

It is assumed that the design variables a and θ are constant within each finite element. This permits us to write optimality conditions independently for each element. The solution for the cell parameters a_i can then be obtained with an iterative procedure based on a first order Lagrangian method. The formulas to update the cell design variables a_i at the kth iteration are,

$$
\left(a_i^e\right)_{k+1} = \begin{cases} \max\left[(1-\zeta)\left(a_i^e\right)_k, a_{\min}\right] \\ \quad \text{if } \left(a_i^e\right)_k + d\left(D_i^e\right)_k \leq \max\left[(1-\zeta)\left(a_i^e\right)_k, a_{\min}\right] \\ \left(a_i^e\right)_k + d\left(D_i^e\right)_k \qquad \text{otherwise} \\ \min\left[(1+\zeta)\left(a_i^e\right)_k, 1\right] \\ \quad \text{if } \left(a_i^e\right)_k + d\left(D_i^e\right)_k \geq \min\left[(1+\zeta)\left(a_i^e\right)_k, 1\right], \end{cases}
\tag{17}
$$

where e ranges over all finite elements and $i = 1, 2, 3$.

In the previous update scheme, the vector D_k, the descent direction at the kth iteration, is the negative of the Lagrangian gradient with respect to the design variables a, eqn (15). The component of the direction vector D for the design variable a_i^e (hole dimension i for the eth element) is,

$$
D_i^e = \sum_{P=1}^{NC}\left\{\int_{\Omega^e}\left[\frac{\partial E_{klmn}^H}{\partial a_i^e}e_{mn}\left(u^P\right)e_{kl}\left(v^P\right)\right]d\Omega\right\} + \kappa\int_{\Omega^e}m\mu^{m-1}\cdot\frac{\partial\mu}{\partial a_i^e}d\Omega.
\tag{18}
$$

The parameter $\zeta > 0$ defines the active upper and lower boundary constraints and the real number d is the step length. This step length is constant and selected by the user at the beginning of the process.

Initially, the interface conditions are set to contact with friction on the coated area and contact without friction on the noncoated zone. After the first iteration, the interface conditions are updated based on the absolute value of the relative displacement. For each contact node the relative displacement is computed, if the value verifies the condition for bone ingrowth, the node is connected with a spring. For the next contact analysis (iterations or time steps), the ingrowth conditions are tested and if they are still verified the spring stiffness is increased, until the condition is set to fully bonded. Thus, the contact surface definition must be updated at each iteration of the optimization process.

6 Results

The remodeling model was applied to a three-dimensional model of an implanted femur. The finite element mesh was created using the same bone geometry used for intact femur in Section 2.3 (the "Standardized Femur" [30]). Two different stem geometries were considered, one based on the Tri-Lock prosthesis by DePuy (Warsaw, Indiana, USA) and the second based on an AML stem of the same manufacturer. In the text we refer to the Tri-Lock stem as *the tapered stem* and to the AML as *the circular section stem*. Figure 10 shows the finite element model for both stem geometries. Stems were considered in totally coated, partially coated, and uncoated versions. The light grey on stem surfaces in fig. 10(c) and (f) correspond to the coated portions of a partially coated stem. Two different materials were tested for each stem, titanium and Co−Cr alloy. For initial bone density distribution two approaches were considered; uniform distribution with relative density $\mu = 0.7$ and non uniform distribution to simulate compact bone ($\mu = 0.8$)

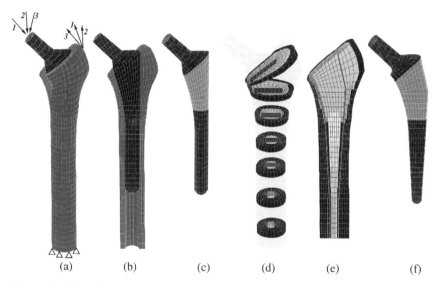

(a)   (b)   (c)   (d)   (e)   (f)

Figure 10: 3D finite element model for a left implanted femur. Prosthesis is represented in black, compact bone in black and trabecular bone in grey. (a) Global view of bone and circular section stem – initial uniform homogeneous solution, (b) sagittal cross section of bone and cylindrical section implant – initial uniform homogeneous solution, (c) cylindrical section stem - light grey on stem surface correspond to the coated portion, (d) Set of transverse cross sections for the tapered stem – non uniform initial solution, (e) sagittal cross section of bone to implant the tapered stem – the distribution of density for non uniform initial solution is shown, (f) Tapered stem – light grey on stem surface corresponds to the coated portion.

and trabecular bone ($\mu = 0.2$), as shown in fig. 10(d) and (e). The medullar cavity anterior and posterior to the tapered stem was filled with a very weak material ($\mu = 0.06$), minimum density value allowed in the numerical formulation) to permit remodeling, in this case densification (fig. 10(d) and (e)). In all cases a perfect fit was assumed between bone and stem. With respect to load application a multiple load analysis was performed with the three load cases shown in table 1 (Section 2.3).

The material properties for bone are the same properties used to test the bone remodeling model for intact femur (Section 2.3), while stems were considered a non-design area with Young modulus equal to 115 GPa for Titanium and equal to 230 GPa for the Co−Cr alloy.

With respect to the biological optimization parameters they are set to $\kappa = 0.02 \times 10^6$ and $m = 2$. The amount of bone mass and trabecular bone are highly influenced by these parameters, and due to its nature we are not able to have $a priori$ evaluation. A parametric study of the metabolic cost κ of bone formation can be found in Fernandes et $al.$ [10]. The displacement threshold value in the ingrowth scheme was set to $0.25\,\mu$m and $0.50\,\mu$m. Since the literature does not provide a definitive value for this parameter, testing the model with different values permits to study the bone ingrowth sensitivity with respect to the relative tangential displacement. For the interface stiffness, before the ingrowth condition is set to bonded, two stages are considered with spring stiffness of 10^5 and 10^8 N/mm. For the friction coefficient on coated surfaces it was assumed a value of 0.6 [40]. The step length factor is $d = 0.05$ and is maintained constant through the iterative process.

6.1 Bone remodeling results

To illustrate the bone remodeling process, the following cases were selected: titanium and Co−Cr cylindrical section stems, as shown in figs 11 and 12, respectively. Figures 11 and 12 show results for totally coated (a), partially coated (b), and uncoated (c) stems. The initial solution for all of these cases is a uniform density distribution ($\mu = 0.7$), and the threshold value for ingrowth is $50\,\mu$m. It should be noted that for the uncoated stem the possibility of ingrowth is not considered and, consequently, the interface conditions do not change during the optimization process.

If these results are analyzed based on extent of coating, uncoated stems presents the lowest level of resorption, while the totally coated stems presents the highest level. The evolution of bone mass is graphically depicted (fig. 13) confirming this observation. The final amount of bone mass is greatest with uncoated and least with fully coated stems. Moreover, overall bone resorption was greater for the Co−Cr compared with the titanium stems; specifically, material-dependent bone mass differences were most apparent around the fully coated stems in each group. These results were anticipated due to a stress shielding effect, and are consistent with published results [41]. Furthermore, it should be noted that differences in bone mass between materials became increasingly evident with the surface

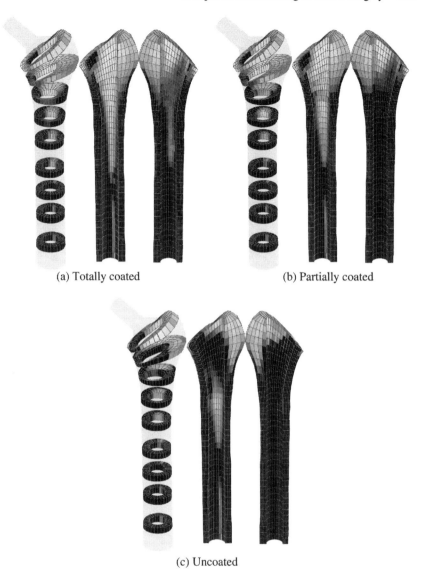

(a) Totally coated   (b) Partially coated

(c) Uncoated

Figure 11: Bone remodeling solution for a **titanium** circular section stem (initial
uniform solution). Black zone is compact bone while grey is trabecular bone. (a) Totally coated solution, (b) Partially coated solution, (c)
Uncoated solution. For each case are shown transverse cross sections, a
sagittal anterior, and a sagittal posterior cross cut.

coating length; the greatest difference in bone loss was observed between the two
fully coated cylindrical stems. Hypertrophy was observed at the distal tip of stems
and for the partially coated stems at the coated zone end, reproducing clinical
observations.

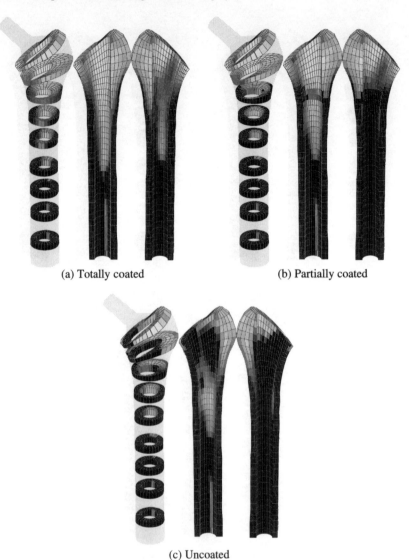

(a) Totally coated   (b) Partially coated

(c) Uncoated

Figure 12: Bone remodeling solution for a **Co−Cr** circular section stem (initial
          uniform solution). Black zone is compact bone while grey is trabecu-
          lar bone. (a) Totally coated solution, (b) Partially coated solution, (c)
          Uncoated solution. For each case are shown transverse cross sections,
          a sagittal anterior, and a sagittal posterior cross cut.

6.2 Bone ingrowth results

The bone ingrowth patterns obtained by the computational model are presented in
figs 14 and 15 for partially coated stem and fully coated stem, respectively. Both the

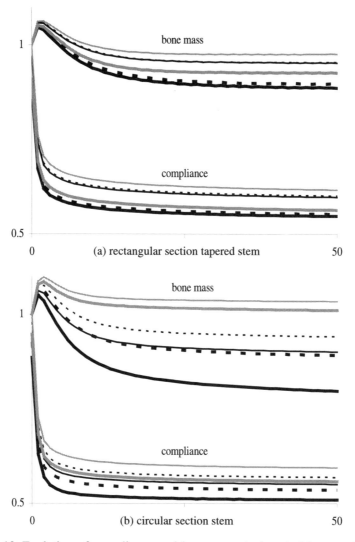

Figure 13: Evolution of compliance and bone mass (volume). (a) tapered stem, (b) circular section stem. Grey is the uncoated stem, black dashed line the partially coated and black full line the totally coated stem. Thick (Co−Cr) and thin (titanium) lines refer to the different stem materials.

partially and fully coated stems are shown in medial/anterior and lateral/posterior views. In each instance one can compare the solution obtained for the different geometries and materials, and also when the threshold value is changed. The starting point is non uniform density distribution. The light grey regions indicate areas without bone ingrowth (separation or relative displacement greater than threshold value), and the dark grey zones depict regions of bone ingrowth.

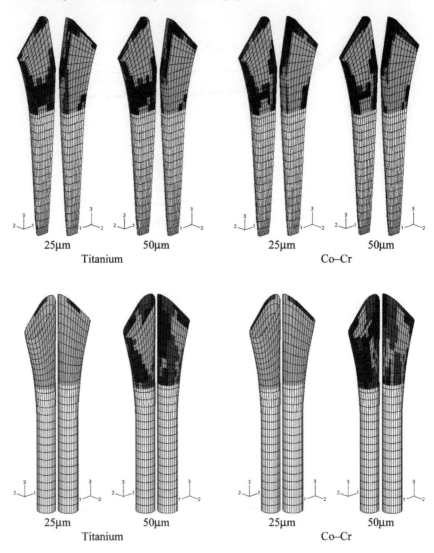

Figure 14: Bone ingrowth results for **partially coated** stems, non uniform initial
densities (threshold value 25 μm and 50 μm, titanium and Co−Cr material, rectangular tapered and circular section). Light grey zones indicates
regions without ingrowth, dark grey zones are regions of bone ingrowth.

A common observation for all configurations tested is that in a given region coating is not a sufficient condition for ingrowth. This result confirms the hypothesis
of this model as well as observations from retrieved specimens; bone ingrowth
does not occur over the entire coated surface area, even with a high friction
coefficient. Bone ingrowth patterns for the tapered geometry are very similar for
fully and partially coated stems. Furthermore, this similarity is maintained for

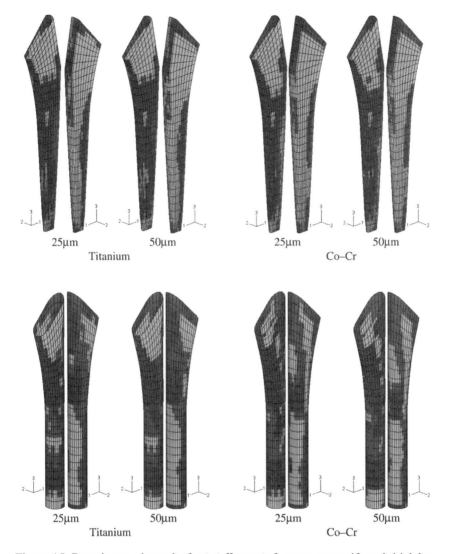

Figure 15: Bone ingrowth results for **totally coated** stems, non uniform initial densities (threshold value 25 μm and 50 μm, titanium and Co−Cr material, rectangular tapered and circular section). Light grey zones indicate regions without ingrowth, dark grey zones are regions of bone ingrowth.

displacement threshold values of both 25 μm and 50 μm. This similarity was not expected *a priori*. In contrast, this independence of ingrowth pattern with respect to extent of coating was not observed with the cylindrical stem. Ingrowth patterns on the cylindrical stem varied with the extent of coating. In fact a lack of ingrowth is observed for the partially coated circular stem for a threshold value of 25 μm. Under these conditions, fibrous tissue (or fibrous cartilage tissue) must appear and loosening can occur. A possible explanation for this observation is the greater inherent stability of the tapered stem. Such stability would result from lower dependence of global displacement on such parameters as coating length and preoperative bone conditions (initial density distribution) as reflected in the mechanical model. Additional displacement analysis was conducted to specifically investigate the issue of stability of stems of different geometry.

6.3 Initial interface relative displacement

Since the criterion to predict bone ingrowth is based on relative interface displacements, the prosthesis stability dependence on stem shape is better understood from a displacement analysis. This analysis was performed for the displacement value at the starting point and only for load case 1. It should be remembered that the ingrowth condition should be verified for all load cases. However for the purpose of this displacement analysis one load case is sufficient, since a similar conclusion will be obtained for the remaining cases. Figures 16 and 17 shows the interface displacement. The normal displacement, separation/no separation zones are identified respectively in dark grey and white. For the tangential displacement three levels of displacements are distinguished: dark grey for displacement above $50\,\mu m$, light grey for displacement between 25 and $50\,\mu m$ and white for displacement below $25\,\mu m$.

Analyzing these results the difference between circular and tapered stem is apparent. For the circular stem the displacement patterns change more significantly when the coating extension is changed. On the other hand for the tapered stem we can note the low level of tangential displacement, which implies a better initial stability. Furthermore, for the tapered stem, the main regulator of the ingrowth process is the contact status (separation/no separation) instead of the tangential (slip) displacement.

The results for remodeling, ingrowth and displacements, show that models such as the one presented in this work, which predict bone ingrowth and subsequent remodeling are useful for analysis of coated stems. Furthermore, the existence of bone ingrowth is an indication that displacements are limited within a range that permits the prosthesis stabilization.

7 Discussion

This chapter discussed the bone behavior after a total hip arthroplasty. A computational model for bone remodeling around cementless stems with ingrowth control was developed. The remodeling model is obtained by the solution of a material optimization problem where the trabecular bone was modeled as an orthotropic material, with relative density at each point computed by minimization of a cost function, which is assumed to be a linear combination of global compliance and total bone volume.

Firstly, the remodeling model was developed for bone without implants. Although this model reproduces the bone adaptation to mechanical demands, a contact

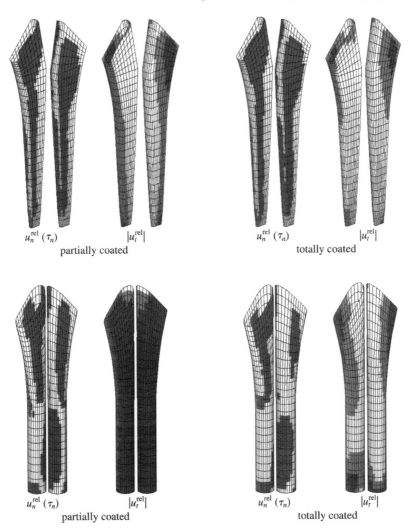

$u_n^{rel}\ (\tau_n)$ $|u_t^{rel}|$
partially coated

$u_n^{rel}\ (\tau_n)$ $|u_t^{rel}|$
totally coated

$u_n^{rel}\ (\tau_n)$ $|u_t^{rel}|$
partially coated

$u_n^{rel}\ (\tau_n)$ $|u_t^{rel}|$
totally coated

Figure 16: Initial interface displacements analyze, non-uniform initial density, load
case 1, **titanium** material stems (normal and tangential displacements,
partial and totally coated, rectangular tapered and circular section). For
normal displacements, dark grey zones represent separation and white
zones close contact. For tangential displacements, dark grey zones represent displacements above 50 μm, light grey zones tangential displacements between 25 μm and 50 μm and white zones below 25 μm.

formulation is needed when a prosthesis is present. In fact, bone and prosthesis
are initially in contact and ingrowth only happens for favorable mechanical conditions. To accomplish this, a new model with the bone/stem interface modeled using
a contact formulation was developed and it was combined with an algorithm based

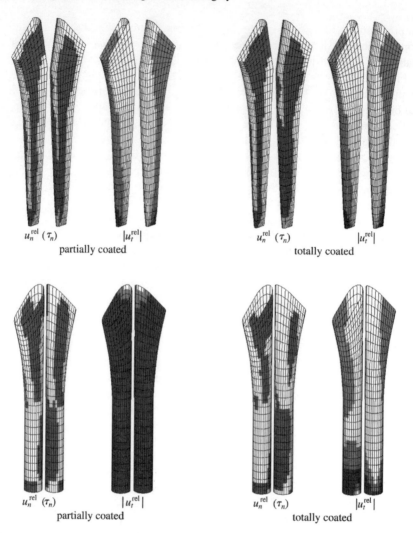

Figure 17: Initial interface displacements analyze, non-uniform initial density, load case 1, **Co−Cr** material stems (normal and tangential displacements, partial and totally coated, rectangular tapered and circular section). For normal displacements, dark grey zones represent separation and white zones close contact. For tangential displacements, dark grey zones represent displacements above $50\,\mu$m, light grey zones tangential displacements between $25\,\mu$m and $50\,\mu$m and white zones below $25\,\mu$m.

on the relative displacement to predict regions of bone ingrowth. This is a relevant point of the model since it involves solving a contact problem that is non-linear. The computational procedure was tested for a 3D element mesh of an implanted femur. Different stem geometries and material were tested in order to compare its performance. Results give us information about the distribution of bone ingrowth on prosthetic stem surfaces as well as the predicted remodeling behavior of those bony attachment sites. A displacement analysis was also done to study the primary stability of stem (postoperative) and to better understand long term ingrowth results.

Final results reproduce clinical observations and, although the model presented in this chapter is theoretical, it would appear to have a useful and sound clinical biological correspondence. However a full clinical validation, step by step, is difficult, in particular with respect to bone ingrowth evolution and remodeling. The distribution of bone densities obtained predicts the loss of bone in proximal femur. These results agree with the clinically observed bone loss under such conditions and with computational results presented by other authors [2]. From the bone remodeling results we can conclude that the uncoated stem leads to less resorption in the proximal femur than the coated one with similar shape. Furthermore, for coated stems, results show that remodeling in tapered stem was less sensitive to the coating length than the circular stem. In other words, the final amount of bone mass is very close for fully and partially coated, in the case of tapered stem. Also the Co−Cr stem leads to more bone resorption than the titanium stem. This is also expected since the stress shielding effect is bigger for stiffest stems. The clinical results of bone ingrowth distribution on the porous coated surface agrees with the hypothesis that motivates this formulation. Bone ingrowth does not occur all over the coated surface, even for high friction coefficients. Indeed, one can observe regions where separation or high relative displacement occurs that prevents bone ingrowth attachment. This model prediction is consistent with clinical observations where bone ingrowth over 20% of the porous coated surface has been observed in retrieved stems. Thus, models such as the one described in this work, which detect bone ingrowth and allow modification of the interface conditions responsible for its remodeling, are useful for analysis of existing stems as well as design and optimization of the coating extent and location. Also some unexpected results were obtained, namely in the tapered stem which reveals a non-dependence of ingrowth patterns on parameters such as coat length, threshold value and initial density distribution. Comparing with a circular section stem, which presents different patterns, these results are possibly due to a higher stability of tapered stem. Such stability implies a minor global displacement dependence on coat length. From the displacement analysis one can conclude that the main regulator of the ingrowth process for the tapered stem is the contact status (separation/no separation).

In the examples shown in this chapter, a multiple load formulation is used and the results were obtained for three load cases, which correspond to the most significant loads on the real femur. However, a larger number of loads should be considered for a better accuracy of the results. Indeed, the high bone resorption observed at the posterior side of the implant may be in part a consequence of the number of load cases. In addition, a larger number of load cases could reduce the amount of bone ingrowth, since the condition for ingrowth has to be verified for all these new load cases. The computational model presented in this chapter is both practical and clinically relevant and will allow for a more knowledgeable approach to design of cementless femoral stems.

Acknowledgments

The authors want to acknowledge and thank Prof. Helder Rodrigues and Prof. José Miranda Guedes – Technical University of Lisbon, Portugal, Dr. Vincent Pellegrini, University of Maryland School of Medicine, USA and Prof. Cristopher Jacobs, Stanford University, USA, for a very rewarding collaboration in the development of the models and results presented in this chapter. The work described here was supported by the Portuguese Foundation for Science and Technology through projects PRAXIS/P/EME/12002/1998 and POCTI/38367/EME/2001.

References

[1] Huiskes, R., Weinans, H., Grootenboer, H., Dalstra, M., Fudala, B. & Slooff, T., Adaptive bone-remodeling theory applied to prosthetic-design analysis. *Journal of Biomechanics*, **20**, pp. 1135–1150, 1987.

[2] Huiskes, R. & Rietbergen, B., Preclinical testing of total hip stems, the effects of coating placement. *Clinical Orthopaedics and Related Research*, **319**, pp. 64–76, 1995.

[3] Harrigan, T.P., Hamilton, J.J., Reuben, J.D., Toni, A. & Viceconti, M., Bone remodelling sdjacent to intramedullary stems: an optimal structures approach. *Biomaterials*, **17**, pp. 223–232, 1996.

[4] Terrier, A., Rakotomanana, R.L., Ramaniraka, A.N. & Leyvraz, P.F., Adaptation models of anisotropic bone. *Computer Methods in Biomechanics and Biomedical Engineering*, **1**, pp. 47–60, 1997.

[5] Doblaré, M. & Garcia, J.M., Application of a bone remodelling model based on a damage-repair theory to the analysis of the proximal femur before and after total hip replacement. *Journal of Biomechanics*, **34**, pp. 1157–1170, 2001.

[6] Keaveny, T. & Bartel, D., Effects of porous coating, with and without collar support, on early relative motion for a cementless hip prosthesis. *Journal of Biomechanics*, **26**, pp. 1355–1368, 1993.

[7] Hollister, S., Kikuchi, N. & Goldstein, A., Do bone ingrowth process produce a globally optimized structure? *Journal of Biomechanics*, **26**, pp. 391–407, 1993.

[8] Keaveny, T. & Bartel, D., Mechanical consequences of bone ingrowth in a hip prosthesis inserted without cement. *Journal of Bone and Joint Surgery*, **77-A**, pp. 911–923, 1995.

[9] Viceconti, M., Muccini, R., Bernakiewicz, M., Baleani, M. & Cristofolini L., Large-sliding contact elements accurately predict levels of bone-implant micromotion relevant to osseointegration. *Journal of Biomechanics*, **33**, pp. 1611–1618, 2000.

[10] Fernandes, P., Rodrigues, H. & Jacobs, C., A model of bone adaptation using a global optimization criterion based on the trajectorial theory of Wolff. *Computer Methods in Biomechanics and Biomedical Engineering*, **2**, pp. 125–138, 1999.

[11] Trevisan, C., Bigoni, M., Randelli, G., Marinoni, E.C., Peretti, G. & Ortolani S., Periprosthetic bone density around fully hydroxyapatite coated femoral stem. *Clinical Orthopaedics and Related Research*, **340**, pp. 109–117, 1997.

[12] Fernandes, P.R., Folgado, J., Jacobs, C. & Pellegrini, V., A contact model for bone remodelling on total hip arthroplasty. *Computer Methods in Biomechanics and Biomedical Engineering-3*, eds. J. Middleton, M.L. Jones & N.G. Shrive, Gordon and Breach, London, pp. 123–128, 2001.

[13] Fernandes, P.R., Folgado, J., Jacobs, C. & Pellegrini, V., A contact model with ingrowth control for bone remodelling around cementless stems. *Journal of Biomechanics*, **35**, pp. 167–176, 2002.

[14] Wolff, J., *The Law of Bone Remodelling*, Maquet P. & Furlong R. (trads.), Springer-Verlag, 1986 (*Das Gesetz der Transformation der Knochen*, Verlag von August Hirschwald, Berlin 1892).

[15] Treharne, R.W., Review of Wolff's law and its proposed means of operation. *Orthopaedic Review*, **10**, pp. 35–47, 1981.

[16] Cowin, S.C. & Hegedus, D.H., Bone Remodeling I: Theory of adaptive elasticity. *Journal of Elasticity*, **6(3)**, pp. 313–326, 1976.

[17] Weinans, H., Huiskes, R. & Grootenboer, H.J., The behavior of adaptive bone-remodeling simulation models. *Journal of Biomechanics*, **25**, pp. 1425–1441, 1992.

[18] Beaupré, G.S., Orr, T.E. & Carter, D.R., An approach for time-dependent bone modeling and remodeling – application: A preliminary remodeling simulation. *Journal of Orthopaedic Research*, **8(5)**, pp. 662–670, 1990.

[19] Mullender, M.G., Huiskes, R. & Weinans, H., A physiological approach to the simulation of bone remodeling as a self-organisational control process. *Journal of Biomechanics*, **27**, pp. 1389–1394, 1994.

[20] Jacobs, C., Simo, C., Beaupré, G. & Carter, D., Adaptive bone remodelling incorporating simultaneous density and anisotropy considerations. *Journal of Biomechanics*, **30(6)**, pp. 603–613, 1997.

[21] Garcia, J.M., Martinez, M.A. & Doblaré, M., An anisotropic internal-external bone adaptation model based on a combination of CAOS and continuum damage mechanics. *Computer Methods in Biomechanics and Biomedical Eng.*, **4(4)**, pp. 355–378, 2001.

[22] Doblaré, M. & Garcia, J.M., Application of a bone remodelling model based on a damage-repair theory to the analysis of the proximal femur before and after total hip replacement. *Journal of Biomechanics*, **34(9)**, pp. 1157–1170, 2001.

[23] Fyhrie, D. & Carter, D., Femoral head apparent density distribution predicted from bone stresses. *Journal of Biomechanics*, **23(1)**, pp. 1–10, 1990.

[24] Pedersen, P., On optimal orientation of orthotropic material. *Structural Optimization*, **1**, pp. 101–106, 1989.

[25] E. Sanchez-Palencia. *Non-Homogeneous Media and Vibration Theory*, Lecture Notes in Physics, **127**, Springer, 1980.

[26] Guedes, J.M. & Kikuchi, N., Preprocessing and postprocessing for materials based on the homogenisation method with adaptive finite elements methods.

Computer Methods in Applied Mechanics and Engineering, **83**, pp. 143–198, 1990.

[27] Cowin, S.C., *Bone Mechanics*, CRC Press, Boca Raton, Fl., 1989.

[28] Luenberger, D.G., *Linear and Nonlinear Programming*, Addison-Wesley, 2nd edn., 1989.

[29] Rodrigues, H. & Fernandes, P.R., Optimization models in the simulation of bone adaptation process. *Computational Bioengineering – Current Trends and Applications*, eds. M. Cerrolaza, M. Doblaré, G. Martínez & B. Calvo, pp. 135–161, ICP, London, 2004.

[30] Viceconti, M., Casali, M., Massari, B., Cristofolini, L., Bassini, S. & Toni, A., The 'standardized femur program' proposal for a reference geometry to be used for the creation of finite element models of the femur. *Journal of Biomechanics*, **29(9)**, p. 1241, 1996.

[31] Kuiper, J.H., *Numerical Optimization of Artificial Joint Designs*, Ph.D. Thesis, Katholieke Univ. Nijmegen, 1993.

[32] Currey, J., *The Mechanical Adaptation of Bones*, Princeton University Press, 1984.

[33] Fernandes, P., Rodrigues, H., Jacobs, C. & Pellegrini, V., A material optimization model for bone remodeling around cementless hip stems. *Proceedings of the European Conference on Computational Mechanics – ECCM-99*, Munich, Germany, 1999.

[34] Rodrigues, H., A mixed variational formulation for shape optimization of solids with contact conditions. *Structural Optimization*, **6**, pp. 19–28, 1993.

[35] Engh, C., Bobyn, J. & Glassman, A., Porous-coated hip replacement – the factors governing bone ingrowth, stress shielding, and clinical results. *Journal of Bone and Joint Surgery*, **69-B(1)**, pp. 45–55, 1987.

[36] Kuiper, J. & Huiskes, R., Friction and stem stiffness affect dynamic interface motion in total hip replacement. *Journal of Orthopaedic Research*, **14(1)**, pp.36–43, 1996.

[37] Engh, C.A., O'Connor, D., Jasty, M., McGovern, T.F., Bobyn, J.D. & Harris, W.H., Quantification of implant micromotion, strain shielding, and bone resorption with porous-coated anatomic medullary locking femoral prostheses. *Clin. Orthop.*, **285**, pp. 13–29, 1992.

[38] Jasty, M., Bragdon, C., Burke, D., O'Connor, D., Lowenstein, J. & Harris, W.H., In vivo skeleton responses to porous-surfaced implants subjected to small induced motions. *Journal of Bone and Joint Surgery*, **79-A**, pp. 707–714, 1997.

[39] ABAQUS, Version 6.3, Hibbit, Karlsson & Sorensen, Inc., RI, USA, 2002.

[40] Dammak, M., Shirazi-Adl, A., Schwartz, M. & Gustavson, L., Friction properties at the bone-metal interface: comparison of four different porous metal surfaces. *Journal of Biomedical Materials Research*, **35**, pp. 329–336, 1997.

[41] Rietbergen, B., Huiskes, R., Weinans, H., Sumner, D. R., Turner, T.M. & Galante, J.O., The mechanism of bone remodeling and resorption around press-fitted THA stems. *Journal of Biomechanics*, **26(4/5)**, pp. 369–382, 1993.

CHAPTER 6

Numerical simulations can influence and undermine the reliability of results in THR

J.A. Simões and A. Ramos
Departmento de Engenharia Mecânica,
Universidade de Aveiro, Portugal.

Abstract

Finite element analysis (FEA) is an important design tool for the analysis of engineering problems. It has been extensively applied in the assessment of prostheses performance in total hip replacements (THR). Due to the nature of this numerical tool, simulation parameters can influence and undermine the reliability of results. This chapter discusses several aspects related to the simulation of biomechanics of the intact and implanted femur. Finite element type (hexahedral versus tetrahedral), mesh refinement (number of degrees of freedom), relevance of muscle forces (bending versus compression), constrained versus unconstrained femoral head and the determination of physiological loading in THR are analyzed and discussed.

1 Introduction

Numerical pre-clinical testing is becoming more important as alternatives to animal testing become an ethical requirement and as patients become more informed about involvement in clinical trials [1]. In this sense, computational modeling will be one of the most important forms to ensure that an implant is safe. Even though finite element simulation has been criticized because of the lack of validation, it is the only way forward to explore 'possible' solutions, even if quantitative results cannot be obtained due to the missing of biological information [2, 3]. Besides other merits, finite element models can be applied to distinguish and predict the performance of implants. However, numerical or experimental simulation can influence and undermine the results of biomechanical analyses because it depends on many factors.

There are many issues in finite element analysis (FEA) of which one must be aware and numbers resulting from commercial FEA applications must be faced with criticism, since they depend on simulation parameters like tissue geometry replication, material properties, boundary conditions (loading and fixation) and finite element selection. Musculoskeletal tissues have irregular geometry and so finite element modeling is increasingly carried out using digitized images generated from computer tomography scanning [2]. Bone materials are normally assumed to be isotropic and homogeneous medias, whereas it is known that they are highly anisotropic and inhomogeneous, in particular cancellous bone [see e.g. 4]. Time-dependent mechanical properties of tissues are also seen as critical to the improvement of biomechanical models [2, 5]. Loading and fixation conditions are relevant input data that can strongly change and undermine the reliability of results [6, 7]. Loads applied to finite element models have been strongly simplified and many published papers have analyzed all sorts of loading configurations, namely in total hip and knee replacements [see e.g. 8, 9] and seem to be a strong limitation on the quantitative accuracy of finite element results. Some researchers have focused on the development of improved geometric precision, whereas others have focused on improved representations of material behavior [2].

Besides the problems previously focused, there are others intrinsically related to the FEA itself. The finite element mesh is a key factor for an efficient analysis and much research has been done on meshing and element performance [see e.g. 10–52]. Finite element models must be sufficiently refined to accurately represent the geometry and mechanical behavior of the bone structure [18, 19, 21]. The results of these models are mesh sensitive and ideally a convergence test should be performed to test the model accuracy [17]. Convergence tests can be done comparing nodal displacements and/or total strain energy [20, 21], or stresses and strains [21]. Following Stolk et al. [17], a completely converged stress-strain distribution can almost never be obtained, since stress singularities locally cause stresses and strains to diverge with increasing mesh refinement. Literature show identical numerical studies using either coarse or very refined finite element models.

Other simulation difficulty is related to the biomechanical forces applied to the hip and how important they are to replicate physiological loading. The biomechanics of the hip is an extremely complex problem and the correct knowledge of the functioning of muscles, ligaments and the hip force contact (HCF) is unknown. Many authors have studied this problem using numerical and experimental models [9, 53–56]. Simulation of physiological loading of the hip is of considerable importance to improve prostheses design, bone remodeling simulations and mechanical testing of implants [56]. There has been considerable debate relatively to the loading of the intact femur. The majority of experimental and analytical studies assume the femur to be simplistically loaded, with the application of just a HCF or the HCF plus the abductors (ABD), which generates a characteristic bending stress/strain pattern at the diaphyseal femur. There is growing evidence to suggest that mechanisms exist which act to minimize bending and produce a predominately compressive stress/strain distribution. The various mechanisms have been comprehensively reviewed by several authors [9, 57–59]. Combinations of muscle forces have been modeled in vitro in an attempt to simulate femoral loading [54]. Telemetry studies of the implanted hip have given reliable data concerning the magnitude and direction of the HCF. Although the direction of the muscle forces can be estimated, their true magnitude during gait or any other activity has yet to be properly defined. The best estimates of the muscle forces have been supplied from muscle optimization studies, such as those of Crowninshield *et al.* [60]. Seireg *et al.* [61], Röhrle *et al.* [62] and Bergmann *et al.* [63]. All of the optimization studies predict some abductor activity. Röhrle *et al.* [62] predicted significant abductor muscle activity, of approximately two times body weight. Apart from the abductors, there is little consensus on the other major muscles that are active during gait. Prediction of muscle forces should be treated with caution since numerous assumptions are made in their calculation. Other sources of error include the location of the centre of mass of skeletal segments, the use of skin markers to track the motion of underlying bone during kinematics studies and the assumption of no antagonistic or synergistic muscle activity. Thus, there is a degree of uncertainty in the selection of which muscles are important, and their relevance to mechanical testing.

Other debatable aspect has to do with the way the femoral head is loaded. How relevant is it to consider a free horizontally constrained femoral head on the strain distribution within the intact femur? Simões *et al.* [56] and Américo *et al.* [64] showed that a horizontally constrained femoral head produces smaller variation in the strain levels when muscle forces are applied. *In vivo* data, demonstrating negligible movement of the femoral head in one-legged stance, support the results of the study and suggest that in the absence of comprehensive muscle force data, a constrained femoral head may provide a more physiologically loading situation [56].

Another aspect on the loading of the implanted femur is related to the change of the biomechanical forces (magnitude and direction) of the hip when a replacement is performed. The HCF and muscle forces are modified due to geometric alterations, as for example changes of the position of the head or that of the great trochanter, provoked by surgery. The prosthesis does not exactly restore the original head centre and the lever arms are different. Although the effect of a femoral head displacement is important from a surgical point of view [6], this variable must be controlled when numerical or experimental studies are performed and since the head location cannot be restored exactly, it is necessary to analyze how it can be misleading in assessing the performance of different designs [6, 65, 66].

This chapter describes different aspects of numerical simulations and how they can change and undermine the output results in total hip replacements (THR). The following issues were assessed:

- Influence of finite element and mesh density;
- Physiological loading and relevance of muscle forces;
- Constrained versus unconstrained femoral head;
- Physiological loading of the implanted femur.

2 Influence of finite element and mesh density

Finite element analyses have been made within a diversity of biomechanical investigations and very complex three-dimensional model (3D) structures have been studied. Prendergast [2] gives an excellent overview on finite element modeling for the analysis of the skeleton, for the analysis and design of orthopaedic devices and for the analysis of tissue growth, remodeling and degeneration, and the contribution of finite element modeling to the scientific understanding of joint replacement is reviewed. In Mackerle [67], one can find a detailed bibliography between 1985 and 1999 on finite element analyses and simulations in biomedicine. From the same author, ref. [68] contains 2188 citations on finite element bibliography for biomechanics from 1987 to 1997.

The biomechanics of the hip is a complex system resulting partly from the geometry of the femur and muscle forces. It is therefore difficult to obtain theoretical expressions of the stress-strain or displacement distributions of the femur and results of numerical models are normally compared with experimental ones, most of the times using strain gauges. The influence of parameters like element type, degree of refinement of the mesh, boundary conditions and hip contact force and muscle forces can be assessed using simplified models, since these allow the determination of theoretical values. Simplified models have been used in very different types of biomechanical studies.

2.1 Materials and methods

2.1.1 Simplified femur model

To assess the influence of finite element and degree of refinement of the mesh, stress and displacement fields of a simplified geometric model as described in Viceconti *et al.* [11] was used [7, 69]. This simplified proximal femur model is an approximation, in shape and dimensions of a femur and was loaded with forces comparable to those found *in vivo* to create a similar stress field [11]. For the loading configuration, $|HCF| = 1976\,N$ ($HCF_x = -1745\,N$ and $HCF_y = -928\,N$) and $|ABD| = 1240\,N$ ($ABD_x = 797\,N$ and $ABD_y = 950\,N$) were considered, being HCF the hip contact force and ABD the abductor force. A Young's modulus of 14,200 MPa and a Poisson's ratio of 0.3 were the assigned material properties. The nodes at the distal end of the model were constrained in all directions and the von Mises equivalent stress and displacement distributions were determined at the inner radius of the curved beam (fig. 1) and compared with theoretical ones.

2.1.1.1 Von Mises equivalent stress Considering the equilibrium forces of a curved beam as illustrated in fig. 2, and for $\theta \le 60°$, the bending moment (M_θ), shear force (F_s) and normal force (F_n) can be obtained respectively by:

$$M_\theta = -HCF_y\, r \sin\theta + HCF_x(r_e - r\cos\theta), \qquad (1)$$

$$F_s = HCF_y \cos\theta - HCF_x \sin\theta, \qquad (2)$$

$$F_n = -HCF_y \sin\theta - HCF_x \cos\theta. \qquad (3)$$

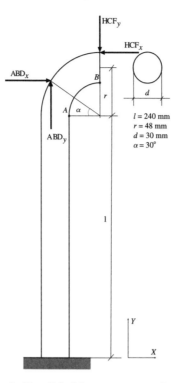

Figure 1: Simplified femur construction [11].

The equivalent von Mises stress (σ_{eq}) can therefore be obtained using the following equation:

$$\sigma_{eq} = \sqrt{\left(\frac{F_n}{A} + \frac{M_\theta \, (r_i - r_n)}{A \, e \, r_i}\right)^2 + \left(\frac{F_s}{A}\right)^2},$$
(4)

where r_i and r_n are the inner and neutral radius (fig. 2), e is the difference between the neutral and middle radius and A is the area of the section at position θ. Replacing eqns (1), (2) and (3) in (4), the equivalent von Mises stress for $\theta \leq 60°$ is:

$$\sigma_{eq} = \sqrt{\begin{array}{l} \left(\dfrac{-HCF_y \, \sin\theta - HCF_x \, \cos\theta}{A}\right. \\ \left. + \dfrac{(-HCF_y \, r\sin\theta + HCF_x \, (r_e - r\cos\theta)) \, (r_i - r_n)}{A \, e \, r_i}\right)^2 \\ + \left(\dfrac{HCF_y \, \cos\theta - HCF_x \, \sin\theta}{A}\right)^2. \end{array}}$$
(5)

For $\theta > 60°$, the bending moment, shear force and normal force are:

$$M_\theta = - HCF_y \, r\sin\theta + HCF_x \, (r_e - r\cos\theta)$$
$$- ABD_y \left(r_e \sin\frac{\pi}{3} - r\sin\theta\right) - ABD_x \left(r_e \cos\frac{\pi}{3} - r\cos\theta\right),$$
(6)

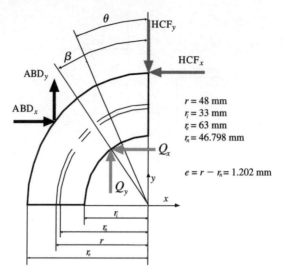

Figure 2: Schematic drawing of a curved beam with relevant dimensions.

$$F_s = \text{HCF}_y \cos \theta - \text{HCF}_x \sin \theta - \text{ABD}_y \cos \theta + \text{ABD}_x \sin \theta, \qquad (7)$$

$$F_n = -\text{HCF}_y \sin \theta - \text{HCF}_x \cos \theta + \text{ABD}_y \sin \theta + \text{ABD}_x \cos \theta. \qquad (8)$$

The von Mises stress distribution can be obtained using:

$$\sigma_{eq} = \sqrt{\begin{pmatrix} \dfrac{-\text{HCF}_y \sin\theta - \text{HCF}_x \cos\theta + \text{ABD}_y \sin\theta + \text{ABD}_x \cos\theta}{A} \\ + \dfrac{(-\text{HCF}_y \, r\sin\theta + \text{HCF}_x (r_e - r\cos\theta))(r_i - r_n)}{A e r_i} \\ + \dfrac{(-\text{ABD}_x (r_e \cos\frac{\pi}{3} - r\cos\theta))(r_i - r_n)}{A e r_i} \\ + \dfrac{(-\text{ABD}_y (r_e \sin\frac{\pi}{3} - r\sin\theta))(r_i - r_n)}{A e r_i} \end{pmatrix}^2 + \left(\dfrac{-\text{HCF}_y \cos\theta - \text{HCF}_x \sin\theta + \text{ABD}_y \cos\theta - \text{ABD}_y \sin\theta}{A} \right)^2}. \qquad (9)$$

To obtain the von Mises stress distribution at the outer surface of the beam, r_i must be replaced by r_e. The equivalent strain distribution can be obtained applying Hooke's Law.

2.1.1.2 Equivalent displacement distribution   To determine the equivalent displacement distribution, a fictitious force $Q(Q_x, Q_y)$ at a point localized by β angle (fig. 2) was considered and the moment provoked by this force is:

$$M_\beta = -\text{HCF}_y \, r\sin\theta + \text{HCF}_x(r_e - r\cos\theta) - \text{ABD}_y \left(r_e \sin\frac{\pi}{3} - r\sin\theta \right)$$

$$- \text{ABD}_x \left(r_e \cos\frac{\pi}{3} - r\cos\theta \right) + Q_{x\beta}(r_i \cos\beta - r\cos\theta)$$

$$+ Q_{y\beta}(r\sin\theta - r_i \sin\beta). \qquad (10)$$

Applying the Castigliano theorem, the x displacement for each θ can be obtained using the following equation (for $\theta > \beta$ and $\theta > 60°$):

$$x\beta = \frac{1}{EI} \int\limits_0^\theta \left[\begin{pmatrix} -\,\text{HCF}_y\, r \sin\theta \\ +\,\text{HCF}_x\, (r_e - r\cos\theta) \\ -\,\text{ABD}_y\, \left(r_e \sin\frac{\pi}{3} - r\sin\theta\right) \\ -\,\text{ABD}_x\, \left(r_e \cos\frac{\pi}{3} - r\cos\theta\right) \\ +\,Q_{x\beta}\, (r_i \cos\beta - r\cos\theta) \\ +\,Q_{y\beta}\, (r\sin\theta - r_i \sin\beta) \end{pmatrix} (r_i \cos\beta - r\cos\theta) \right] r d\theta. \quad (11)$$

For the inner radius, the x displacement of any point can be determined using the following equation:

$$x\beta = \frac{1}{EI} \left[\begin{array}{l} -\,\text{HCF}_y\, r^2 \left(r_i \cos\beta - \tfrac{1}{2}r\right) \\[4pt] +\,\text{HCF}_x\, \left(\tfrac{\pi}{2} r_e\, r_i \cos\beta - r_e r - r r_i \cos\beta + r^2 \tfrac{\pi}{4}\right) \\[4pt] -\,\text{ABD}_y r \left[\begin{array}{l} \tfrac{\pi}{6} r_e r_i \sin\tfrac{\pi}{3} \cos\beta - r_e r \sin\tfrac{\pi}{3}\left(1 - \sin\tfrac{\pi}{3}\right) \\ -\,r r_i \cos\beta \cos\beta\, \tfrac{\pi}{3} \\ +\,\tfrac{1}{2}r^2 \left[1 - \left(\sin\tfrac{\pi}{3}\right)^2\right] \end{array} \right] \\[14pt] -\,\text{ABD}_x r \left[\begin{array}{l} \tfrac{\pi}{6} r_e r_i \cos\tfrac{\pi}{3} \cos\beta \\ -\,(r_e r \cos\tfrac{\pi}{3} + r r_i \cos\beta)\left(1 - \sin\tfrac{\pi}{3}\right) \\ +\,r^2 \left(\tfrac{\pi}{12} - \tfrac{1}{2}\sin\tfrac{\pi}{3}\cos\tfrac{\pi}{3}\right) \end{array} \right] \end{array} \right] + K_x, \quad (12)$$

being K_x an integration constant, E the Young's modulus and I the second moment of area.

Following the same procedure for the displacement in the y-direction, the following equation can be derived:

$$y\beta = \frac{1}{EI} \int\limits_0^\theta \left[\begin{pmatrix} -\,\text{HCF}_y\, r \sin\theta \\ +\,\text{HCF}_x\, (r_e - r\cos\theta) \\ -\,\text{ABD}_y\, \left(r_e \sin\frac{\pi}{3} - r\sin\theta\right) \\ -\,\text{ABD}_x\, \left(r_e \cos\frac{\pi}{3} - r\cos\theta\right) \\ +\,Q_{x\beta}\, (r_i \cos\beta - r\cos\theta) \\ +\,Q_{y\beta}\, (r\sin\theta - r_i \sin\beta) \end{pmatrix} (r\sin\theta - r_i \sin\beta) \right] r d\theta \quad (13)$$

and therefore:

$$y\beta = \frac{1}{EI} \left[\begin{array}{l} -\,\text{HCF}_y\, r^2 \left(\tfrac{\pi}{2}r - r_i \sin\beta\right) \\[4pt] +\,\text{HCF}_x\, \left(r_e r - \tfrac{\pi}{2} r_e r_i \sin\beta - \tfrac{1}{2}r^2 - r r_i \sin\beta\right) \\[4pt] -\,\text{ABD}_y r \left[\begin{array}{l} r_e r \sin\tfrac{\pi}{3} \cos\tfrac{\pi}{3} - \tfrac{\pi}{6} r_e r_i \sin\tfrac{\pi}{3} \sin\beta \\ -\,r r_i \sin\tfrac{\pi}{3} \sin\beta \sin\beta\, \tfrac{\pi}{3} \\ -\,r^2 \left(\tfrac{\pi}{12} + \tfrac{1}{2}\sin\tfrac{\pi}{3}\cos\tfrac{\pi}{3}\right) \end{array} \right] \\[14pt] -\,\text{ABD}_x r \left[\begin{array}{l} r_e r \left(\cos\tfrac{\pi}{3}\right)^2 - \tfrac{\pi}{6} r_e r_i \cos\tfrac{\pi}{3} \sin\beta \\ -\,\tfrac{1}{2}r^2 \left[1 - \left(\sin\tfrac{\pi}{3}\right)^2\right] \\ +\,r r_i \sin\beta \left(1 - \sin\tfrac{\pi}{3}\right) \end{array} \right] \end{array} \right] + K_y, \quad (14)$$

being K_y an integration constant.

The integration constants, K_x and K_y, are obtained for $\beta = 90°$ and the displacement using the following equations (resulting from the equilibrium forces of the linear part of the beam):

$$x_l = \frac{M_{90°}\, l^2}{2EI} - \frac{F_c l^3}{3EI},\qquad(15)$$

$$y_l = \frac{Pl}{AE},\qquad(16)$$

where P is the resultant force in the y direction and l is the length of the linear part of the beam (fig. 1). These displacements must be added to the ones obtained for the curved part of the beam. Again, to obtain the displacements at the outer surface of the beam, r_i must be replaced by r_e.

If the displacement in the z-direction is not considered, the equivalent displacement (δ) can be obtained using:

$$\delta = \sqrt{\left(x_\beta^2 + y_\beta^2\right)}.\qquad(17)$$

The numerical stresses and displacements obtained using the finite element method were compared with identical theoretical ones, these obtained using the above-derived equations. For the finite element analysis, four different element types were tested: 4-node linear tetrahedral elements; 10-node quadratic tetrahedral elements; 8-node linear hexahedral elements; and 20-node quadratic hexahedral elements. These finite elements are frequently used in typical biomechanical analysis. The influence of the number of degrees of freedom (NDOF) and CPU time (computational weight) were also assessed.

The simulations were preformed with Hyperworks® 5.1 (Altair Engineering, Inc.), using pre and post processor Hypermesh® 5.1 and solver Hyperstruct® 5.1 and were performed on a PC Pentium IV @ 2.53 MHz with 2 GByte of RAM memory. The maximum NDOF possible to be solve was of the order of 600,000. Meshes higher than these were impossible to run with the available hardware resources.

2.1.2 Femur model

A proximal geometry of a femur was used in the simulations to assess the influence of mesh density and element type. The "Standardized Femur" model (3rd generation, model number 3103) was used as reference geometry. It is a 3D solid model made available in public domain derived from CT-scan dataset of a composite human femur replica [70]. This new design has a cortical bone analogue consisting of short-glass-fibre-reinforced epoxy, rather than the fibre glass-fabric-reinforced epoxy of the 2nd generation femur. The new cortical analogue offered the possibility of improving the uniformity of mechanical properties within a composite replicate bone, allowed for greater anatomic detail to be added to the bones, and simplified the fabrication process [71].

The material properties were assigned with reference to those indicated by the manufacturer and assumed to be isotropic and linearly elastic. The Young's modulus of the cortical (fibre glass reinforced epoxy cortex) and cancellous (polyurethane

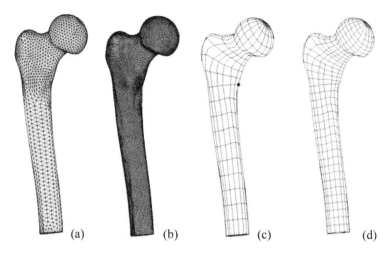

Figure 3: Tetrahedral ((a) model Tetra_A and (b) model Tetra_C) and hexahedral ((c) model Hexa_A and (d) model Hexa_G) meshes of the proximal femur. Results were picked at the dot shown in Hexa_A model.

core) analogues was 19 GPa and 0.26 GPa, respectively. A Poisson's ratio of 0.3 was assigned for both materials. The boundary conditions were set-up to accurately reproduce those used in the experimental set-up described in Heiner and Brown [71].

Figure 3 shows model Tetra_A (coarse mesh), model Tetra_C (strongly refined mesh), model Hexa_A (coarse mesh) and model Hexa_G (refined mesh). The von Mises stresses and principal strains were assessed at a node localized at the proximal-medial periosteal surface of the femur (dot in fig. 3). Except for model Hexa_A, all others presented more than NDOF = 20,000, which accordingly to Stolk *et al.* [22] can be sufficient to obtain convergent results.

Two tetra models (Tetra_A and Tetra_B) were generated to obtain similar results to the ones obtained with hexahedral models. A third model (Tetra_C) was greatly refined (until the maximum capacity of the hardware). The Hexa_B model is a duplication of elements of model Hexa_A; model Hexa_C is a model obtained from the refinement of the cancellous bone structure of model Hexa_A; Model Hexa_D is a duplication of the cortical bone elements of model Hexa_A; meshes of models Hexa_E, Hexa_F and Hexa_G are mesh refinements of the cancellous bone structure of the Hexa_D model.

2.2 Results and discussion

2.2.1 Simplified femur model

Table 1 contains the theoretical and numerical results (equivalent von Mises, strains and displacements) obtained at nodes at the inner radius of the beam. Since different NDOF were simulated, the results presented in this table are for the ones whose differences to the theoretical values were minimum. Figure 4 illustrates the von

Table 1: Results of the simplified femur (curved beam).

Point		Theoretical	Finite element analysis			
			Tetra_4	Tetra_10	Hexa_8	Hexa_20
A	von Mises (MPa)	29.0	24.8	24.3	24.8	23.9
	Strain (με)	2042	1510	1482	1513	1456
	Displacement (mm)	1.832	1.816	1.832	1.861	1.370
	NDOF	–	591543	562845	565580	595200
B	von Mises (MPa)	6.0	2.1	2.7	2.7	2.8
	Strain (με)	423	125	105	162	143
	Displacement (mm)	2.065	2.441	2.637	2.723	2.633
	NDOF	–	5874	4944	5475	5570

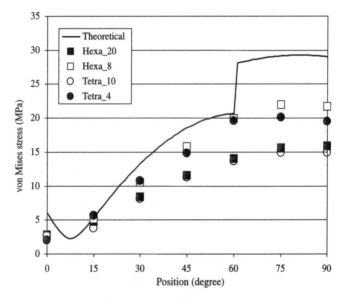

Figure 4: Equivalent von Mises stress distribution for coarse meshes (Tetra_4:
NDOF = 5874; Tetra_10: NDOF = 4944; Hexa_8: NDOF = 5475;
Hexa_20: NDOF = 5570).

Mises stress distribution along the inside radius of the beam for the coarsest meshes.
Figure 5 shows identical results for meshes very highly refined.

The von Mises stress distributions evidence, for the problem simulated, different tendencies, and results must be analyzed at points A and B of the beam and
in between them. At points A and B (15° and 75°), high-refined meshes, independently of the element type, provoked stress values of the same order of theoretical

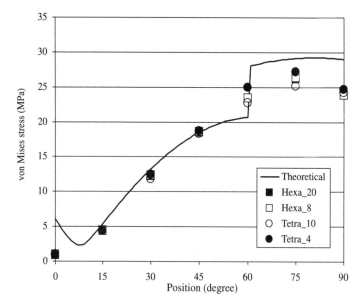

Figure 5: Equivalent von Mises stress distribution for refined meshes (Tetra_4: NDOF = 591543; Tetra_10: NDOF = 562845; Hexa_8: NDOF = 565580; Hexa_20: NDOF = 595200).

ones. For coarser meshes, the differences were significant (fig. 4), and for this case, quadratic elements (Hexa_20 and Tetra_10) provoked, relatively to the other elements (Hexa_8 and Tetra_4), higher differences. From the point of the abductor force (60°) to point A, the differences in stresses are higher than those obtained for the rest of the beam.

The stress values at point A for all elements were similar, ranging from 24.3 MPa (Tetra_10) to 23.9 (Hexa_20). Tetra_4 and Hexa_8 allowed same stress values. The relative strain difference was of the order of 26%. Except for the Hexa_20 element, the equivalent displacements were identical to the theoretical ones. The relative difference for the Hexa_20 was of the order of 25%. However, simulating the same model with 551400 NDOF (less 43800 NDOF), a relative difference of 2% was observed, which shows that results are very dependent on mesh density and a small variation on the number of nodes and elements can give better results. For higher refined meshes, stresses, strains and displacements at point A were identical to theoretical ones.

At point B, due to its singular characteristic, the relative stress differences were significantly higher, 65% for Tetra_4, 55% for Tetra_10 and Hexa_8 and 53% for Hexa_20. Differences in strain were significant, ranging from 62% (Hexa_8) to 75% (Tetra_10). For the equivalent displacement, differences were smaller, but still significant, ranging from 18% (Tetra_4) to 32% (Hexa_8). These results were considered for coarse meshes (NDOF from 4944 to 5874), which provoked lower relative differences. It was also observed that results at this point were very sensible

Table 2: Numerical results of the proximal composite femur bone.

Model	N_elements	N_nodes	NDOF	CPU (s)	Strain (μɛ)	Stress (MPa)	Displacement (mm)
Tetra_A	23197	35433	99763	236	−740.1	15.20	0.3327
Tetra_B	34733	53200	158496	360	−759.0	14.39	0.3874
Tetra_C	143904	212737	635724	5117	−945.0	17.99	0.4857
Hexa_A	1158	5379	15570	11	−780.4	15.22	0.3966
Hexa_B	2222	10185	29988	29	−691.7	13.95	0.3825
Hexa_C	4562	20966	61332	244	−730.9	13.98	0.3793
Hexa_D	2962	13180	38811	105	−749.1	14.20	0.3938
Hexa_E	3664	16800	49479	180	−749.8	14.21	0.3936
Hexa_F	4522	20945	61674	290	−751.2	14.23	0.3936
Hexa_G	5224	23825	70152	409	−751.5	14.24	0.3936

to mesh density. In fact, using a Tetra_4 mesh with only 476 NDOF, the von Mises stress obtained was 5.4 MPa, a relative difference of 10%.

Results strongly depend on mesh density and element type. It was observed that less refined meshes provoked stresses and displacements more closely to the theoretical ones at point B; on the other way round, very high density meshes provoked better results at point A. Overall, the results of the simplified model showed that none of the elements used in the simulations evidenced to be best, or the most suitable for the problem studied. However, linear element type and coarse meshes seem to be more effective to generate reliable results at characteristic and singular points of the structure. Refined meshes can give adequate results, however there seems to be an optimum value for the NDOF for which results do not change significantly, increasing unnecessarily the computational effort. Analyzing the problem as a whole, it seems that tetrahedral and hexahedral linear elements generated results more closely to theoretical ones.

2.2.2 Femur model

Table 2 shows the von Mises stresses, equivalent strains and equivalent displacements (picked at a node localized at dot of fig. 3) on the medial aspect of the femur. The hexahedral meshes of models D to G allowed very similar results. Contrarily, the tetrahedral Tetra_C mesh provoked significantly different results. It can be seen that relative to the Tetra_A mesh, the increase of NDOF was 537% and the relative differences were respectively 28%, 18% and 46% for the principal strain, von Mises stress and equivalent displacements. When comparing the results obtained with tetrahedral and hexahedral elements, higher density meshes with tetrahedral elements are necessary to obtain results identical to the ones obtained with hexahedral element meshes.

The Hexa_A, the coarsest mesh of all hexahedral meshes, produced results which are comparatively different from those obtained with higher NDOF meshes. This can partly be explained by the low NDOF = 15570 used, less than 20000, which,

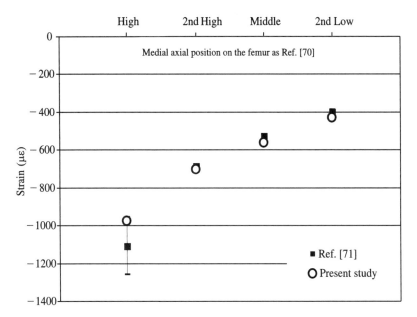

Figure 6: Comparison between numerical and experimental [70] femoral strains.

following Stolk *et al.* [22] is the minimum necessary to obtain the convergence of a mesh of the proximal femur.

No theoretical values of stress, strain and displacement are known at the point on the femur were results were picked, and therefore it is impossible to determine their deviations relatively to the finite element ones. Heiner and Brown [70] have published an experimental study concerning the axial strain distribution of a 3rd generation composite femur, similar to the numerical model used. Based on their results, fig. 6 shows the comparison of strains obtained with model Hexa_A (the coarsest mesh) and experimental strains obtained by Heiner and Brown [70]. As one can see, the numerical strains do not differ much from experimental strains, the highest difference being at the level of the lesser trochanter, which is a region of irregularity in strain distribution.

3 Physiological loading and relevance of muscle simulation

3.1 Materials and methods

According to several published studies, stress and strain distributions within the intact femur seem to be a controversial subject. In fact, the choice of muscle forces, as well as the HCF, in both experimental and finite element studies, has been somewhat arbitrary, with large variations between authors. The characterization of loading regimes that produce physiological strain distribution is yet to be assessed. The principal question is to know if the intact femur is predominately loaded in

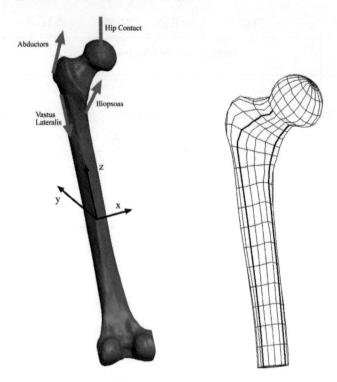

Figure 7: Applied HCF and muscle forces; curve of nodes where results were obtained.

bending or in compression? Within the present study, accordingly to Taylor *et al.* [9], two typical pseudo bending and compression load cases were simulated using finite element analysis.

The strain distribution at the diaphyseal region of the femur was assessed simulating two loading configurations: HCF plus abductors (load case 1) and HCF plus the abductors, vastus lateralis and iliopsoas (load case 2) [9]. A numerical model of a commercial composite femur (2nd generation, Pacific Research Labs) was used. The material properties were assumed to be isotropic and linearly elastic. The Young's modulus of the cortical (fibre glass reinforced epoxy cortex) and cancellous (polyurethane core) analogues was 19 GPa and 0.26 GPa, respectively. A Poisson's ratio of 0.3 was assigned for both materials. The femur was rigidly constrained at a distance of 200 mm from the condyles. Preliminary analysis was performed to evaluate the influence of the femur constraining distance and it was observed that results did not change for lower distances (nearer to the condyles). The 3-D finite element mesh consisted of 13184 nodes and 2962 hexahedral elements (quadratic 20-node), which corresponded to 38559 DOF.

Figure 7 shows the vector forces applied to the femur and the nodes (figure shows only the medial and posterior aspects) where the results were assessed. The direction and magnitude of the hip force contact and muscle forces are given in table 3.

Table 3: Muscle and HCF of the two load cases simulated [9].

Vector forces (N)		x	y	z
LOAD CASE 1	HCF	−616	−171	−2800
	Abductors	430	0	1160
LOAD CASE 2	HCF	−1062	−0.130	−2800
	Abductors	430	0	1160
	Vastus Lateralis	0	0	−1200
	Iliopsoas	78	525	525

3.2 Results and discussion

For both load cases, the displacement, axial strain and equivalent von Mises stress distributions were determined at the anterior, posterior, lateral and medial aspects of the femur. Figure 8 illustrates the axial strain distributions. The deformed geometries of the femur for the load cases simulated were not significantly different. The equivalent maximum displacements was 6.9 mm (5.8 mm laterally and 3.2 mm distally) for load case 1 and 5.6 mm (4.9 mm laterally and 2.6 mm distally) for load case 2. Interesting to note that for load case 1, the femur moved 2 mm in the posterior direction while for the other load case it moved 1 mm in the anterior direction. Considering the characteristics of the direction and magnitude of the forces, the bending of the femur was mainly provoked by the HCF, which seems to be the main responsible for stress-strain distribution of the femur. The abducting muscle force increases the bending of the femur, inducing a higher displacement at the front plane.

For both load configurations analyzed, not taking into account the lateral aspect, the peak stresses were not much different and occurred proximally at the neck of the femur. Differences were observed at the lateral aspect, were the peak stress for load case 1 was 56.5 MPa and for load case 2 was 38.6 MPa, a decrease of 17.9 MPa, which corresponds, relatively to load case 1, a decrease of 32%. Considering the average of the stresses, the highest differences were at the medial aspect, around 10 MPa, with an increase of stress from load case 1 (46 MPa) to load case 2 (56 MPa), and a more compression stress distribution was observed. For all the other aspects, differences of peak stresses were very small, 4 MPa, 9 MPa and 1 MPa, respectively at the lateral, anterior and posterior aspects. A decrease of stresses from load case 1 to load case 2 was observed by introducing the vastus lateralis and iliopsoas forces.

Overall, the strains were much higher for load case 1, a predominantly bending load case. As expected, tensile and compressive strains occurred at the lateral and medial aspect respectively. At the anterior aspect, tensile strains were the most predominant, while for the posterior aspect, compressive strains occurred in about two thirds of the femur.

The average strain value for load case 1, at the medial aspect, was approximately −3200 $\mu\varepsilon$. The peak strain was −3968 $\mu\varepsilon$ for load case 1 and −3774 $\mu\varepsilon$ for load case 2 and occurred at the same region of the medial aspect of the femur. Relatively to

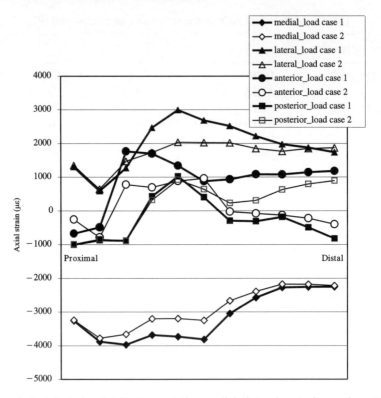

Figure 8: Axial strain distributions at the medial, lateral, anterior and posterior aspects of the femur.

the lateral aspect, the average strain value was 1960 με for load case 1 and 1700 με for load case 2, a difference of 260 με. The peak strain values were 2997 με and 2039 με, respectively.

Strains were comparatively lower at the anterior and posterior aspects. The average strain at the anterior aspect was 913 με and 206 με for load case 1 and load case 2, respectively. At the posterior aspect, a negative average value of –275 με was observed for load case 1, while and for load case 2 the value was 143 με, partially provoked by the iliopsoas force direction (towards the anterior direction).

To obtain a typical compression strain distribution at all aspects of the femur, the differences of strains should be small, which was not observed with the load configurations simulated. It is therefore questionable if load case 2 provokes a predominantly compressive stress-strain distribution at all aspects of the femur. The bending effect was still effective and visible for load case 2. These results show that muscle simulation is relevant in the characterization of stress patterns on the diaphyseal of the femur. By simulating together the HCF with the abductors, vastus lateralis and iliopsoas, a less bending effect was noted. Even though, it is questionable whether load conditions that create a predominantly bending stress distribution accurately represent the *in vivo* biomechanics of the hip. Selection of muscle forces, their magnitude and direction, as well as the HCF must be carefully done to assess their influence on the stress-strain distribution and reactions with other boundary structures.

The results of this investigation do not support the hypothesis that the femur is loaded markedly in compression, not for the loading configurations analyzed.

4 Constrained versus unconstrained femoral head

4.1 Materials and methods

The applied boundary conditions are of equal importance when modeling the femur as an isolated structure, but this has rarely been considered. The femoral head can be simulated as being either unconstrained or horizontally constrained. Most finite element analyses have simulated the femoral head to be unconstrained [9, 53, 63, 65–67, 72]. In contrast, the majority of experimental studies have assumed the femoral head to be horizontally constrained [54] except for some studies like Christofolini et al. [55] and Rohlmann et al. [72] who simulated the femoral head as unconstrained. The reason for this division between finite element studies and experimental studies, using unconstrained and horizontally constrained femoral heads, respectively, is not clear in the literature. Is the effect of constrained or unconstrained femoral head simulation on the strain distribution relevant?

An in vivo radiological study performed by Taylor et al. [9] suggested that there is minimal medial deflection of the loaded femoral head during one-legged stance (approximately 1.5 mm). Therefore, in an attempt to simplify experimental set-ups and in the absence of comprehensive muscle force data, the question arises whether it is reasonable to simulate the femoral head as horizontally constrained.

The same numerical model of the femur was used to analyze the influence of constraining, or not, the femoral head movement in the anterior-posterior direction. For both cases simulated, the HCF, the abductors, the vastus lateralis and iliopsoas were considered as the system forces.

4.2 Results and discussion

Figure 9 shows the strain distribution at the medial, lateral, anterior and posterior aspects of the femur simulating a free and horizontally constrained head. The x, y and z components of the displacement vector of the unconstrained femoral head were −4.867 mm in the x-direction, −1.007 mm in the y-direction and −2.649 mm in the z-direction. For the constrained head these were −4.823 mm in the x-direction, 0 mm in the y-direction (head movement constrained) and −2.677 mm in the z-direction. For the load case considered, differences of strain distribution and magnitude were minimal in all aspects of the femur. It was observed that for the medial aspect, the results for both cases were similar; for the lateral aspect the differences were small. Only at the posterior aspect of the femur pronounced differences were seen at the distal and proximal regions of the femur, although the magnitude of strains are also were small. Overall, it seems that either simulating the femoral

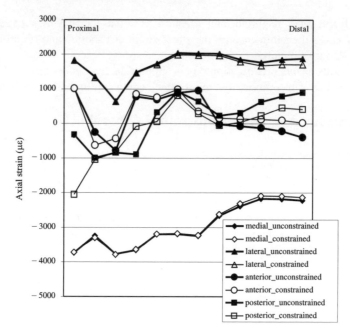

Figure 9: Constrained versus unconstrained femoral head.

head horizontally constrained or unconstrained it does not change significantly the strain patterns and magnitudes of these.

5 Physiological loading of the implanted femur

5.1 Materials and methods

The intact femur is subjected to a system of loads and moments that cannot be applied to the implanted femur. We must remember that the femur is overconstrained by the joint forces, the ligaments, and the muscle forces. There is no perfect solution when one tries to replicate the three forces and three moments as in the intact femur with identical femora implanted with different stems. Following Cristofolini and Viceconti [6] there are two main options: one that applies the same force magnitude for the hip joint and the abducting force (same forces) and a different moment will be applied due to the changed lever arms; and one that applies the same bending moment to the femur (same moment) and different force values are required. In this case, the magnitude, direction, and position of the resultant vector force must stay constant with respect to the femoral diaphysis [6].

There seems to be no agreement in the literature on the preferred solution. However, Cristofolini and Viceconti [6] refere that to compensate for the unavoidable geometry changes, the implanted femur should be loaded in such a way as to apply

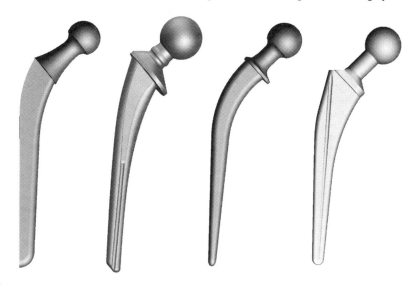

Figure 10: CAD models of the Charnely, Lubinus SPII, Stanmore and Müller
Straight cemented prostheses.

the same bending moment, rather than the same forces as in the intact femur. If
this is not done, errors can be expected in the strain measurement that possibly
overshadow existing differences between implants, or give the impression that the
difference exists when, in fact, the variations observed depend merely on the loading
setup [6].

A detailed numerical study was performed to determine how loading configurations of the implanted femur can undermine the reliability of strain measurements.
Based on the intact femur loading configurations of walking during gait, different
implanted femur loading configurations were analyzed. These were derived keeping constant some of the load components and allowing others to vary. A set of
plausible combinations of forces with bending and torsion moments in the median,
frontal and horizontal planes were considered. The difference of strain in all aspects
of the intact and the implanted femur was the parameter used to select the suitable
loading configuration for the Charnely, Lubinus SPII, Stanmore and Müller Straight
cemented prostheses (fig. 10). The strain values were picked at a distance of 20 mm
from the tip of the longest prosthesis (Lubinus SPII), which was at a distance of
20 mm from the region where the femur was constrained. The prosthesis simulated
allowed offsets ranging from 28.25 mm (Charnley) to 35.48 mm (Stanmore).

Figure 11 contains the geometric dimensions (table 4) of the implanted femur
used to derive the implanted femur force system. These dimensions were used to
derive the moments provoked either only by the HCF or together with the abductor
(glutei) force. Dimension c and d (distances from the glutei insertion point) were
kept constant in the simulations.

To apply the same system of loads to the intact and to the implanted femur
it was necessary to derive the summation of moments and forces somewhere

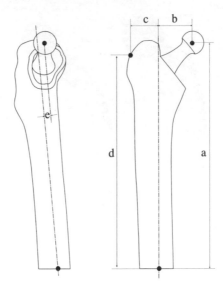

Figure 11: Geometric and dimensional variables of the implanted femur.

Table 4: Dimensions of the intact and implanted femur.

	a	b	c	d	e
Intact femur	230	44	25	205	0
Charnley	227.16	28.25	25	205	0.50
Lubinus SPII	223.55	33.37	25	205	−1.51
Stanmore	230.48	35.48	25	205	0.61
Müller Straight	221.83	32.79	25	205	−4.71

at the cortex of the intact femur, far enough from the tip of the prosthesis and from the region were the femur was constrained. Figure 12 shows schematically the loading configuration considered and forces and moments generated. These forces and moments are modified after a prosthesis implantation, and depend on the surgical procedure, geometry and dimensions of the implant itself. Do determine the new biomechanical forces of the implanted femur it is necessary to firstly determine the moments and forces transmitted through the intact femur. For the purpose of the study, the hip joint and muscle force magnitudes were taken from Stolk *et al.* [73] (table 5, fig. 12) which reference Bergmann *et al.* [63], and to generate the new HCF and abductors force, the following conditions were considered:

- Equilibrium of forces and moments considering only the HCF;
- Equilibrium of forces and moments considering the HCF and the abductors (force direction maintained unchanged).

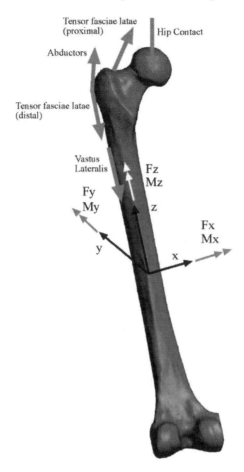

Figure 12: Moments and forces transmitted (Mz-horizontal plane; My-coronal plane and Mx-median plane); x (medially), y (anteriorly) and z (proximally).

Table 5: Moments and forces of the intact femur [73].

Vector forces (N)	xx	yy	zz
Hip force contact	−405	−246	−1719
Abductors (glutei)	435	32	649
Tensor fasciae latae (proximal part)	54	87	99
Tensor fasciae latae (distal part)	−4	−5.3	−143
Vastus Lateralis	−7	139	−697

Table 6: Systems of moments and forces analyzed.

	Fx	Fy	Fz	Mx	My	Mz
Case_0	Intact femoral force system					
Case_1*			X		X	X
Case_2*	X				X	X
Case_3*			X	X	X	
Case_4*	X			X	X	
Case_5	X	X	X		X	
Case_6			X	X	X	X
Case_7	X		X	X	X	
Case_8		X	X	X	X	
Case_9	X		X	X		X

*Abductors force magnitude and direction unchanged

The magnitude and direction of the tensor fasciae latae (distal), tensor fasciae latae (proximal) and the vastus lateralis were maintained unchanged. Considering the equilibrium somewhere at the distal part of the femur, the following set of equations can be set-up:

$$
\begin{aligned}
\sum Fx_{\text{int\_femur}} &= \text{ABD}_x + \text{HCF}_x \\
\sum Fy_{\text{int\_femur}} &= \text{ABD}_y + \text{HCF}_y \\
\sum Fz_{\text{int\_femur}} &= \text{ABD}_z + \text{HCF}_z \\
\sum Mx_{\text{int\_femur}} &= \text{HCF}_y a - \text{HCF}_z e + \text{ABD}_y d \\
\sum My_{\text{int\_femur}} &= -\text{HCF}_x a - \text{HCF}_z b - \text{ABD}_x d + \text{ABD}_z c \\
\sum Mz_{\text{int\_femur}} &= -\text{HCF}_y b - \text{ABD}_y c
\end{aligned}
\tag{18}
$$

If the abductor direction force is considered unchanged:

$$
\begin{aligned}
\text{ABD}_y &= \alpha \text{ABD}_z, \\
\text{ABD}_x &= \beta \text{ABD}_z.
\end{aligned}
\tag{19}
$$

For the abductors direction force considered, $\alpha = -1.490$ and $\beta = -0.0741$. These equations lead to interminable solutions, some impossible to be implemented since they are non-physiological. The loading cases analyzed are presented in table 6. For load Case_1, load Case_2, load Case_3 and load Case_4, the HCF was allowed to change in magnitude and direction. For the other cases studied, the HCF was allowed to change as well as the magnitude of the abductor force. Table 7 contains the HCF and abductor forces simulated and analyzed.

The loading of the intact femur was applied to the different implanted configurations, which corresponds to load Case_0. The other load cases were analyzed to evidence the importance of the components of the HCF on the moments provoked. Some of the cases aimed to evidence that non-physiological loading can be generated.

Table 7: Derived HCF and abductors force directions and magnitudes.

Force(N)		Lubinus SPII			Charnley			Müller Straight			Stanmore		
		Med.	Ant.	Prox.	Med.	Ant.	Prox.	Med.	Ant.	Prox.	Med.	Ant.	Prox.
Case_0	HFC	-405	-246	-1719	-405	-246	-1719	-405	-246	-1719	-405	-246	-1719
	ABD	435	32	649	435	32	649	435	32	649	435	32	649
Case_1	HFC	-291	-383	-1719	137	-349	-1719	117	-328	-1719	142	-355	-1719
	ABD	435	32	649	435	32	649	435	32	649	435	32	649
Case_2	HFC	-405	-383	-2637	-405	-349	-5347	-405	-328	-5108	-405	-355	-5420
	ABD	435	32	649	435	32	649	435	32	649	435	32	649
Case_3	HFC	-291	-253	-1719	-335	-265	-1719	-341	-250	-1719	-333	-292	1719
	ABD	435	32	649	435	32	649	435	32	649	435	32	649
Case_4	HFC	-405	-255	-2637	-405	-268	-2188	-405	-251	-2137	-405	-302	-2206
	ABD	435	32	649	435	32	649	435	32	649	435	32	649
Case_5	HFC	-858	-280	-2394	-634	-263	-2060	-634	-263	-2061	-635	-263	-2062
	ABD	888	66	1324	664	49	990	664	49	991	665	49	992
Case_6	HFC	-1492	-320	-3150	-1289	-284	-2808	-918	-282	-2391	-1901	-263	-3500
	ABD	1394	103	2080	1166	87	1738	886	66	1321	1630	121	2430
Case_7	HFC	-1461	-324	-2071	2851	-4	-4016	-972	-288	-1949	-5362	-614	-887
	ABD	1491	111	2223	-2821	-209	-4207	1002	74	1494	5392	400	8042
Case_8	HFC	-2465	-375	-4309	29	-225	-1304	-1558	-316	-3136	633	-192	-622
	ABD	2172	161	3239	157	12	234	1385	103	2066	-301	-22	-449
Case_9	HFC	-1365	-320	-3150	-1136	-284	-2808	-856	-282	-2391	-1600	-263	-3500
	ABD	1394	103	2080	1166	87	1738	886	66	1321	1630	121	2430

The HC and abductor forces derived using eqns (18) and (19) show that, although the system forces are in equilibrium, non-physiological loading can be derived, either due to very high magnitude forces or to direction forces that are physiological contrarily. For example, for load Case_7 and for the Charnley design, the direction of the abductor force is different than the physiological one. The same was observed for load Case_8 for the Stanmore prosthesis. For load Case_7 and for the same prosthesis, we can observe that the direction of the HCF is towards proximally, which is naturally impossible. Other load cases show considerable high magnitude forces which are also improbable to occur *in vivo*.

5.2 Results and discussion

For the load cases studied, the absolute difference of strains in the x, y and z direction between the intact and implanted femur were determined and are presented in table 8. Ideally, the loading configuration of the implanted femur should provoke same strains as the ones provoked by the intact femur; however, this is not possible, unless extra forces are added to the force system. Therefore, the more suitable loading configuration is the one that minimizes the differences in strains in all aspects of the femur. Due to the magnitudes of strains (namely ε_z) at the lateral and medial aspects of the femur, it seemed much more relevant to look at the z component of the strains to select the suitable loading configuration. Many conclusions can be drawn based on the strains presented at table 8.

For the prostheses loaded with the loading configuration of the intact femur, it can be seen that the Lubinus SPII provoked higher strain differences in all aspects of the femur. The Charnley and the Stanmore provoked identical differences; the Müller Straight was, of the four prostheses, the one that provoked the smallest differences in strain.

Load Case_4 was of all loading configurations the one that provoked the less strain deviation for all designs. Other loading configurations, such as load Case_1 and load Case_2, provoked significant differences in strains and are not suitable implantable loading configurations. Therefore, load Case_4 that considers Fx, Mx and My (with the abductor force direction unchanged) is apparently a suitable loading configuration for the THR analyzed and seem to be independent of prosthesis design (geometry and material). However, there is a possibility that for other hip prosthesis designs the suitable loading configuration can probably not be the one as load Case_4. It is necessary to previously perform identical study to select the loading that minimizes the differences of strains to the intact femur.

The study showed that it is important to derive correctly the implanted femur-loading configuration, especially if different designs are being compared. For a certain design, the bending in the front plane can be sufficient; for others probably not. It is necessary to understand which is the most critical load component and then try to restore the constant conditions for that one, having in mind that for others the deviations are less relevant. The correct determination of the load configuration for implanted femurs has been neglected in many published studies.

Table 8: Strains in the three orthogonal directions.

Strain (με)		Lubinus SPII				Charnley				Müller Straight				Stanmore			
		Med.	Post.	Ant.	Lat.	Med.	Post.	Ant.	Lat.	Med.	Post.	Ant.	Lat.	Med.	Post.	Ant.	Lat.
Case_0	εx	161	62	52	116	92	37	39	75	102	44	23	49	129	6	1	70
	εy	153	6	45	126	89	44	28	77	82	44	22	54	109	2	3	82
	εz	524	210	168	389	301	138	107	242	315	149	98	180	405	19	4	247
Case_1	εx	65	115	115	24	444	85	123	455	427	1111	142	667	387	115	176	481
	εy	45	115	105	27	469	68	108	455	483	47	98	490	443	120	151	451
	εz	192	378	259	92	1528	263	381	1551	1498	185	342	1641	1374	393	1644	1473
Case_2	εx	24	180	122	29	633	406	207	423	600	314	196	503	538	524	332	445
	εy	1	176	115	34	681	378	200	438	683	300	158	503	626	518	309	423
	εz	51	585	1513	90	2180	1317	1612	3717	2105	1037	531	1655	1905	1686	1060	1455
Case_3	εx	45	56	30	1	22	44	37	2	36	41	10	20	54	42	279	10
	εy	30	52	32	8	18	51	29	5	12	41	14	14	33	38	19	5
	εz	127	184	115	9	64	162	106	2	89	134	66	49	149	139	73	19
Case_4	εx	3	12	20	4	3	6	29	6	14	7	1	20	32	1	11	8
	εy	15	11	19	14	9	15	20	7	13	8	6	15	8	2	9	7
	εz	14	4	75	8	20	39	77	7	14	24	38	51	74	5	38	10

Table 8: Continued.

Strain (με)		Lubinus SPII				Charnley				Müller Straight				Stanmore			
		Med.	Post.	Ant.	Lat.	Med.	Post.	Ant.	Lat.	Med.	Post.	Ant.	Lat.	Med.	Post.	Ant.	Lat.
Case_5	εx	32	75	45	14	17	38	33	3	27	48	15	29	54	1	16	11
	εy	16	70	47	8	10	46	25	4	2	48	21	25	26	4	14	1
	εz	84	245	167	58	44	146	93	23	59	159	87	82	144	2	44	23
Case_6	εx	20	81	50	28	2	60	52	23	21	48	14	37	21	55	29	45
	εy	2	77	52	24	8	69	44	29	7	47	20	36	17	50	35	57
	εz	40	267	185	107	8	223	159	96	34	157	84	110	25	187	118	163
Case_7	εx	72	174	65	36					48	99	27	41				
	εy	60	163	71	35					24	97	34	39				
	εz	218	564	245	139					129	325	130	124				
Case_8	εx	0	101	66	48	38	27	29	27	3	56	19	55				
	εy	20	95	68	48	36	35	20	33	28	53	26	60				
	εz	29	333	241	183	120	106	77	93	26	182	104	177				
Case_9	εx	112	85	33	160	151	63	37	181	45	49	5	105	274	64	4	360
	εy	136	79	44	158	165	73	36	185	75.5	49	17	101	326	56	14	359
	εz	408	271	154	556	529	232	122	626	187	161	68	334	986	405	42	1204

6 Concluding remarks

The main objective of this study was to analyze different issues in the simulation of THR. First, a study was presented and the influence of element type and NDOF in stresses, strains and displacements generated using a simplified femur construction and a realistic one was discussed. Conclusions are somehow difficult to draw and it is not possible to clearly suggest the use of an element type to model the biomechanical behavior of the proximal femur. However, comparing results obtained with the simplified model and the "realistic" proximal femur, we conclude that it is not possible to extrapolate these from the simple model to the proximal femur. For the former one, tetrahedral linear elements allowed results more closely to theoretical ones, but hexahedral quadratic elements seem to be more stable and less influenced to the degree of refinement of the mesh when modeling the proximal femur. To generate numerically reliable results and to have confidence in the models used in simulations, it is necessary to correlate them with valid experimental data. However, if the study is of comparative nature, it is prudent to simulate numerical models with identical finite element type and NDOF.

The importance of muscle force simulation was discussed and for the load configurations analyzed, although the use of the vastus lateralis and iliopsoas provoked lower strain magnitudes at the medial and lateral aspects of the femur, these were still significantly higher than ones observed at the anterior and posterior aspects. Therefore, it is questionable if the *in vivo* femur is loaded pronouncedly in compression.

The simulation of boundary conditions plays an important key role to obtaining reliable results. The simulation of constraining the horizontal (anterior-posterior) movement of the femoral head showed insignificant differences in strain relative to the ones observed for an unconstrained head. This fact raises a question whether in the absence of comprehensive muscle force data if it is reasonable to simulate the head as horizontally constrained.

Finally, a study was performed to derive adequate loading configurations for implanted femurs with different hip femoral components. If it is not done, errors can be expected in the strain distributions that possibly hide differences between different femoral designs. For the designs analyzed, the adequate implanted system force was generated by using in the equilibrium the Fx (medially direction) of the HCF and the bending moments (Mx and My) provoked by the HCF and abductors force (vector direction maintained unchangeable). At least the bending moment at the coronal plane must be restored in the implanted femur loading configuration.

Acknowledgments

The authors gratefully acknowledge the Fundação para a Ciência e a Tecnologia do Ministério da Ciência e do Ensino Superior for funding António Ramos with grant SFRH/BD/63217/2002. Part of the work was supported by project POCTI/EME/38367/2001.

References

[1] Prendergast, P.J. & Maher, S.A., Issues in pre-clinical testing of implants. *J. Mat. Proc. Tech.*, **118**, pp. 337–342, 2001.

[2] Prendergast, P.J., Finite element models in tissue mechanics and orthopaedic implant design. *Clin. Biomech.*, **12(6)**, pp. 343–366, 1997.

[3] Huikes, R., The law of adaptive bone remodeling: a case for crying Newton? *Bone Structure and Remodeling*, eds. A. Odgaaard & H. Weinans, World Scientific, Singapore, pp. 15–24, 1995.

[4] van Rietbergen, B., Odgaard, A., Kabel, J. & Huiskes, R., Direct mechanics assessment of elastic symmetries and properties of trabecular bone. *J. Biomech.*, **29**, pp. 1653–1657, 1996.

[5] Fung, Y.C., On the foundations of biomechanics. *J. Appl. Mech.*, **50**, pp. 1003–1009, 1983.

[6] Cristofolini L. & Viceconti M., In-vitro stress shielding measurements can be affected by large errors. *J. Arthroplasty*, **14(2)**, pp. 215–219, 1999.

[7] Ramos, A. & Simões, J.A., HYPERMESH® finite element model of the proximal femur: some considerations, *International Congress on Computational Bioengineering*, eds. M. Doblaré, M. Cerrolaza & H. Rodrigues, 24–26 September, Zaragoza, pp. 321–327, 2003.

[8] Berelmans, W.A.M., Poort, H.W. & Slooff, T. J., A new method to analyse the mechanical behavior of skeletal parts. *Acta Orthop. Scand.*, **43**, pp. 301–317, 1972.

[9] Taylor, M., Tanner, K.E., Freeman, M.A.R. & Yettram, A.L., Stress and strain distribution within the intact femur: compression or bending? *Med. Eng. Phys.*, **18**, pp. 122–131, 1995.

[10] Polgar, K., Viceconti, M. & O'Connor, J.J., A comparison between automatically generated linear and parabolic tetrahedral when used to mesh a human femur. *Proc. Instn. Mech. Engrs. H*, **215**, pp. 85–94, 2001.

[11] Viceconti, M., Bellingeri, L., Cristofolini, L. &. Toni, A., A comparative study on different methods of automatic mesh generation of human femurs. *Med. Eng. Phys.*, **20**, pp. 1–10, 1998.

[12] Merz, B., Lengsfeld, M., Müller, M.R., Kaminsky, J., Rüegsegger, P. & Niederer, P., Automated generation of 3D Fe-models of the human femur – comparison of methods and results, *Computer Methods in Biomechanics and Biomedical Engineering*, eds. J. Middleton, M.L. Jones & G.N. Pande, Gordon and Breach, Amsterdam, pp. 125–134, 1996.

[13] Marks, L., Mesh density problems and solutions, *Tips and workarounds for CAD Generated Models*, NAFEMS Limited, Glasgow, pp. 21–27, 1999.

[14] Keyak, J.H. & Skinner, H.B., Three-dimensional finite element modeling of bone: effects of element size. *J. Biomed. Eng.*, **14**, pp. 483–489, 1992.

[15] Ladd, A.J.C. & Kinney, J.H., Numerical errors and uncertainties in finite-element modeling of trabecular bone. *J. Biomech.*, **31**, pp. 941–945, 1998.

[16] Vander Sloten, J. & Van Der Perre, G., The influence of geometrical distorsions of three-dimensional finite elements, used to model proximal femoral bone. *Proc. Instn. Mech. Eng. H.*, **209**, pp. 31–36, 1993.

[17] Stolk, J., Verdonschot, N. & Huiskes, R., Management of stress fields around singular points in a finite element analysis, *Computer Methods in Biomechanics and Biomedical Engineering*, eds. J. Middleton, M.L. Jones, N.G. Shrive & G.N. Pande, Gordon and Breach Science Publishers, London, pp. 57–62, 2001.

[18] Huiskes, R. & Chao, E.Y.S., A survey of finite element analysis in orthopaedic biomechanics: the first decade. *J. Biomech.*, **16**, pp. 385–409, 1983.

[19] Verma, A. & Melosh, R.J., Numerical tests for assessing finite element model convergence. *Int. J. Numer. Meth. Eng.*, **24**, pp. 843–857, 1987.

[20] Hart, R.T., Hennebel, V., Thongpreda, N., Van Buskirk, W.C. & Anderson, R.C., Modeling the biomechanics of the mandible: A three-dimensional finite element study. *J. Biomech.*, **25**, pp. 261–286, 1992.

[21] Marks, L.W. & Gardner, T.N., The use of strain energy as a convergence criterion in the finite element modeling of bone and the effect of model geometry on stress convergence. *J. Biomed. Eng.*, **15**, pp. 474–476, 1993.

[22] Stolk, J., Verdonschot, N. & Huiskes, R., Sensitivity of failure criteria of cemented total hip replacements to finite element mesh density. In 11th *Conf. Of the European Society of Biomechanics*, July 8–11, Toulouse, France, pp. 165, 1998.

[23] Sakamoto, J., Tawara, D. & Oda, J., Large-scale finite element analysis based on CT images considering inhomogeneousness of bone. *2003 Summer Bioengineering Conf.*, June 25–29, Florida, pp. 49–50, 2003.

[24] Jeffers, J.R.T. & Taylor, M., Mesh considerations for adaptive finite element analyses of cement failure in total hip replacement. *2003 Summer Bioengineering Conf.*, June 25–29, Florida, pp. 729–730, 2003.

[25] Muccini, R., Baleani, M. & Viceconti, M., Selection of the best element type in the finite element analysis of hip prostheses. *J. Med. Eng. Technol.*, **24(4)**, pp. 145–148, 2000.

[26] Zachariah, S.G., Sanders, J.E. & Turkiyyah, G.M., Automated hexahedral mesh generation from biomedical image data: applications in limb prosthetics. *IEEE Trans. Rehabil. Eng.*, **4(2)**, pp. 91–102, 1996.

[27] Viceconti, M., Zannoni, C., Testi, D. & Cappello, A., A new method for the automatic mesh generation of bone segments from CT data. *J. Med. Eng. Technol.*, **23(2)**, pp. 77–81, 1999.

[28] Camacho, D.L.A., Hopper, R.H., Lin, G.M. & Myers, B.S., An improved method for finite element mesh generation of geometrically complex structures with application to the skullbase. *J. Biomech.*, **30(19)**, pp. 1067–1070, 1997.

[29] Li, H. & Cheng, G., New method for graded mesh generation of all hexahedral finite elements. *Compt. Struct.*, **76**, pp. 729–740, 2000.

[30] Lo, S.H. & Ling, C., Improvement on the 10-node tetrahedral element for three-dimensional problems. *Comput. Methods Appl. Mech. Engrg.*, **189**, pp. 961–974, 2000.

[31] Owen, S.J. & Saigal, S., Formation of pyramid elements for hexahedra to tetrahedral transitions. *Comput. Methods Appl. Mech. Engrg.*, **190**, pp. 4505–4518, 2001.

[32] Jimack, P.K., Mahmood, R., Walkley, M.A. & Berzins, M., A multilevel approach for obtaining locally optimal finite element meshes. *Adv. Eng. Soft.*, **33**, pp. 403–415, 2002.

[33] Chabanas, M., Luboz, V. & Payan, Y., Patient specific finite element model of the face soft tissues for computer-assisted maxillofacial surgery. *Medical Image Analysis*, **7**, pp. 131–151, 2003.

[34] Globisch, G., Practical aspects and experiences. On an automatically parallel generation technique for tetrahedral meshes. *Parallel Computing*, **21**, pp. 1979–1995, 1995.

[35] Biswas, R. & Strawn, R.C., Mesh quality control for multiply-refined tetrahedral grids. *App. Num. Math.*, **20**, pp. 337–348, 1996.

[36] Lee, C.K. & Lo, S.H., Automatic adaptive refinement finite element procedure for 3D stress analysis. *Finite Elements in Analysis and Design*, **25**, pp. 135–166, 1997.

[37] Krejèi, R., Bartoš, M., Dvořăk, J., Nedoma, J. & Stehlik, J., 2D and 3D finite element pre- and post-processing in orthopaedy. *Int. J. of Medical Informatics*, **45**, pp. 83-89, 1997.

[38] Lo, S.H., Optimization of tetrahedral meshes based on element shape measures. *Comput. Struct.*, **63(5)**, pp. 951–961, 1997.

[39] Berzins, M., A solution-based triangular and tetrahedral mesh quality indicator. *J. Sci. Comput.*, **19(6)**, pp. 2051–2060, 1998.

[40] Tang, K., Chou, S.Y., Chen, L.L. & Woo, T.C., Tetrahedral mesh generation for solids based on alternating sum of volumes. *Computer in Industry*, **41**, pp. 65–81, 2000.

[41] Benzley, S.E., Merkley, K., Blacker, T.D. & Schoof, L., Pre- and post-processing for the finite element method. *Finite Elements in Analysis and Design*, **19**, pp. 243–260, 1995.

[42] Field, D.A., The legacy of automatic mesh generation from solid modeling. *Computer Aided Geometric Design*, **12**, pp. 651–673, 1995.

[43] Biswas, R. & Strawn, R.C., 1998, Tetrahedral and hexahedral mesh adaptation for CFD problems. *App. Num. Math.*, **26**, pp. 135–151, 1998.

[44] Chiba, N., Nishigaki, I., Yamashita, Y., Takizawa, C. & Fujishiro, K., A flexible automatic hexahedral mesh generation by boundary-fit method. *Comput. Methods Appl. Mech. Engrg.*, **161**, pp. 145–154, 1998.

[45] Yoshimura, S., Wada, Y. & Yagawa, G., Automatic mesh generation of quadrilateral elements using intelligent local approach. *Comput. Methods Appl. Mech. Engrg.*, **179**, pp. 125–138, 1999.

[46] Zachariah, S.G. & Sanders, J.E., Finite element estimates of interface stress in the trans-tibial prosthesis using gap elements are different from those using automated contact. *J. Biomech.*, **33**, pp. 895–899, 2000.

[47] Tsuboi, H., Tanaka, M., Ikeda, K. & Nishimura, Computation results of the TEAM workshop Problem 7 by finite element methods using tetrahedral and hexahedral elements. *J. Mat. Proc. Tech.*, **108**, pp. 237–240, 2001.

[48] Owen, S.J., Hex-dominant mesh generation using 3D constrained triangulation. *Computer-Aided Design*, **33**, pp. 211–220, 2001.

[49] Dhondt, G.D., Unstructured 20-node brick element meshing. *Computer-Aided Design*, **33**, pp. 233–249, 2001.

[50] Muller-Hannemann, M., Quadrilateral surface meshes without self-intersecting dual cycles for hexahedral mesh generation. *Computational Geometry*, **22**, pp. 75–97, 2002.

[51] Parthasarathy, V.N., Graichen, C.M. & Hathaway, A.F., A comparison of tetrahedron quality measures. *Finite Elements in Analysis and Design*, **15**, pp. 255–261, 1994.

[52] Cifuentes, A.O. & Kalbag, A., A performance study of tetrahedral and hexahedral elements in 3-D finite element structural analysis. *Finite Elements in Analysis and Design*, **12**, pp. 313–318, 1992.

[53] Bergmann, G., Graichen, F. & Rohlmann, A. Hip joint loading during walking and running measured in two patients. *J. Biomechanics*, **26**, 969–990, 1993.

[54] Colgan, D., Trench, P., Slemon, D., McTague, D., Finlay, J.B. & O'Donell, P., A review of joint and muscle simulation relevant to in-vitro stress analysis of the hip. *Strain*, May, pp. 47–61, 1994.

[55] Cristofolini, L., Viceconti, M., Toni, M. & Giunti, A., Influence of thigh muscles on the axial strains in a proximal femur during early stance in gait. *J. Biomechanics*, **28(5)**, 617–624, 1995.

[56] Simões, J.A., Vaz, M.A., Blatcher, S. & Taylor, M., Influence of head constraint and muscle forces on the strain distribution within the intact femur. *Med. Eng. Phys.*, **22**, 453–459, 2000.

[57] Pauwels, F., *Biomechanics of the locomotor apparatus*, Springer Verlag, Berlin/Heidelberg/New York (1980).

[58] Currey, J.D., *The mechanical adaption of bones*, Princeton University Press, Princeton, NJ (1984).

[59] Frost, H.M., *Bone remodeling and skeletal modeling errors*, Orthopaedics Lecturers, Springfield (IL) (1973).

[60] Crowninshield, R.D., Johnston, R.C., Andrews, J.G. & Brand, R.A., A biomechanical investigation of the human hip. *J. Biomech.* **11** (1978), pp. 75–85.

[61] Seireg, A. & Kempke, W., Behavior of *in vivo* bone under cyclic loading. *J. Biomech.* **2**, pp. 455, 1975.

[62] Röhrle, H., Scholten, R., Sigolotto, C., Sollbach, W. & Kellne, H., Joint forces in the human pelvis–leg skeleton during walking. *J. Biomech.* **17**, pp. 409–424, 1984.

[63] Bergmann, G., Heller, M. & Duda, G.M., Preclinical testing of cemented hip replacement implants: Pre-normative research for a European Standard; Final report of Workpackage 5: Development of the Loading Configuration, ed. G. Bergamann. HIP98. Free University, Berlin, 2001.

[64] Américo, J., Moreira, R. & Simões, J., Numerical studt of the biomechanics of the hip. 6th Portuguese Conference on Biomedical Engineering, 11–12 June, University of Algarve, pp. 135, 2001.

[65] Cristofolini L., A critical analysis of stress shielding evaluation of hip prostheses. *Critical Reviews in Biomedical Engineering* **25** (**4&5**): 409–483, 1997.

[66] Ramos, A.M. & Simões, J.A., Physiological loading in Total Hip Replacements, *J. Arthroplasty* (submitted), 2004.

[67] Mackerle, J., Finite element analyses and simulations in biomedicine: a bibliography (1985–1999). *Engng. Comput.*, **17(7)**, pp. 813–856, 2000.

[68] Mackerle, J., A finite element bibliography for biomechanics (1987–1997). *App. Mech. Rev.*, **51(10)**, pp. 587–634, 1998.

[69] Ramos, A.M. & Simões, J.A., Tetrahedral versus hexahedral finite elements in modeling the intact femur. *Med. Eng. Phys.* (submitted), 2004.

[70] www.cineca.it/hosted/LTM-IOR/back2net/ISB_mesh/isb_ mesh.html.

[71] Heiner, A.D. & Brown, T.D., Structural properties of a new design of composite replicate femurs and tibias. *J. Biomech.*, **34**, pp. 773–781, 2001.

[72] Rohlmann, A., Mossner, U., Bergamann, G. & Kolbel, R., Finite-element-analysis and experimental investigation of stresses in a femur. *J. Biomed. Eng.*, **4**, pp. 241–247, 1982.

[73] Stolk, J., Verdonshot, N. & Huiskes R., Stair Climbing is More Detrimental to the Cement in Hip Replacement than Walking. *Clin. Orthop. Rel. Res.*, **1(405)**, pp. 294–305, 2002.

CHAPTER 7

Structural analysis for pre-surgery planning: two applications in dentistry and urology

C. Bignardi[1], E. Zanetti[2] & G. Marino[3]
[1]Department of Mechanics, Politecnico di Torino, Italy.
[2]Department of Industrial and Mechanical Engineering,
University of Catania, Italy.
[3]Department of Urology, Ospedale Mauriziano, Torino, Italy.

Abstract

The chapter focuses on current problems and developments in two areas where biomechanics, and numerical structural analysis in particular, could be useful: designing dental prostheses and implants, and conducting structural evaluations of the pelvic floor.

For the first area, different types of dental implants and prosthetic designs used for partially or totally edentulous patients were considered in order to analyze the strain-stress state in bone, which determines whether the biomechanical system will succeed or fail.

In the second area of investigation, our aim was to demonstrate the importance of restoring pelvic organ supporting structures (the urethro-pelvic and pubovesical ligaments) following resection surgery performed for uterine or bladder neoplasias, etc.

1 Introduction

Biomechanics is a part of bioengineering that can be defined as the application of mechanical engineering concepts and methods to the investigation and solution of problems in medicine and biology.

While the scope of biomechanics is straightforward enough, the ways and means it uses to pursue its aims vary widely.

Though the field abounds with abstrusely theoretical basic research, which we respect since not to do so would be to set limits on intellectual enquiry, there are very few practical applications. Apart from these theoretical efforts, certain investigations call for some form of clinical follow-up, though without working out the details. What little has been done to solve clinical problems has invariably sprung from interdisciplinary work, and goes hand in hand with methodological advances.

We elected to study biomechanics because of its ability to support research and clinical applications. Thus seen, biomechanics can make an enormous contribution to surgical practice.

The turning point in establishing engineering's potential role in biological and clinical studies came towards the end of the 1960's, when it was realized that the theoretical and experimental methods of mechanical engineering could be focused on biological structures in general, and on bone in particular [1, 2].

Thus, a biological structure could potentially be treated as a normal engineering material. This is particularly true of its ability to withstand stresses, including fatigue stresses, and its structural behavior. To handle biological structures in this way, it was necessary to be able to calculate the forces acting throughout the system, to characterize materials, to perform structural analysis and, consequently, to introduce numerical techniques such as the finite element method [3].

Investigations of the "human system" and the prosthetization of any of its parts must thus start from an awareness that any form of surgical intervention will invariably affect the strain-stress state of the structures involved, either directly or indirectly.

Even with the approximations that most numerical models introduce for the mechanical properties of biological tissues (e.g., their isotropy, homogeneity and linear behavior), for the conditions at the interface with prosthetic devices, and for loading and constraint conditions, structural analysis has made significant progress since 1960. For orthopedic implants in particular, structural analysis has made it possible to formulate general rules that now enable us to understand which approaches should be ruled out before proceeding with actual prosthesis design.

The experience gained in one of the most mature areas of structural biomechanics, viz., orthopedic biomechanics, encourages us to apply the methods of numerical structural analysis to assessing the behavior of other biological structures that undergo structural changes following surgery designed to restore a failed function or to remove, for example, neoplastic formations.

2 Dental biomechanics

2.1 Question: what influence do different prosthesis configurations have on bone stress/strain pattern?

The implant-supported prosthesis is an alternative to conventional removable dentistry: while conventional dentures may meet the needs of many patients, others require more retention, stability, function and aesthetics. A review of recent literature [4] indicated that implants used to support an overdenture have a very high success rate, and are thus likely to become more and more widespread.

Today, similar clinical situations can be handled using a variety of prosthetic solutions: in particular, the implant support can differ according to the type of implants used and their layout. Clinical comparisons of different surgical treatments are difficult, as each patient's biomechanical situation is unique, and the scientific literature provides no clear guidance to the alleged benefits claimed for specific types of dental implant and their morphological characteristics [5].

It is known, however, that the success or the failure of implants interfaced with bone (e.g., orthopedic and dental implants) depends on the structural condition of the biomechanical system made up of the bone structure and the implant [1, 6], providing that the biological reaction is favorable. A good understanding of the strain/stress pattern makes it possible to establish whether bone maintenance, resorption or addition is more likely to take place [7]. Hoshaw *et al.* [8] applied a dynamic axial tensile load for 500 cycles per day for five consecutive days to Brånemark implants inserted in rabbit tibiae. The result was bone loss around the implant neck, a region where finite element analysis showed high strains. Duyck *et al.* [9] found crater-like bone defects as a result of a dynamic transverse load applied on Brånemark implants inserted bicortically in rabbit tibiae. The interpretation was that the bone loss had been caused by excessive stresses. Roberts *et al.* [10] reported a high remodeling rate around the tops of implant threads.

All of these studies confirm that analyzing stress patterns can provide useful guidance in selecting the type of implant to be used.

Analyzing a biomechanical system of this kind is complicated because of the different structures involved (compact bone, cancellous bone, gum, implant, prosthesis), which feature complex geometries and dissimilar mechanical properties. This makes load transmission from the teeth to the bone difficult to evaluate intuitively. As a result, the finite element method (FEM) is needed in order to perform comparative evaluations whereby different surgical approaches to the same bone situation can be simulated.

2.2 Analyzed prosthesis configurations and the findings of structural analysis

By way of example, we will illustrate two cases of partial or full edentulism that can be treated with different prosthetic solutions.

2.2.1 Case I

Two different kinds of implant supports for overdenture retention were compared. The two types differed in number of implants, size, location in the mandible and in whether or not a bar is used to connect the implants.

The first solution (fig. 1(a)) for overdenture retention will be referred to below as the 'conventional' design, and simulates the insertion of two mutually parallel Brånemark implants in the chin area. An acrylic saddle serves as the base for the prosthesis and is attached to these implants.

The second solution (fig. 1(b)) will be designated as the 'modified' design, and simulates the insertion of four screw-type rootform implants anchored to the chin area with bicortical fixation. These implants differ in orientation, and are connected

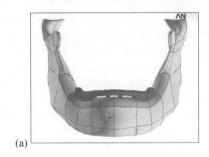 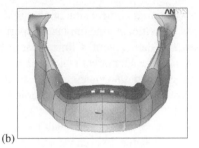

(a)   (b)

Figure 1: FEM models of (a) mandible with a 'conventional' implant support design, (b) mandible with a 'modified' implant support design.

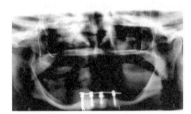 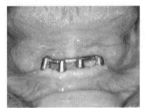

Figure 2: X-ray image (left) and picture (right) of the 'modified' implant support design.

Table 1: Mechanical properties of materials.

Materials	Young's modulus (MPa)	Poisson's ratio
Cortical bone	13,000	0.3
Trabecular bone	300	0.3
Gum	20	0.3
Titanium	100,000	0.3
Resin	2000	0.4
Damping layer	500	0.4

to each other by a metal wire by means of a syncrystallization process (fig. 2) [11]. The acrylic saddle used as a base for the prosthesis is attached to this metal wire. A plastic layer is placed between the wire and the saddle to perform a damping function.

A fully osseointegrated condition was simulated (secondary stability). The numerical models consisted of approximately 33,000 4-node tetrahedron elements. Modeled materials are listed in table 1, while mechanical properties agree with data found in the literature [12, 13].

The two models were asymmetrically loaded at the second premolar. Loads were distributed, simulating occlusal contact with the corresponding upper tooth.

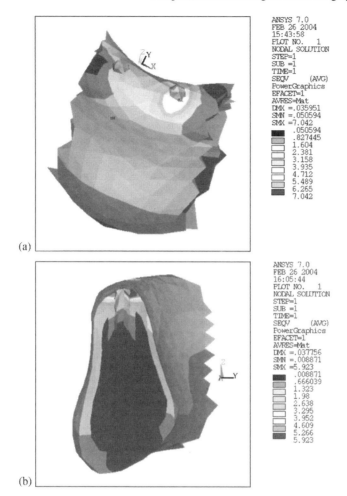

Figure 3: von Mises stress pattern in cortical bone for 'conventional' implant support design: (a) external view, (b) cross section. Stress values are in MPa.

The vertical component of the load was 50 N, while the distal-mesial component was 50 N [9]. Constraints simulate muscle action during mastication.

Analysis focused on identifying the cortical and trabecular bone stress/strain pattern and thus determining whether the structural condition was favorable to bone remodeling. von Mises stresses were first considered in order to locate the most highly stressed areas. A more detailed analysis was then carried out to assess the major direction of stress in these areas.

The analysis of von Mises stresses in cortical bone indicated that the peak stress occurs at the implant nearest to the applied load (figs 3(a), (b) and 4(a), (b) in both implant support designs. Peak stress was located on the distal side at the point of implant insertion into cortical bone.

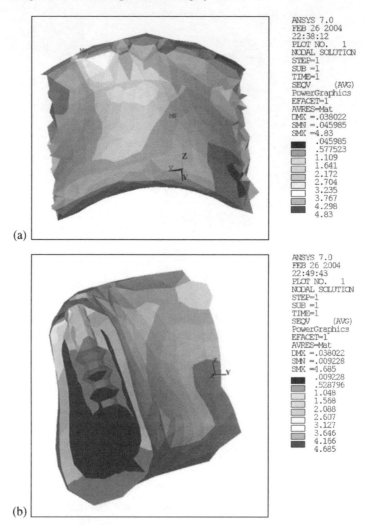

Figure 4: von Mises stress pattern in cortical bone for 'modified' implant support design: (a) external view, (b) cross section. Stress values are in MPa.

A more detailed stress analysis indicated that the peak stress is due to a notch effect: the stress field is typically triaxial, while the stressed area is very small and matches the clinical evidence of conical resorption [8]. The analysis also showed that the most influential force component is exerted along the y (distal-mesial) direction, given that the force application point was nearly aligned with one of the constraint points, along the z (vertical) direction.

On the whole, the 'modified' overdenture produced smaller stresses than the 'conventional' design, as von Mises stresses were 34% lower.

This can be explained by the fact that load is distributed over a larger number of implants. In addition, the notch effect is reduced whenever there is more than one discontinuity: stress is more evenly distributed, even if the average stress level rises.

The numerical results are corroborated by clinical experience [14] and by radiographic images showing larger alveolar bone losses (typical resorbed cones) at the point of Brånemark implant insertion in the bone. These observations are borne out elsewhere in the literature [15].

A more detailed analysis was performed in order to assess the structural importance of the metal wire connecting all implants in the 'modified' solution. A hypothetical model without wire was developed for this purpose. The numerical analysis demonstrated that eliminating a 2 mm diameter wire produces a 5% higher peak stress. The reduction in implant-bone system stiffness was moderate: assuming that secondary stability has been achieved, the implants are linked to each other by means of cortical bone, which has a lower Young's modulus than the metal wire but provides a much better geometry because of its larger size.

The results would have differed had we considered primary stability: as the implant would not yet be osseointegrated, it would be constrained in the cortical bone by contact forces alone, thus making the wire's role in restricting implant bending more important.

Analysis of the stresses in the trabecular bone indicated that the most highly stressed area for the 'conventional' implant was located at the distal tip of the implant opposite the loaded area. These stresses can be disregarded for two main reasons: their magnitude was low [16], and their location was far from the proximal implant area, which is the most critical as regards bone remodeling.

For the 'modified' implant, the most highly stressed area was adjacent to the point of implant insertion. On the whole, these stresses were quite well distributed over the entire implant area, and never reached critical levels [16].

2.2.2 Case II

Over the years, it has been necessary to develop appropriate orthodontic techniques in order to restore fully or partially edentulous maxillae with thin cortical bone, as has been demonstrated the quality and amount of bone plays a fundamental part in reducing strains in the bone adjacent to the implant under load [17]. The most commonly used techniques include maxillary sinus cerclage and lateral insertion [18], while sinus lifting, i.e., elevating the floor of the maxillary sinus, has recently attracted considerable attention [19]. However, this type of surgery is fairly invasive, involves a long waiting time before the implant structures can be used and, above all, leads to severe sequelae should the implant fail. Adding to all of these drawbacks is the fact that the endosteal membrane is extremely fragile, and can sometimes tear during the operation solely as a result of the patient's breathing, even without being stressed by poor surgical procedures. As another immediate or long-term complication, the implant may shift into the sinus if there is little or no periimplant ossification.

For all of these reasons, attempts have been made to develop alternative techniques that conserve the physiological anatomical structure. The first to develop

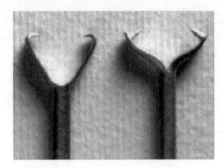

Figure 5: Two-phase integration brackets.

such an alternative approach was Apolloni [20], who used a technique based on cortical support outside the sinus area. However, the Apolloni implant has several disadvantages, including a lack of primary stability, anchorage similar to that provided by subperiosteal implants and the fact that the buccal mucoperiosteal flap may be positioned in an area where it is often subject to tensile stresses from muscle insertions.

The 'two-phase' implant technique is a further evolution of this method which provides good primary stability, as the implant can be retained immediately to the bone by means of the teeth at the outside edges (fig. 5) [11]. In addition, it is covered by a bone graft that not only makes it a bicortical endosseous implant, but also provides a sufficient support surface for the mucoperiosteal flap.

As this technique would appear to be less invasive and easier to implement, we proceeded to verify whether it was also biomechanically valid. The sinus lifting technique was compared with the 'two-phase' implant approach. Specifically, the first technique considered employs conventional implants following an autologous bone graft from the palate, while the second involves inserting screw-type rootform implants and innovative bracket-type implants rigidly connected by a wire by means of a syncrystallization process. Implants anchored with bicortical fixation were chosen in order to increase primary stability, thus reducing micromovements and optimizing stress distribution.

Comparing different surgical treatments is by no means easy, as there is no universally accepted method for defining the patient's degree of bone atrophy, and each patient constitutes a unique biomechanical system. We thus chose to conduct a finite element analysis, as this makes it possible to simulate different surgical treatments on the same patient.

The geometrical models are shown in figs 6 and 7. Full osseointegration was simulated, since all implants are surrounded by 1 mm thick cortical bone in both models. The volumes indicated in fig. 6 were divided into 49,000 ten-node tetrahedron elements, while those in fig. 7 were divided into 15,000 ten-node tetrahedron elements (simpler geometry made it possible to use larger elements). A finer mesh was used where results indicated high stress gradients. Each model is constituted by four different materials, whose properties are shown in table 2 [21].

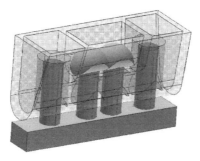

Figure 6: Model of a portion of maxilla with conventional implants.

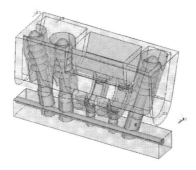

Figure 7: Model of a portion of maxilla with screw-type rootform implants and innovative bracket-type implants rigidly connected by a wire.

Table 2: Mechanical properties of materials.

Materials	Young's modulus (MPa)	Poisson's ratio
Cortical bone	11,000	0.3
Trabecular bone	300	0.3
Implants	100,000	0.3
Teeth	110,000	0.3

To simplify modeling, all materials were assumed to be homogeneous and isotropic, even though bone is known to show marked anisotropy. A recent study demonstrates that anisotropy, when considered, can lead to a 20% to 30% rise in mandible stress levels, suggesting that careful consideration should be given to its use in finite element studies of dental implants [22]. In the authors' opinion, considering that bone patient mechanical characteristics are not known, it is not worthy to further complicate the numerical model and this assumption should not invalidate the comparison between the two surgical approaches.

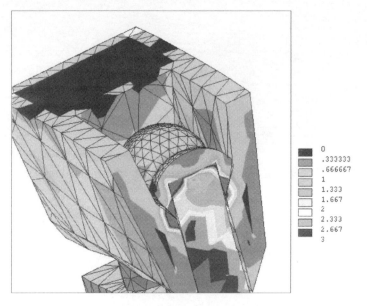

Figure 8: von Mises stress pattern for the second case of load: conventional implant design. Stress values are in MPa.

The maxillar portion was fully constrained at both ends.

Two heavily loaded situations were simulated where load is concentrated at the middle of the bone segment. In the first case, a pure vertical load of 200 N was applied, while a 40 N posteriorly-directed horizontal component was added in the second case.

Three different areas were analyzed: the external surface of the cortical bone, the transition between cortical and trabecular and implant longitudinal and cross sections.

Close attention was devoted to bone in all cases. The von Mises equivalent stress is shown in order to provide a clearer overview and to identify the most highly stressed areas.

Load is quite well distributed in both cases of load, as stresses are spread over the entire bone even if the load is applied on one single node. Dangerous stresses are reached in very small areas, viz., the bone-implant interface in the case of conventional implants (fig. 8) and the points where the retaining pins enter the bone for more innovative subperiosteal implants (fig. 9).

Though stress levels are quite similar for both surgical approaches, there are certain differences. First, the external cortical surface is subject to higher stresses when the subperiosteal implant is used (figs 10 and 11), as this type of implant sits atop the cortical bone; though no dangerous stresses are reached, this is because the geometrical model simulates a perfect fit between the implant and cortical bone.

Second, trabecular bone is not highly stressed, because most of the load is carried by the stiffer cortical bone. Some stress concentration occurs where angled

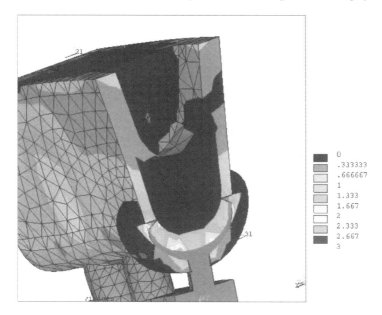

Figure 9: von Mises stress pattern for the second case of load: subperiosteal implant design. Stress values are in MPa.

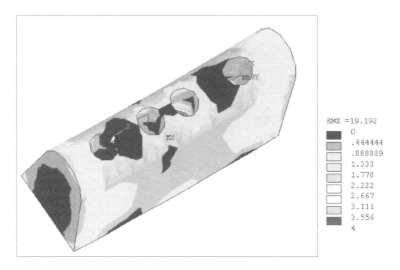

Figure 10: von Mises stress pattern in cortical bone for the second case of load: conventional implant design. Stress values are in MPa.

screws exit trabecular bone and sit against cortical bone, though stress still remains low. Third, cross-sectional views show that stress levels are similar at both ends, while stress concentrations occur in the middle sections in the case of conventional implants (fig. 8).

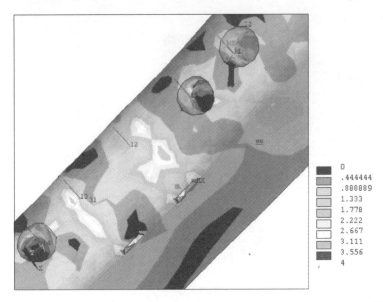

Figure 11: von Mises stress pattern in cortical bone for the second case of load: subperiosteal implant design. Stress values are in MPa.

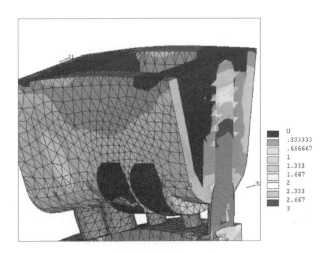

Figure 12: von Mises stress pattern for the second case of load and when the sub-periosteal implant design is adopted. Stress values are in MPa.

These stress concentrations are found at the implant's point of emergence, at the cortical bone-grafted bone interface (fig. 9), and at the distal ends of the screws (fig. 12). This is in good agreement with Meyer *et al.* [17], who identified the same critical areas in the case of a solitary implant and found similar stress levels in the case of an atrophic maxilla with good trabecular bone quality. According to the same author, larger stress should be expected in the case of poor trabecular bone quality because most load is carried by cortical bone, whereas an average maxilla has a thicker cortical layer which would result in lower stress.

3 Pelvic floor biomechanics

3.1 Question: how important is it to restore the supporting structures for pelvic organs, i.e., the urethro-pelvic and pubo-vesical ligaments, after resection surgery?

Image diagnosis of bladder conditions has long been entrusted to urethro-cystography.

This examination shows the degree of rotation and deflection of the cervico-urethral tract, and the degree of opening and closing of the neck of the bladder at rest, during micturition and under stress. In some examination centers, it has been replaced by ultrasonography to evaluate relationships between the cervico-urethral angle and neighboring structures.

Urodynamic investigation, by itself, provides analytical manometric information concerning the detrusor and its relationships with the sphincter mechanisms. It reveals bladder and sphincter dysfunction, but cannot supply a picture of pelvic support. CT and MRI are regarded as second-level examinations. They provide a 3D reconstruction of the muscles, fasciae and ligaments, both at rest and during a Valsalva's manoeuvre [23].

At present, however, no diagnostic examination is capable of providing a true 3D dynamic picture in orthostatism and under load, together with a description of the extent of stresses and deflections of the pelvic floor [24–26].

3.2 Structural analysis and findings

A CT image from a 24-year-old woman was used to create a 3D geometrical model of the pelvic bone, muscles and organs. Mimics graphics software was employed to reconstruct the surfaces, while Rhinoceros software was used to refine the images and save them in the IGES format compatible with the pre-post processor and the finite element solver used. Geometries of different organs were saved in individual subsystems. Each subsystem (pelvis, obturator muscles, levator ani muscle, colon, uterus, vagina, bladder, urethra, pelvic fascia, sphincter, perineum) was meshed with triangular shell elements to provide a good simulation of surfaces with abrupt changes in section. The model consisted of a total of 10,084 nodes and 21,250 elements (fig. 13).

Obturator muscles with their origins on foramina and their postero-lateral insertions on femurs were first inserted in the pelvic bone system. The elevator ani group (LA) was inserted anteriorly on the pubis, laterally on the tendon of each internal obturator muscle and posteriorly on the sacro-coccygeal tract. The pelvic fascia was inserted in the central space above the LA and attached anteriorly to the pubis,

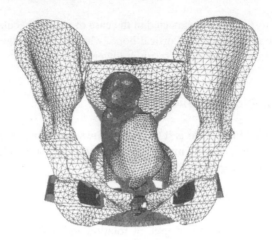

Figure 13: Numerical model of the pelvic bone, muscles and organs.

laterally to the tendinous arch and posteriorly on the sacro-coccygeal insertion. Anterior perineum, urethral sphincter, tendon center and posterior perineum with anal sphincter and ano-coccygeal ligament were positioned in an underlying plane.

These muscles and ligaments were joined to each other and to the pelvis by their own ligaments and fibrous insertions. The anterior perineum was attached to ischio-pubic rami by means of hinges, allowing it to deflect when loaded. Urethro-pelvic ligaments running transversely into the endopelvic fascia and pubo-urethral ligaments running longitudinally into periurethral fascia were represented.

Urethro-pelvic and pubo-vesical ligaments were reconstructed in the same way. Periurethral and perivesical parts of endopelvic fascia were inserted into the anterior segment of pubis and laterally to obturator tendons.

The vescico-urethral tract was interposed in the anterior hiatus of the pelvic fascia and the underlying perineum by describing connections between pubourethral ligaments, the pelvic fascia and the pubis. In the same way, the vagina and uterus were positioned in the openings on the pelvic fascia and perineum. Utero-sacral, cardinal pubo-rectal and utero-sacral ligaments were completed.

Since the space between the viscera is small, fasciae and ligaments were realistically represented as fused together. Lastly, the ano-rectal tract was inserted in the anal sphincter.

The sphincter was adjacent to the medial margin of the LA and connected to coccyx by the corpus ano-coccygeum.

The link between pelvic fascia and perineum was established by inserting several vertical tie-rods or struts designed to shorten when loaded and act as shock absorbers.

Each structure was assigned a specific Young's modulus (E) and Poisson's ratio (ν) (table 3). These mechanical properties were obtained from experimental testing for the bladder [27], and were taken from the literature for the other structures [28–30].

All materials involved were considered to be isotropic with linear behavior.

Table 3: Mechanical properties of materials.

Materials	Young's modulus (MPa)	Poisson's ratio
Bone	20,000	0.3
Ligaments	1000	0.3
Muscles	0.400	0.4
Bladder	0.028–0.150	0.4
Pelvic fascia	0.030	0.4
Colon	0.025	0.4
Uterus and vagina	0.020	0.4

The subject was assumed to be in orthostatic position. Pressure and gravity loads were applied.

The average pressures exerted on bladder and colon by urine and faeces were 10 and 50 cm H_2O, respectively. A gravity load of 60 N was selected to represent the weight of the intestines and pelvic organs estimated from donor bladder measurements.

Structural analysis indicated that the highest stresses for this load situation are in the anterior tract of the pelvic fascia and the anterior perineum adjacent to the sphincter area. Some changes occurred when the urethro-pelvic and the pubo-vesical ligaments were not included in the model. In this simulation, the prepubic tract of the pelvic fascia deflected significantly. The load is concentrated on the underlying perineum near the urethra and sphincteric tracts that become unsteady under to excessive stress.

These findings support the validity of surgical procedures designed to reconstruct stress-relieving lines of force and bearing constraints.

4 Conclusions

Combining the analytical techniques of engineering with clinical experience, and orthopedic experience in particular, has enabled us to avoid major biomechanical errors and significantly reduce the number of short-term prosthesis failures – provided, of course, that no problems arise as a result of surgical quality or biological causes.

Our analysis of the experimental and theoretical methods used to solve biomechanical problems of a structural nature in concrete applications has led us to conclude that the only practicable approach consists of combining the finite element method with clinical verification

We have outlined several FEM applications drawn from our experience to show how this method can make a far from negligible contribution to clinical practice.

Currently, the frontiers of structural biomechanics lie both in customized studies of biomechanical systems which take the unique biological properties and configurations found in each individual into account, and in studies which do not stop short with the immediate post-operative period, but also investigate how the bio mechanical system created by implanting a prosthesis changes over time. When the biological structure affected by surgery is bone, this type of long-term analysis necessarily involves observing and evaluating the biostructural role played by bone remodeling. Bone remodeling is the phenomenon whereby bone tissue adapts its structure, morphology and mechanical properties to changing mechanical stresses. The remodeling equations are constitutive in nature, and determine the rate of change in bone density and form in response to the mechanical stimulus that guides the structural alteration. The nature of the remodeling stimulus is not fully understood, and there are various theories linking remodeling to changes in mechanical parameters.

The objective is to investigate the changes in the structure and mechanical properties of the new bone tissue that occur as it is remodeled around the prosthesis, and determine whether the new biomechanical system thus created is capable of reaching equilibrium.

In the future, it is likely that computer aided surgery (CAS) methods will be developed which, together with increasingly sophisticated imaging techniques, will make it possible to perform customized, interdisciplinary studies of individual cases that combine preoperative planning with structural analysis and virtual surgery. There are also good prospects for using robots in surgery.

References

[1] Lorenzi, G.L. & Calderale, P.M., Problemi meccanici delle artroprotesi. *Proc. of the LIX SIOT Congress*, Cagliari, pp. 1–107, 1974.

[2] Calderale, P.M., Biomechanics of load-bearing human joints and arthro-prostheses. *Proc. of the 2nd Italian-Polish Symp. Bioengineering*, Udine, pp. 215–229, 1975.

[3] Calderale, P.M. & Bignardi, C., Biomechanics needs FEM. *The Finite Element Method in the 1990's*, Book dedicated to O.C. Zienkiewicz, eds. E. Oñate, J. Periaux & A. Samuelsson, Springer-Verlag/CIMNE, pp. 367–376, 1991.

[4] Doundoulakis, J.H., Eckert, S.E., Lindquist, C.C. & Jeffcoat, M.K., The implant-supported overdenture as an alternative to the complete mandibular denture. *J Am. Dent. Assoc.*, **134(11)**, pp. 1455–1458, 2003.

[5] Jokstad, A., Braegger, U., Brunski, J.B., Carr, A.B., Naert, I. & Wennerberg, A., Quality of dental implants. *Int. Dent. J.*, **53(6 Suppl 2)**, pp. 409–443, 2003.

[6] Calderale, P.M., Fasolio, G. & Mongini F., Experimental analysis of strains influencing mandibular remodelling. *Acta Orthopaedica Belgica*, **46(5)**, pp. 601–610, 1980.

[7] Frost, H.M., Skeletal structural adaptions to mechanical usage (SATMU): 1. Redefining Wolff's law: the bone remodelling problem. *Anatomic Records*, **226**, pp. 403–413, 1990.

[8] Hoshaw, S.J., Brunski, J.B. & Cochran G.V.B., Mechanical loading of Brånemark implants affects interfacial bone modeling and remodeling. *Int. J. Oral and Maxillofacial Implants*, **9**, pp. 345–360, 1994.

[9] Duyck, J., Ronold, H.J., Van Oosterwyck, H., Naert, I., Vander Sloten, J. & Ellingsen, J.E., The influence of static and dynamic loading on marginal bone reactions around osseointegrated implants: an animal experimental study. *Clin. Oral Implants Res.*, **12(3)**, pp. 207–218, 2001.

[10] Roberts, W.E., Hohlt, W.F. & Analoui, M., Implant-anchored space closure as a viable alternative to fixed prostheses. *Biological Mechanisms of Tooth Movement and Craniofacial Adaptation*, eds. Z. Davidovitch & L.A. Norton, Harvard Society for the Advancements of Orthodontics, Boston, pp. 617–621, 1996.

[11] Surgical Centre, www.glorenzon.it

[12] Haribhakti, V.V., The dentate adult human mandible: an anatomic basis for surgical decision making. *Plast. Reconstr. Surg.*, **97(3)**, pp. 536–541, 1996.

[13] Terheyden, H., Muhlendyck, C., Sprengel, M., Ludwig, K. & Harle, F., Self-adapting washer system for lag screw fixation of mandibular fractures. Part II: *In vitro* mechanical characterization of 2.3 and 2.7 mm lag screw prototypes and *in vivo* removal torque after healing. *J. Craniomaxillofacial Surg.*, **27(4)**, pp. 243–251, 1999.

[14] Lorenzon, G., Bignardi, C., Zanetti, E.M. & Pertusio R., Analisi BIOMECCANICA di sistemi implantari. *Dental Cadmos*, **10**, pp. 63–86, 2003.

[15] Luo, X., Ouyang, G. & Ma, X., Three dimensional finite element analysis on the mandibular complete overdenture supported by nature roots or implants, *Zhonghua Kou Qiang Yi Xue Za Zhi*, **33(5)**, pp. 303–305, 1998.

[16] Giesen, E.B., Ding, M., Dalstra, M. & Van Eijden, T.M., Changed morphology and mechanical properties of cancellous bone in the mandibular condyles of edentate people. *J. Dent. Res.*, **83(3)**, pp. 255–259, 2004.

[17] Meyer, U., Vollmer, D., Runte, C., Bourauel, C. & Joos, U., Bone loading pattern around implants in average and atrophic edentulous maxillae: a finite-element analysis. *J. Craniomaxillofacial Surg.*, **29**, pp. 100–105, 2001.

[18] Zitzmann, N.U. & Scharer, P., Sinus elevation procedures in the resorbed posterior maxilla. Comparison of the crestal and lateral approaches. *Oral Surg. Oral Med. Oral Pathol. Oral Radiol. Endod.*, **85(1)**, pp. 8–17, 1998.

[19] Smiler, D.G., Holmes, R.E., Sinus lift procedure using porous hydroxiapatite: A preliminary clinical report. *J. Oral Implantology*, **13**, pp. 239–253, 1987.

[20] Apolloni, M., *Atlante Pratico di Implantologia Dentale*, Edi-Ermes, Milano, 1989.

[21] Hart, R.T., Hennebel, V.V., Thongpreda, N., Van Buskirk, W.C. & Anderson, R.C., Modeling the biomechanics of the mandibole: a three-dimensional finite element study. *J. Biomechanics*, **25(3)**, pp. 261–286, 1992.

[22] O'Mahony, A.M., Williams, J.L. & Spencer P., Anisotropic elasticity of cortical and cancellous bone in the posterior mandible increases peri-implant stress and strain under oblique loading. *Clin. Oral Implants Res.*, **12(6)**, pp. 648–657, 2001.

[23] Christensen, L.L., Djurhuus, J.C. & Constantinou, C.E., Imaging of pelvic floor contraction using MRI. *Neurourol. Urodyn.*, **14(3)**, pp. 209–216, 1995.

[24] Hoyte, L., Fielding, J.R., Versi, E., Mamisch, C., Kolvenbach, C. & Kikinis, R., Variations in levator ani volume and geometry in women. The application of MR based 3D reconstruction in evaluating pelvic floor dysfunction. *Arch. Esp. Urol.*, **54(6)**, pp. 532–539, 2001.

[25] Myers, R., Cahill, D., Devine, R. & King, B., Anatomy of radical prostatectomy as defined by magnetic resonance imaging. *J. Urol.*, **159(6)**, pp. 2148–2158, 1998.

[26] Poore, R.E., Cullough, D.L. & Jarow. J.P., Puboprostatic ligament sparing improves urinary continence after radical retropubic prostatectomy. *Urology*, **51(1)**, pp. 67–72, 1998.

[27] Marino, G. & Bignardi, C., Urological surgery needs biomechanics. *Proc. of the 2nd European Uro-Oncological Forum*, Fontanafredda, in press, 2004.

[28] Regnier, C.H., Kolsky, H., Richardson, P.D., Ghoniem, G.M. & Susset, J.G., The elastic behaviour of the urinary bladder for large deformations. *J. Biomechanics*, **16(11)**, pp. 915–922, 1983.

[29] Asped, R.M., Larsson, T., Svenson, R. & Heinegard, D., Computer controlled mechanical testing machine for small samples of biological viscoelastic materials. *J. Biomed. Eng.*, **13(6)**, pp. 521–526, 1991.

[30] Yahia, L.H., Audet, J. & Drouin, G., Rheological properties of the human lumbar spine ligaments. *J. Biomed. Eng.*, **13(5)**, pp. 399–406, 1991.

CHAPTER 8

A numerical evaluation of the posterior cruciate ligament reconstruction on the biomechanics of the knee joint

N.A. Ramaniraka[1], A. Terrier[1], N. Theumann[2] & O. Siegrist[3]

[1] *Division of Orthopaedics Research, Swiss Federal Institute of Technology, Lausanne, Switzerland.*
[2] *Radiology Department, Centre Hospitalier Universitaire du Canton de Vaud, Lausanne, Switzerland.*
[3] *Hôpital Orthopédique de la Suisse Romande, Lausanne, Switzerland.*

Abstract

Previous clinical studies suggested that a nonoperative treatment of a posterior cruciate ligament (PCL) tear might induce late knee arthrosis, despite its good short-term results. Nevertheless, the results of operative treatment of PCL injuries remains unclear, the kinematics of the knee is not always restored. Knee arthrosis has been reported in 20% to 60% of patients after operative treatment.

Many investigations have focused on PCL surgical techniques to restore the function of the knee after PCL reconstruction. Clinical follow-up and experimental measurements were conducted to investigate the effectiveness of PCL reconstruction techniques. These studies have shown that, in the short-term, both single and double bundles PCL reconstruction can restore the kinematics of the knee. However, in these studies, the kinematics only were measured with anteroposterior loads or knee flexion. Nowadays, few data have been reported on the biomechanical behavior of the knee after PCL reconstruction under functional loading conditions. The lack of a biomechanical basis may in part explain the poorer clinical outcomes following PCL injury and surgery. A better knowledge of the biomechanics of the knee after PCL reconstruction may bring new insights for a better surgical reconstruction.

We propose a numerical model of a knee joint to evaluate the effects of PCL reconstruction techniques on the biomechanics of the knee joint, namely the compressive force in the tibiofemoral and patellofemoral compartments, and the tensile stress generated inside the PCL bundles.

1 Introduction

The PCL is one of the primary ligament stabilizers of the knee. Its main role is to prevent a posterior translation of the tibia. A rupture of the PCL is source of laxity, which may induce a disabling function of the knee joint. In the long-term, this leads to abnormal cartilaginous wear and then to premature knee arthritis. PCL injuries are less common than anterior cruciate ligament (ACL) injuries, and they often go unrecognized. In the literature [1] their incidence ranges 3–20% of all ligament injuries versus 45–90% for ACL tears. Despite its relative importance, the PCL has received much less attention regarding its anatomical and biomechanical roles in the knee joint function. The insufficiency of biomechanical basis may in part explain the poorer clinical outcomes following PCL injury and surgery [2]. Basically, the replacement of the deficient ligament is expected to restore the initial knee stability. Although this surgical technique is widespread, long-term clinical results are still inconsistent and the knee joint function is unfortunately not always restored [3]. A main cause of this inconsistency is the deterioration of the mechanical properties of the graft due to the nonphysiologically high tension applied to the graft [4, 5]. A high tension induces poor vascularity and focal myxoid degeneration in the patellar tendon graft used for cruciate ligament reconstruction [5]. A plastic deformation of the ligament occurs and involves a molecular reorganization and a tissue weakening. The microfractures, generated by abnormal loading, cannot be repaired sufficiently quickly, then the structure disaggregates and weakens.

The inconsistency of PCL replacement motivated the present study. A PCL replacement may be improved if the biomechanical behavior and the kinematics of the knee joint are better controlled. To improve current surgical results, it is essential to look further into the interaction of the PCL with the other joint elements. Namely, the knowledge of the joint bearing forces (tibiofemoral and patellofemoral compartments) and the forces inside different structures of the knee is required to better understand the biomechanical behavior of the joint.

In this study, a numerical model was developed to evaluate the effects of PCL reconstruction techniques on the biomechanics of the knee. In a first step, we have generated the numerical model of an individualized knee joint including bones and major soft tissues. The *second step* consisted to evaluate the influence of surgical reconstruction techniques on the force generated in the femorotibial and patellofemoral compartments, and on the stress induced in the PCL with the developed model.

2 Previous works on PCL

2.1 Anatomy and biomechanical properties of the PCL

The PCL is a ligament extended from the lateral surface of the medial femoral condyle to the posterior part of the tibia [3, 4, 6, 7]. The PCL is composed of anterolateral (AL) and posteromedial (PM) fibres bulks [8–10]. The geometries of the PCL were also evaluated [11, 12]. Each fibre bulk has different functions over the range of flexion: the AL component is tight in flexion and lax in extension; conversely, the PM component is tight in extension and lax in flexion.

Mechanical properties of the PCL were reported in previous studies [2, 13–16]. Prietto *et al.* [14] proposed one value to define the PCL linear stiffness (204 N/mm) for the two bundles whereas Harner *et al.* [2] found that the linear stiffness of the AL fibre bulk was significantly larger (2.6 times) than that of PM one. Mechanical properties of PCL are then often approximated by these stiffness values despite its evident non-linearity. In the recent studies, Pioletti *et al.* [15] have developed an experimental setting to identify the viscoelastic behavior of the ACL and PCL. They have fitted the viscoelastic constitutive law, obtained from experimental measurements, with hyperelastic law. Weiss *et al.* [16] has represented the ligament as a fibre-reinforced composite with transversely isotropic material symmetry using a hyperelastic strain energy uncoupling deviatoric and dilatational behavior.

2.2 Reconstruction techniques

Two different techniques are usually adopted for PCL reconstruction: (a) reconstruction with one bundle graft replacing the AL fibre bulk, and (b) reconstruction with two bundles graft replacing the AL and PM fibre bulks. The one bundle reconstruction was thought to control the posterior translation over the entire range of knee flexion [17, 18], but abnormal posterior translation frequently appeared in the long term due probably to graft elongation [19, 20]. Two-bundles reconstructions were then investigated to prevent graft elongation.

The abilities of these PCL reconstruction techniques have been compared in previous studies [21, 22]: (a) a one bundle reconstruction, and (b) a two bundles reconstruction. They concluded that a double-bundle PCL reconstruction restored better the normal knee laxity than the one bundle isometric reconstruction. In the same way, Harner *et al.* [19] have shown that the kinematics behavior of intact knee with a "native" PCL and a knee with double bundles reconstruction are similar. The posterior tibia translation with double bundles did not significantly differ from the intact knee, while a sensible difference of behavior was found with a one bundle reconstruction. Reconstruction with double bundles also restored the *in situ* forces more closely than did the single-bundle reconstruction: the force generated in the graft with one bundle reconstruction was lower than force in the intact knee [19]. Mannor *et al.* [23] experimentally investigated the influence of the insertion sites on the graft tension during a knee flexion. They performed the measurements of posterior tibia translation during knee flexion in four cases: (a) intact knee, (b) PCL resection, (c) one-bundle reconstruction, and (d) two-bundles reconstruction by using 12 cadaveric knee joints. PCL tension in the intact knee and graft tensions with one and two-bundles reconstruction were also measured. They concluded that two-bundles reconstruction controlled better the posterior tibial translation. Moreover, bundles tension during knee flexion depended on the femoral insertion sites.

Despite improvement of PCL reconstruction with two-bundles grafts, the long-term resistance to posterior translation remains unknown. Further biomechanical analysis is still needed for rational choice between these two techniques.

2.3 Influence of graft insertion

The location of the PCL insertion was already evaluated in previous studies. Bois-gard *et al.* [24] have reconstructed a 3D computed model of the knee joint from *in vivo* MRI acquisitions. They have used the model to perform an anatomical study of the PCL during flexion (0° to 75°), and an assessment of the optimal location for an intra-articular graft. They took 13 acquisitions from 0 to 75° of flexion and used the Delaunay reconstruction to obtain a 3D geometric model. A matching process to fix one part of the articulation during the movement, allows for the kinematics analysis of the tibia relative to the fixed femur. Their model allows calculating the displacement of a bone point during knee flexion. Knowing the relative displacement of the bone insertions of the ligament, they determine the length of the PCL and its bands and evaluate the length variation during movement. They also determine the optimal location for the insertion of a graft that would lead to the least stretch during flexion. During flexion the posterior band increases its length by 10% at 50°, and by 20% at 75° of flexion. The anterior band stretched more, and might reach 40% elongation at 75° of flexion. The best position for insertion of a graft was in the postero-lateral portion of the anatomical tibia insertion, and posterior to the anatomical femoral insertion. This method confirms the data in the literature and specifies the points of insertion for a graft, which lead to the least variation in length during flexion.

Carlin *et al.* [25] have developed an experimental method of measuring the *in situ* forces in a ligament with a universal force-moment sensor (UFS). They attached a UFS to the tibia and measured *in situ* forces of the human PCL as a function of knee flexion in response to tibia loading. At a 50-N posterior tibia load, the force in the PCL increased from 25 N at 30° to 48 N at 90° of knee flexion. At 100 N, the corresponding increases were to 50 N and 95 N, respectively. Of note, at 30° knee flexion, approximately 45% of the resistance to posterior tibia loading was caused by contact between the tibia and the femoral condyles, whereas, at 90° of knee flexion, no resistance was caused by such contact.

2.4 Pre-tension in the PCL

After PCL reconstruction, a majority of knees present residual anterior-posterior laxity due to inadequate graft pre-tensioning [23, 26].

Markolf *et al.* [27] have measured force generated in the graft as a function of the amount of pre-tension applied to the bone block of the free end of the graft, which is inserted in the tibia tunnel. They applied a pretension at 90° of flexion. The anterior-posterior laxity was then measured at different angles of knee flexion by using a load-cell on the PCL. They found that the level of pre-tension needed to restore normal anterior-posterior laxity at 90° of flexion ranged from 6 to 100 N (mean: 43 N).

A biomechanical study was conducted by Wang *et al.* [28] to investigate the optimal graft tension and the mode of fixation in PCL reconstruction. They measured the PCL tension at different angles of knee flexion with a force transducer, and the optimal tension of the PCL graft that allows a full range of knee motion was studied with a tension-meter in 12 cadaver knees. The modes of fixation failure between interference screw fixation and post fixation were studied with an Instron (Canton, MA) machine in 8 cadaver knees. They found that the optimal tension of PCL graft, which allows full range of knee motion, was 68 N. The average load of graft failure was 417 N with interference screw fixation and 367 N with post fixation when the patellar bone-tendon-bone graft was tested. The sites of failure for interference screw fixation were caused by rupture of ligament substance and bone plug pullout; those of post fixation were caused by rupture of ligament substance, fracture, and as a result of suture breakage. Wang *et al.* [28] suggested that a 367 N tension to the graft at 20° to 30° of knee flexion is optimal in PCL reconstruction.

The initial tension applied to the graft at the time of fixation is one of the most important factors affecting the outcome of cruciate ligaments reconstruction. Orthopaedic surgeons have generally preferred to apply a relatively high degree of initial tension on the autograft during ACL reconstruction surgery. In the field of basic science, however, only a few experimental studies have been conducted to evaluate the effect of high initial tension on the results after ligament reconstruction. Yoshiya *et al.* [29] investigated the effects of initial loads on a patellar tendon graft. They observed poor vascularity and focal myxoid degeneration within the graft pretensioned with a load of 39 N, but not within the graft pretensioned with a load of 1 N. They suggested that a high degree of tension might be detrimental to the patellar tendon autograft during surgical reconstruction of the ACL. In contrast, Arms *et al.* [30] and Fischer *et al.* [31] looked at ultimate failure loads in patellar tendon grafts fixed with high tension and with low tension. One year after reconstruction, the high-tension grafts had inferior failure loads compared with the low-tension grafts. A major reason for the disagreement about the effects of high initial tension on the autograft between studies is that intraoperative and postoperative variables, such as graft volume, strength, isometry, fixation strength, and postoperative management, are varied using free-tendon autografts.

Despite these previous studies, there is no consensus on the range values of prescribed pretension needed to restore the function of the knee. To clarify the effect of pretension on the autograft, it is necessary to develop a numerical model in which the effect of pretension can be isolated from other factors.

2.5 Types of grafts for PCL reconstruction

Different types of grafts are proposed for the PCL reconstruction. These grafts may be autograft (patient's own tissue), allograft (tissue taken from another person) or synthetic graft.

Autografts using hamstring tendons and central third bone patella tendon bone (BPTB) are usually used with good outcomes [32]. The quadriceps tendon is also used as graft and present thick with good biomechanical properties [33]. However, the quadriceps strength may significantly decrease with time.

Allografts provide the graft material in a freeze-dried, fresh-frozen, irradiated or preserved state. The effects of these processes on the mechanical properties of the graft remain unclear [33].

Synthetic ligaments are not currently used for PCL reconstruction, as their long-term follow-up results are not yet well known. Synthetic grafts are stiff with poor elastic properties.

2.6 Numerical models of the knee including the PCL

Previous studies [34–40] have been conducted to measure the knee kinematics and the evolution of the joint contact areas by using 3D numerical models. A 3D mathematical model of the knee was developed in [38]. The model was validated with experimental kinematics measurements on the same knee. They determined the strains of the ligaments by using an optimization procedure based on the minimization of the difference between the kinematics of the model and the experimental data for given values of ligament stiffness. The model was tested with anterior-posterior and varus-valgus laxities. Results were then compared with data in the literature. The model was simplified by considering ligaments as multiple straight-line elements, which connect the femur and the tibia and not with 3D geometries [40]. Friction at the contact surfaces was neglected and the stabilization due to menisci was not taken into account the passive model of the knee was only simulated. Mommersteeg et al. [39] have improved the model by using multi-bundle structures with non-uniform mechanical properties and zero force lengths as ligaments. The model was validated with experimental kinematics measurements data (anterior/posterior and varus/valgus laxities) of the same knees. In the improved 3D numerical reconstructions, the patello-femoral joint was not taken into account.

Li et al. [34] developed a 3D finite element tibio-femoral joint model of a human knee joint. The 3D geometry was reconstructed from magnetic resonance (MR) images of a cadaveric knee specimen. The same specimen was tested using a robotic/UFS system. Knee kinematics data under anterior-posterior tibia loads (up to 100 N) were obtained. Reference lengths (zero-load lengths) of the ligaments and stiffness of the meniscus springs were estimated by using an optimization procedure that involved the minimization of the differences between the kinematics predicted by the model and those obtained experimentally. The joint kinematics and in situ forces in the ligaments in response to axial tibia moments of up to 10 Nm were calculated by using the model and were compared with published experimental data on knee specimens. However, in their model, the ligaments were modeled with non-linear elastic springs, and menisci were simulated by equivalent-resistance springs. This model did not allow calculation of stress in the soft tissues as accurately as desired.

Jilani et al. [35] developed a 3D finite element model of tibio-femoral joint, which includes various elements as femur, tibia, cartilage, meniscus, and ligaments. The model was used to investigate the non-linear response of the tibio-femoral joint during full extension under internal-external torques of up to 10 Nm applied to the femur. The influences of ligaments resection were investigated. They found that under femoral internal torque, there were no significant changes on the tensile forces in the ligaments, while under external torque; important changes were observed in the ligament tension forces. Moreover, a resection of the lateral collateral ligament (LCL) increased the forces inside the ACL and PCL. Similar large cruciate ligament forces were also observed under varus-valgus moments subsequent to a collateral ligament injury [36].

Bendjaballah *et al.* [37] used a 3D finite element model of the human tibiofemoral joint to investigate the mechanics of the knee under drawer forces. They deduced that PCL and ACL were the primary restraints to femoral anterior and posterior drawer forces, respectively. They also found that a resection of one of these ligaments increased drastically the joint anterior-posterior motion. Moreover, section of cruciate ligaments (PCL and ACL) induced large tensile forces in collateral ligaments, which increased the pressure on the tibia plateau transmitted through menisci.

2.7 Effects of loading on the ligament mechanical properties

Initial graft tension is one of the important factors that influence the long-term results of cruciate ligaments reconstruction. Katsuragi *et al.* [41] reported that high initial tension induced poor vascularity and focal myxoid degeneration in a patellar tendon graft used for ACL reconstruction in a canine model. Moreover, an unphysiologically high initial tension caused deterioration of the mechanical properties of the cruciate ligaments. In addition, an excessively high initial graft tension would increase compressive forces at the tibiofemoral joint, inducing damage to the articular cartilage. However, studies have shown that excessively low graft tension also causes rapid deterioration of the mechanical properties of the grafted tendon. Yasuda *et al.* [42] showed that an immobilisation of joints might deteriorate the mechanical properties of tendons and ligaments, and reduced their cross-sectional area. A stress deprivation has been regarded as an essential causative factor in joint disuse. Even if joint motion is allowed, stress deprivation rapidly reduced the mechanical properties of the tendon and ligament tissues, and increased the cross-sectional area of them. Restressing increased the mechanical properties once reduced by stress deprivation. The reduction of the ultimate stress might be explained by the reduction of the total area of collagen fibrils in tendon cross-section and the increase of thin and immature fibrils.

3 Numerical model of the knee joint

3.1 Data acquisitions

Magnetic resonance images (MRIs) and CT-scanner images acquisitions were performed on the right knee of a volunteer. The knee was immobilized in full extension inside a plaster to avoid any movement during acquisition, and was

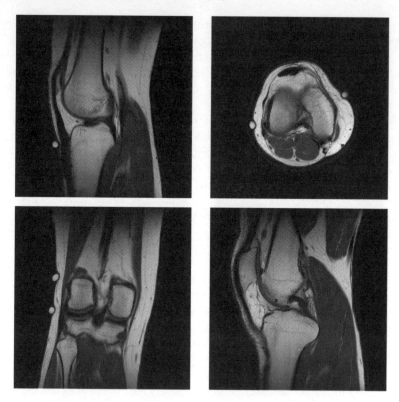

Figure 1: MRIs in the sagittal, coronal, and frontal planes.

fixed on a support radio-transparency. Six points of references (3 points on the femur and 3 points on the tibia) were placed on the lower limb in order to super-impose the 3D geometries models of bone and soft structures reconstructed from MRI and CT-scanner images (figs 1 and 2).

3.1.1 MRIs acquisition
MRIs were used for the geometry reconstruction of soft structures (ligaments, menisci, tendons, cartilage). A MR scanner (Siemens, model Magnetom Symphony) was used for acquisition. The optimal size of the pixels (pixel spacing) was 0.39 mm, with a resolution of 512×512 pixels, with a thickness of cuts of 3 mm. The images were taken in the sagittal, coronal and transverse plans.

3.1.2 CT images acquisition
CT-scanner images were used for 3D geometry reconstruction of bone structures. Acquisition was done in helical mode. The thickness of the cuts was 1.25 mm.

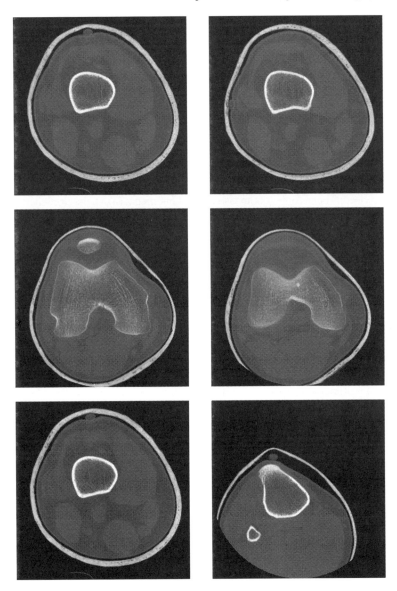

Figure 2: CT images of the knee joint in helical mode. Six points of reference were used to match the MRIs and CT-scanners images.

3.2 Numerical modeling

3.2.1 Constitutive laws of ligaments and patellar tendons

A biomechanical model of cruciate ligaments and patellar tendons of the knee joint was developed in our laboratory [43]. The model accounts for large strains and non-linear viscoelasticity to better understand its biomechanical properties. To this end, a custom-made experimental set-up was developed to measure the stress-strain curves with different rate of deformations and the stress relaxation at different deformations by controlling temperature and humidity.

The constitutive laws of soft tissues were based on the generalized standard material and were developed for large displacements situations, differing to most of material models previously developed. This allowed us to integrate them in 3D numerical model of joints (knee, shoulder or hip joint) in order to calculate the stress inside soft and bone structures as well as the large amplitude kinematics of the joint.

Results from our experimental set-up have shown that cruciate ligaments and patellar tendons exhibit a non-linear elastic behavior in addition to a viscous behavior. The viscous behavior encompassed two phenomena: (a) a behavior where stress depended on strain rate (short-term memory effects), and (b) a behavior where stress relaxed on a longer time scale (long-term memory effects).

In order to describe the different mechanical behaviors of the specimens in a general mechanical framework, a theoretical model was developed by simultaneously taking into account the non-linear elastic behaviors [15, 43], the short-term memory effects and the long-term memory effects. This proceeding satisfied the basic mechanical and thermodynamics requirements [43–45]. The original model, based on the different mechanical behaviors, described in one framework a compact description of different soft tissues. The description of the short-term memory effects was new in situations involving large deformations. Considering the specimens as isotropic, homogeneous and incompressible restricted the model.

The identification process of the different mechanical behaviors was facilitated with the proposed model. The non-linear elasticity was described with two parameters, the short-term memory effects with one parameter and the long-term memory effects with six parameters. No statistical differences were found between the parameters used for the ACLs, the PCLs and patellar tendons.

The non-linear elastic behavior was then implemented in a finite element code. The stress field in an ACL was calculated during a knee flexion and a tibial drawer test. The calculated stress field was inhomogeneous, with the highest stress in the anteromedial part of the ACL. It was found that internal rotation of the knee generally increased the calculated stress in the ACL. These numerical results agreed with *in vitro* studies found in the literature. The numerical results yielded a stress field in the ligament that was complementary to *in vitro* studies, where only the resultant ligament force can be measured.

Several useful clinical conclusions could be drawn from this biomechanical study. Diagnosis of an ACL rupture is generally performed by a contralateral comparison of antero-posterior knee laxity (tibial drawer test) using a quasi-static load. However, diagnosis of an injured knee would be more accurate if the antero-posterior load was dynamically applied to the knee: in this case, a knee with a rupture of the ACL would not show any effect, whereas a knee with an intact ACL would become stiffer when increasing the strain rate. In case of ACL replacement, the graft should be preconditioned in order to diminish the effects of stress relaxation. During the rehabilitation program after an ACL suture or replacement, flexion of the knee in an internal position should be omitted because internal rotation increases the stresses in the ligament.

3.2.2 3D reconstruction of bones and soft tissues

The Amira software was used for semi-automatic segmentation of MRI and CT-scanner images. Bones and soft structures were matched by using the 6 reference points fixed on femur and tibia during image acquisitions. The curves obtained from segmentation were transferred in Patran software to reconstruct the 3D geometry of the joint and to mesh the bone and soft structures with finite elements methods (FEMs) (fig. 3).

Bones were considered as rigid bodies and soft structures were meshed with 8-node hexahedral volume elements. The insertion zones of ligaments (ACL, PCL, LCL, medical collateral ligament (MCL)) on the femoral and tibial bones were obtained from the registration of MRI and CT-slices.

Soft structures were modeled with the non-linear hyperelastic law corresponding to the strain energy developed in [15]. The passive stress-strain law applied to soft tissues is based on this potential recently applied for other joint soft tissues [15].

The MCL, LCL, ACL, and PCL were taken into account. These ligaments and the patellar tendon were modeled with the non-linear hyperelastic law corresponding to the strain energy [46]:

$$W_e = \alpha \exp\left[\beta(I_1 - 3) - \frac{\alpha\beta}{2}(I_2 - 1)\right] \tag{1}$$

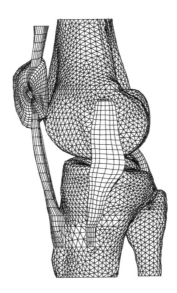

Figure 3: Mediolateral view of the knee joint. The model includes main bones (femur, tibia, patella, fibula) and soft structures (PCL, ACL, collateral ligaments, cartilage layers and the patellar tendon).

Table 1: Values of materials constant α and β for the
ACL, PCL and patellar tendon.

	α (MPa)	β
ACL	0.30	12.20
PCL	0.18	17.35
Patellar tendon	0.09	66.96

W_e is the strain energy, α and β are material constants, and I_1 and I_2 are the strain invariants.

$$I_1 = \operatorname{tr}[C], \tag{2}$$

$$I_2 = \frac{1}{2}\left([\operatorname{tr}C]^2 - \operatorname{tr}[C]^2\right) \tag{3}$$

$C = F^T F$ is the (right Cauchy-Green) material metric tensor, where $F = \partial y/\partial x$ is the gradient deformation tensor.

The mean values of α and β were obtained from experimental measurements and reported in the table 1.

The cartilages layers of the tibia, femur and patella were considered as homogenous isotropic materials (Young's modulus: 12 MPa, Poisson's ratio: 0.45) [47].

3.2.2.1 Contact surface modeling   The tibiofemoral, patellofemoral and meniscofemoral joints were modeled with frictional discontinuous unilateral contact elements allowing large slip. Coulomb friction was used for tangential contact law. The coefficient of friction was set to 0.1.

3.2.2.2 Loading conditions   The loading condition was a full flexion of the knee, from full extension to 90° of flexion. Flexion of 90° was obtained by applying forces in the directions of the biceps femoris and the semi-tendinosus muscles. The femur was fixed and the tibia was free in the 6 degrees of freedom.

The quadriceps muscles were represented with 80 linear springs fixed in the upper part. The biceps muscles were represented with 2 linear springs. The mechanical property of the quadriceps was obtained from literature [33].

3.2.3 Numerical implementation

The numerical simulations were performed with the Finite Element software Abaqus/Standard. The model was applied to calculate the compressive force in the patellofemoral and the tibiofemoral compartments, and the stresses inside soft structures.

In order to evaluate the effects of PCL reconstruction on the biomechanics of the knee, four cases were then simulated. A knee with:

(a) *Native PCL*: The insertion zones of ligaments were obtained by matching the MRIs and CT-scans slices (fig. 4).

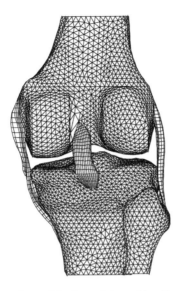

Figure 4: Posteroanterior view of the knee joint with a "native" PCL. The "native" PCL and collateral ligaments are presented.

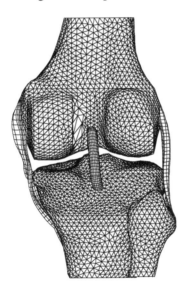

Figure 5: Posterior view of a one bundle reconstructed PCL. Only, the anterolateral bundle was replaced with an autograft.

(b) *Sectioned PCL.*
(c) *Reconstructed PCL with one bundle graft*: The femoral and tibial attachments of the bundle graft were located within the native anterolateral PCL insertion locations (fig. 5).

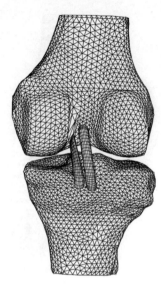

Figure 6: Posterior view of a two bundles reconstructed PCL. The right ligament represent the anterolateral bundle and the left that of the posteromedial ligaments.

(d) *Reconstructed PCL with two bundles graft*: The attachments of the bundles graft were located within the native anterolateral and posteromedial insertion locations (fig. 6). Mechanical property of patellar tendon was used for grafts.

4 Results

4.1 Medial tibiofemoral compartment

The compressive forces in the medial tibiofemoral compartment, during a knee flexion, were calculated in the four cases (native PCL, sectioned PCL, one bundle reconstruction and two bundles reconstruction). The distributions of these compressive forces were shown, for a "native" PCL and sectioned PCL in figs 7 and 8. It was observed that the maximal values of the compressive force in the medial compartment occurred at 65° of flexion.

The maximal values of compressive force in the medial femorotibial compartment are reported in the table 2.

4.2 Lateral tibiofemoral compartment

The compressive force in the lateral tibiofemoral compartment was also calculated during a knee flexion. The behaviors of native PCL and reconstructed PCL were similar; no significant difference was found with the native PCL and reconstructed

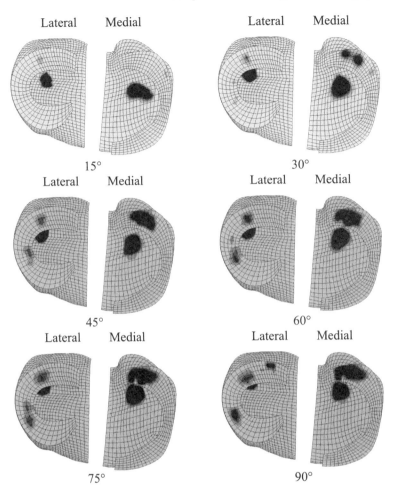

Figure 7: Distribution of the compressive force at the cartilage layer of the tibial compartments of an intact knee with "native" PCL during a knee flexion. The contact surface in the tibiofemoral compartment is composed of the part of the tibia cartilage uncovered by the menisci and the part covered by the menisci. The dark grey represent the zone with high pressure.

PCL at different angles of flexion. A sectioned PCL induced a lower compressive force in the lateral tibiofemoral.

The maximal values of compressive force in the lateral femorotibial compartment are reported in the table 3.

4.3 Patellofemoral compartment

The pressure generated in the patellofemoral compartment by the knee flexion was also calculated (fig. 9). The value of patellar contact force increased with knee

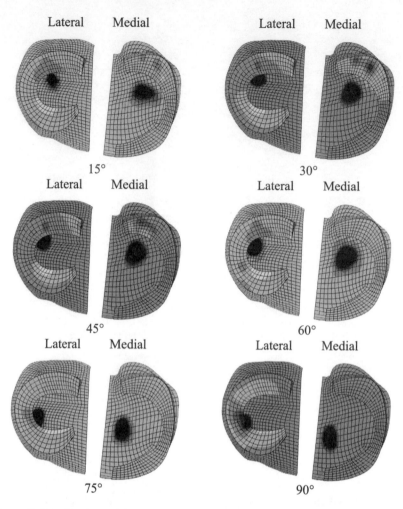

Figure 8: Distribution of the compressive force at the cartilage layer of the tibial
compartments of a knee with sectioned PCL during a knee flexion. The
contact surface in the tibiofemoral compartment is composed of the part
of the tibia cartilage uncovered by the menisci and the part covered by
the menisci.

flexion angle. No significant difference was found between the pressure induced
with a native and reconstructed PCL. A sectioned PCL induced a higher force than
in the other cases. The distribution of the contact pressure at the cartilage layer of
the patella was reported at a different angles of flexion (fig. 10).

The maximal values of compressive force in the patellofemoral compartments
are reported in the table 4.

Table 2: Maximal values of joint bearing forces in the medial tibiofemoral compartment.

	Compressive force (N)
A "native" PCL	338
A sectioned PCL	445
One bundle reconstructed PCL	311
Two bundles reconstructed PCL	378

Table 3: Maximal values of joint bearing forces in the lateral tibiofemoral compartment.

	Compressive force (N)
A "native" PCL	255
A sectioned PCL	183
One bundle reconstructed PCL	238
Two bundles reconstructed PCL	288

Table 4: Maximal values of joint bearing forces in the patellofemoral compartment.

	Compressive force (N)
A "native" PCL	398
A sectioned PCL	440
One bundle reconstructed PCL	402
Two bundles reconstructed PCL	398

4.4 Tensile stress in the PCL

The occurrence of excessive tensile stress inside the PCL graft is a source of failure in the PCL reconstruction. The maximal values of tensile stress inside the native and the reconstructed PCL, during a knee flexion, were calculated. The tensile stress inside the PCL increased with the angle of knee flexion.

The tensile stress inside the PM bundles of the native PCL and of the two bundles reconstructed was compared. The tensile stress inside the two bundles reconstructed PCL is slightly higher than that of the native PCL. The evolutions of tensile stress inside the PCL and grafts are reported in fig. 11.

The tensile stress inside the AL bundle was also calculated with the native and the two bundles reconstructed PCL, the stress inside the AL of the two bundles reconstruction was higher than that of the native PCL.

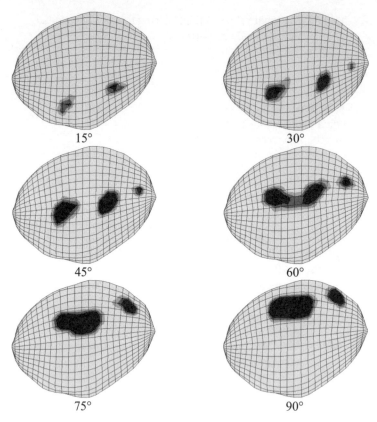

Figure 9: Distribution of the pressure at the cartilage layer of the patello-femoral compartment with an intact knee with a "native" PCL during the knee flexion, from 15° to 90°.

5 Discussion

After a PCL injury, the choice between an operative and a non-operative treatment remains controversial. For a surgical treatment, the surgeon might choose between one-bundle and two-bundles reconstructions. But, the long-term results of this treatment are unclear. The main subjects of studies in the literature were focused on the kinematics effects of PCL deficiency and of PCL reconstruction. To evaluate the effectiveness of surgical treatment, few experimental studies have been conducted in the past to measure the tibiofemoral and patellofemoral forces after PCL surgery [48–50]. No numerical calculations were conducted to evaluate the biomechanical effects of the PCL deficiency and its replacement. A numerical study might bring new insights to better understand the effectiveness of PCL reconstructions. The main goal of our study was to evaluate the biomechanical effects of a sectioning PCL and its replacement. To this end, we have firstly developed a numerical model of an intact knee as a reference model. In a second step, the PCL was replaced with

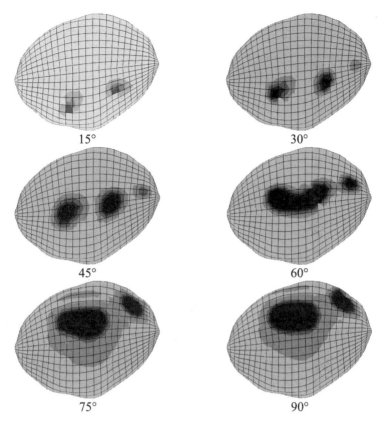

Figure 10: Distribution of the compressive stress at the cartilage layer of the patello-femoral compartment with a sectioned PCL during the knee flexion, from 15° to 90°.

a two-bundles graft, the insertion zones of the bundles were located at the insertion zones of the native PCL. In a third step, the PCL was replaced with a one-bundle reconstructed graft replacing the AL fiber of the PCL. Concerning the type of graft, autograft using central third bone patella tendons bone was usually used with good outcomes [19]. For this reason, the hyperelastic constitutive law of patellar tendon was used in the PCL reconstruction of our study. This law allowed a finite deformation of the soft tissues. In the last step, the PCL was sectioned. The model included the major bony and soft structures of the knee, mainly the ligaments, the cartilage layers, the menisci and the patellar tendon.

5.1 Medial tibiofemoral and patellofemoral compressive force

The medial tibiofemoral compressive force was the first biomechanical parameter calculated in this study. The highest value of compressive force was obtained with a sectioned PCL at 65° of knee flexion.

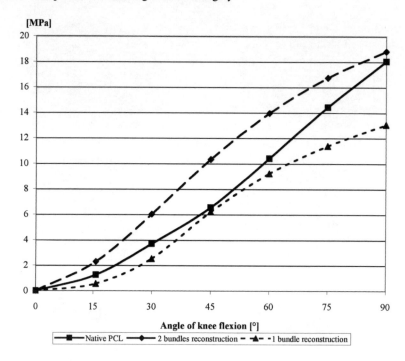

Figure 11: Evolution of the maximum tensile stress inside PCL during a knee flexion from 15° to 90° in (a) "native PCL", (b) two bundles reconstructed PCL, and (c) one bundle reconstructed PCL.

Moreover, Keller *et al.* [48] have suggested that despite a good short-term result of non-operative treatment of the PCL, late knee arthritis might occur. The occurrence of high compressive force in this joint was thought to be an important etiologic factor of late knee arthritis. High incidence of osteoarthritis was reported in the medial and patellofemoral compartments following conservative treatment of PCL injuries. PCL-deficiency was thought to increase high pressures in these compartments. Our results have shown, that a sectioned PCL induced a slightly high compressive force in the medial tibiofemoral compartment during the immediate post-operative period. The difference between the compressive forces induced by the sectioned PCL and by the reconstructed PCL was not significant. However, no numerical study has been conducted to date to evaluate this difference.

The high compressive force, observed in this study, in the medial tibiofemoral and patellofemoral compartments could be related to the pressure measured with a PCL-deficiency in the works of Singerman *et al.* [49] and Skyhar *et al.* [50] and might explain the occurrence of osteoarthritis developed in the long term in these regions with a nonoperatively treated PCL injuries [2]. In fact, it has been shown that a conservative treatment might induce in the long term a degeneration of the tibia cartilage layer. Singerman *et al.* [49] and Skyhar *et al.* [50] have found that a resection of the PCL might result in an approximate 10 percent increase in the medial tibiofemoral compressive force.

5.2 Lateral tibiofemoral compressive force

In our study, the intact knee with native PCL and the knees with reconstructed PCL induced nearly the same force in the lateral compartment. A slightly lower contact force in the patellofemoral compartment was observed with the sectioned PCL. As seen in several studies conducted in the past, the rupture of the PCL did not affect the lateral tibiofemoral compartment.

5.3 Tensile stress

In the cases of native PCL and reconstructed PCL, the high values of tensile stress occurred at the femoral insertion zones of the graft. As observed in the clinical cases, a rupture of the PCL might occur in these zones.

Fox *et al.* [4] have measured the tensile stress inside the PCL at different angles of knee flexion by applying a tibial anterior-posterior force. In this study, we have calculated the tensile stress generated inside the PCL by the movement of the tibia due to the applied force at the biceps and the semitendinosus muscles as described in the loading conditions, no tibial anterior-posterior force was applied.

We have found that the tensile stresses inside the native PCL and inside the two bundles reconstructed PCL were slightly greater than that of the one bundle reconstructed graft. This result corresponded with the work of Harner *et al.* [19]. They suggested that the tibiofemoral contacts and the posterolateral structures might share the load in the case of a one bundle reconstruction. Carlin *et al.* [25] have developed an experimental method of measuring the *in situ* forces in a ligament with a UFS. They measured the *in situ* forces of the human PCL as a function of knee flexion in response to tibia loading. At 30° knee flexion, approximately 45% of the resistance to posterior tibia loading was caused by contact between the tibia and the femoral condyles, whereas, at 90° of knee flexion, no resistance was caused by such contact.

Abdel-Rahman *et al.* [51] developed a complex mathematical model of an intact knee joint to calculate the tibiofemoral contact pressure and the ligament forces during a knee flexion. They have found that the force in the AL fibre of the PCL was maximal around 60° of knee flexion. In their model, the ligamentous structures were represented with spring elements extending from the femoral insertion to the tibial one. Moreover, the tibiofemoral contact surfaces were considered as planar surfaces. As a loading condition, they applied a posterior force at the center of mass of the tibia. Concerning the contact pressure in the tibiofemoral joint, they found that the medial contact force increased until 60° and then decreased until 90°. In the lateral compartment, the contact force decreased from full extension to 90° of flexion. By comparing their results with ours, it was found that the behaviors of the contact pressure in the medial compartment were similar with our results, but a difference of result was detected in the lateral compartment. We have found that the lateral contact force reached the maximum around 65° of flexion as in the medial compartment. We suggested that this difference in their results and our results might be due, on one hand, to the difference in the geometry of the tibial plateau and in the representation of the ligaments, and on other hand, to the difference of loading conditions.

5.4 Limitations of the model

There are several limitations of our model. First, the knee flexion was the only loading condition considered. Others loading conditions such as internal/external rotation or varus/valgus loading should be tested to better understand the biomechanical behavior of the knee with reconstructed PCL. Moreover, as seen in experimental measurements by other authors, the posterior tibial loading in the different angle of the knee flexion should be simulated to test the laxity of the knee after reconstruction or with a sectioned PCL.

The strain energy of the constitutive law was experimentally determined and identified. But, the cartilage constitutive law was that from the literature. In order to improve our model, a more sophisticated model should be used. Moreover, an anatomic biomechanical study should be conducted to investigate the optimal graft pretension during the PCL reconstruction.

5.5 Perspectives

In previous studies [41, 42], the main factors of the graft failure are micro-fractures. So, a new concept of soft tissue, based on the continuum with micro-cracks, is necessary to describe the long-term behavior of the mechanical properties of the PCL graft.

The theories of macroscopic properties of cracked solids predict the modification of the stiffness, the change of anisotropy orientation caused by micro-cracking. The development of a continuum theory dealing with micro-crack distribution has an obvious interest for mechanics of materials, mainly for the ligament in the framework of the present study. The model will be based on continuum mechanics, allowing discontinuity of scalar and vector fields, and on the basis of multi-field descriptors.

The ligament is a material with high anisotropy, due to the direction of the component fibres. Regarding, the structure of the ligament, the shear stress in the direction of the privileged direction is the main cause of micro-fractures.

For an isolated crack in a finite linear and elastic solid, the loading (tension, compression and shear) produces a crack opening displacement of the same mode only (uncoupled). In most situations, it is acceptable to neglect the relative influence of any cracks. In this case, at distances from the first crack that are much larger than the crack size, the expression for stress simplifies. The far-field asymptotes become applicable at a relatively close distance from the first crack and justify the basic assumption of non-interacting cracks. In reality, interactions of cracks may either increase the stiffness or decrease the stiffness of the material.

The distribution of micro-cracks is a function of the orientation of the contacting lips. The damage at each point of the material is quantified by a field of doublets (D, n), where D is the density of micro-cracks with normal n.

The model of damaged continuum is based on the discontinuity of fields (displacement, velocity). In this model, the field of cracks (here scalar and vector discontinuity) is entirely characterized by torsion and curvature tensors [52], considered as constitutive primal variables. It follows that the geometry of a continuum is defined by (a) a metric tensor and volume-form g, and (b) an affine connection D characterized by the torsion and curvature tensors (additional variables for a continuum with micro-cracks) [53].

Constitutive laws of creeping soft tissues will be derived based on the Coleman and Noll [54] class of materials. In this framework, the thermomechanics will be described as below.

The basic theory developed for generalized gradient materials in [52] will be adapted to capture the time evolution of the micro-crack distribution within the tissue, and therefore the changes of its mechanical properties over the time. More precisely, the transverse isotropy symmetry of soft tissue undergoing finite strain will be included in the continuum models of creeping ligaments (artificial or not). Then, the obtained constitutive laws will be discretized to allow implementation in finite element code. Since the increase of micro-crack density, captured by geometric variables, is probably not governed by differentiable evolution laws, some specific time integration (as implicit projection in finite elastoplasticity) should be developed and used e.g. [53] to ensure quadratic convergence of the finite element models and linearization methods.

References

[1] Harner, C.D. & Höher, J., Evaluation and treatment of PCL injuries. *Am. J. Sports Med.*, **26**, pp. 471–482, 1998.

[2] Harner, C.D., Vogrin, T.M. & Woo, S.L.Y., Anatomy and biomechanics of the PCL (Chapter 1). *PCL Injuries: A Practical Guide to Management*, ed. G.C. Fanelli, Springer: Berlin and New York, pp. 3–22, 2001.

[3] Bomberg, B., Acker, J. & Boyle, J., The effects of PCL loss and reconstruction on the knee. *Am. J. Knee Surgery*, **3(2)**, pp. 85–96, 1990.

[4] Fox, R.J., Harner, C.D., Sakane, M., Carlin, G.J. & Woo, S.L.Y., Determination of the in situ forces in the human PCL using robotic technology. A cadaveric stuy. *Am. J. Sports Med.*, **26(3)**, pp. 395–401, 1998.

[5] Pearsal, A.T., Pyevich, M., Draganich, L., Larkin, J.J. & Reider, B., In vitro study of knee stability after posterior cruciate ligament reconstruction. *Clin. Orth. Related Res.*, **327**, pp. 264–271, 1996.

[6] Amis, A., Beynnon, B., Blankevoort, L., Chambat, P., Christel, P., Durselen, L., Friederich, N.F., Grood, E.S., Hertel, P., Jakob, R.P., Muller, W. & O'Brien, M., Proceedings of the EESKA Scientific Workshop on

Reconstruction of the anterior and posterior cruciate ligaments. *Knee Surgery, Sports Traumatology, Arthroscopy*, **2**, pp. 124–132, 1994.

[7] Cooper, D., PCL reconstruction: the anatomic and biomechanical basis. *Oper. Techn. Sports Med.*, **2(1)**, pp. 89–93, 1993.

[8] Race, A. & Amis, A., Loading of the two bundles of the PCL: an analysis of bundle function in A-P drawer. *J. Biomechanics*, **29(7)**, pp. 873–879, 1996.

[9] Burks, R.T., *Knee ligaments: Structure, Function, Injury and Repair*, eds. D. Daniel, W.H. Akeson & J.J. O'Connor, Raven Press: New York, pp. 59–76, 1990.

[10] Kannus, P., Bergfeld, J., Järvinen, M., Johnson, R.J., Pope, M. & Yasuda, K., Injuries to the PCL of the knee. *Sports Med.*, **12**, pp. 110–131, 1991.

[11] Lee, T.Q. & Woo, S.L.Y., A new method for determining cross-sectional area of soft tissues. *J. Biomech. Eng.*, **110**, pp. 110–114, 1988.

[12] Woo, S.L.Y., Danto, M.I., Ohland, K.J., Lee, T.Q. & Newton, P.O., The use of a laser micrometer system to determine the cross-sectional shape and area of ligaments: a comparative study of two existing method. *J. Biomech. Eng.*, **112**, pp. 426–431, 1990.

[13] Kennedy, J.C., Hawkins, R.J., Willis, R.B. & Danylchuck, K.D., Tension studies of human knee ligaments: yield point, ultimate failure, and disruption of the cruciate and tibial collateral ligaments. *J. Bone J. Surgery*, **58A**, pp. 350–355, 1976.

[14] Prietto, M.P., Bain, J.R., Stonebrook, S.N. & Settlage, R.A., Tensile strength of the human PCL. *Trans. ORS*, **13**, p. 195, 1988.

[15] Pioletti, D.P., Rakotomanana, L.R., Benvenuti, J.F. & Leyvraz, P.F., Viscoelastic constitutive law in large deformations: application to human knee ligaments and tendons. *J. Biomechanics*, **31(8)**, pp. 753–758, 1998.

[16] Weiss, J.A., Maker, B.N. & Govindjee, S., Finite element implementation of incompressible, tranversely isotropic hyperelasticity. *Comp. Meth. Appl. Mech. Eng.*, **135**, pp. 107–128, 1996.

[17] Anderson, J. & Noyes, F., Principles of posterior cruciate ligament reconstruction. *Orthopedics*, **18**, pp. 493–500, 1995.

[18] Chen, C., Chen, W. & Shih, C., Arthroscopic PCL reconstruction with quadriceps tendon-patellar bone autograft. *Archives of Orthopaedics and Trauma Surgery*, **119**, pp. 86–94, 1999.

[19] Harner, C.D., Janaushek, M.A., Kanamori, A., Yagi, M., Vogrin, T.M. & Woo, S.L.Y., Biomechanical analysis of a double bundle PCL reconstruction. *Am. J. Sports Med.*, **28(2)**, pp. 144–151, 2000.

[20] Harner, C., Vogrin, T., Hoher, J., Ma, C.B. & Woo, S.L.Y., Biomechanical analysis of a PCL. Deficiency of the posterolateral structures as a cause of graft failure. *Am. J. Sports Med.*, **28**, pp. 32–40, 2000.

[21] Stahelin, A.C., Sudkamp, N.P. & Weiler, A., Anatomic double-bundle PCL reconstruction using hamstring tendons. *Arthroscopy*, **17(1)**, pp. 88–95, 2001.

[22] Race, A. & Amis, A., PCL reconstruction. In vitro biomechanical comparison of 'isometric' versus single and double-bundled anatomic grafts. *J. Bone J. Surgery*, **80B**, pp. 173–179, 1998.

[23] Mannor, D.A., Shearn, J.T., Grood, E.S., Noyes, F.R. & Levy, M.S., Two-bundle PCL Reconstruction: An in vitro analysis of graft placement and tension. *Am. J. Sports Med.*, **28**, pp. 833–845, 2000.

[24] Boisgard, S., Levai, J.P., Saidane, K., Geiger, B. & Landjerit, B., Study of the PCL using a 3D computer model: ligament biometry during flexion, application to surgical replacement of the ligament. *Acta Orthop. Belg.*, **65(4)**, pp. 492–502, 1999.

[25] Carlin, G.J., Livesay, G.A., Harner, C.D., Ishibashi, Y., Kim, H.S. & Woo, S.L.Y., In-situ forces in the human posterior cruciate ligament in response to posterior tibial loading. *Ann. Biomed. Eng.*, **24(2)**, pp. 193–200, 1996.

[26] Galloway, M., Grood, E., Mehalik, J., Levy, M., Saddler, S.C. & Noyes, F.R., PCL reconstruction. An in vitro study of femoral and tibial graft placement. *Am. J. Sports Med.*, **24**, pp. 437–445, 1996.

[27] Markolf, K.L., Slauterbeck, J.R., Armstrong, K.L., Shapiro, M.S. & Finerman, G.A., A biomechanical study of replacement of the PCL with a graft. Part 1: isometry, pre-tension of graft, and antero-posterior laxity. *J. Bone J. Surgery*, **79A**, pp. 375–380, 1997.

[28] Wang, C.J., Chen, H.H., Chen, H.S. & Huang, T.W., Effects of knee position, graft tension, and mode of fixation in posterior cruciate ligament reconstruction: a cadaveric knee study. *Arthroscopy*, **18(5)**, pp. 496–506, 2002.

[29] Yoshiya, S., Andrish, J.T., Manley, M.T. & Bauer, T.W., Graft tension in anterior cruciate ligament reconstruction. An in vivo study in dogs. *Am. J. Sports Med.*, **15**, pp. 464–470, 1987.

[30] Arms, S.W., Pope, M.H., Johnson, R.J., Fischer, R.A., Arvidsson, I. & Eriksson, E., Analysis of ACL failure strength and initial strains in the canine model. *Trans. ORS*, p. 524, 1990.

[31] Fischer, R.A., Arms, S.W. & Joshi, R., In vivo analysis of the strain in normal and reconstructed canine knee ligaments. *Trans. ORS*, p. 198, 1987.

[32] Fu, F.H., Bennett, C.H., Ma, C.B., Menetrey, J. & Lattermann, C., Current trends in ACL reconstruction. Part II. Operative procedures and clinical correlations. *Am. J. Sports Med.*, **28**, pp. 124–130, 2000.

[33] Staubli, H.U., Schatzmann, L., Brunner, P., Rincon, L. & Nolte, L.P., Mechanical tensile properties of the quadriceps tendon and patellar ligament in young adults. *Am. J. Sports Med.*, **27**, pp. 27–34, 1999.

[34] Li, G., Gil, J., Kanamori, A. & Woo, S.L.Y., A validated three-dimensional computational model of a human knee joint. *J. Biomech. Eng.*, **121**, pp. 657–662, 1999.

[35] Jilani, A., Shirazi-Adl, A. & Bendjaballah, M.Z., Biomechanics of human tibio-femoral joint in axial rotation. *The Knee*, **4**, pp. 203–213, 1997.

[36] Bendjaballah, M.Z., Shirazi-Adl, A. & Zukor, D.J., Finite element analysis of human knee joint in varus-valgus. *Clin. Biomech.*, **3**, pp. 139–148, 1997.

[37] Bendjaballah, M.Z., Shirazi-Adl, A. & Zukor, D.J., Biomechanical response of the passive human knee joint under anterior-posterior forces. *Clin. Biomech.*, **13**, pp. 625–633, 1998.

[38] Blankevoort, L. & Huiskes, R., Validation of a three-dimensional model of the knee. *J. Biomechanics*, **29(7)**, pp. 955–961, 1996.

[39] Mommersteeg, T.J.A., Huiskes, R., Blankevoort, L., Kooloos, J.G.M., Kauer, J.M.G. & Maathuis, P.G.M., A global verification study of a quasi-static knee model with multi-bundle ligaments. *J. Biomechanics*, **29(12)**, pp. 1659–1664, 1996.

[40] Mommersteeg, T.J.A., Blankevoort, L., Huiskes, R., Kooloos, J.G.M. & Kauer, J.M.G., Characterization of the mechanical behavior of knee ligaments: a numerical-experimental approach. *J. Biomechanics*, **29(2)**, pp.151–160, 1996.

[41] Katsuragi, R., Yasuda, K., Tsujino, J., Keira, M. & Kaneda, K., The effect of nonphysiologically high initial tension on the mechanical properties of in situ frozen ACL in canine model. *Am. J. Sports Med.*, 2000.

[42] Yasuda, K. & Hayashi, K., Changes in biomechanical properties of tendons and ligaments from joint disuse. *J. Osteo. Res. Soc. Int.*, pp. 122–129, 1999.

[43] Pioletti, D.P., Rakotomanana, L.R. & Leyvraz, P.F., Non linear viscoelastic model and experimental identification of the ACL. *ASME Advances in Bioengineering*, **31**, pp. 35–36, 1995.

[44] Pioletti, D.P., Rakotomanana, L.R. & Leyvraz, P.F., Strain rate effects on the mechanical behavior of the ACL-bone complex. *Med. Eng. Phys.*, **21**, pp. 95–100, 1999.

[45] Pioletti, D.P. & Rakotomanana, L.R., On the independence of time and strain effects in the stress relaxation of soft tissues. *J. Biomechanics*, **33**, pp. 1729–1732, 2000.

[46] Pioletti, D.P. & Rakotomanana, L.R., Non-linear viscoelastic law for soft biological tissues. *Europ. J. Mech.*, **5**, pp. 749–759, 2000.

[47] Moglo, K.E. & Shirazi-Adl, A., On the coupling between anterior and posterior cruciate ligaments, and knee joint response under anterior femoral drawer in flexion: a finite element study. *Clin. Biomech.*, **18**, pp. 751–759, 2003.

[48] Keller, P.M., Shelbourne, K.D., McCarroll, J.R. & Rettig, A.C., Non operatively treated isolated PCL injuries. *Am. J. Sports Med.*, **21**, pp. 132–136, 1993.

[49] Singerman, R., Berilla, J., Archdeacon, M. & Peyser, A., In vitro forces in the normal and cruciate-deficient knee during simulated squatting motion. *J. Biomech. Eng.*, **121**, pp. 234–242, 1999.

[50] Skyhar, M.J., Warren, R.F., Ortiz, G.J., Schwartz, E. & Otis, J.C., The effects of sectioning of the posterior cruciate ligament and the posterolateral complex on the articular contact pressures within the knee. *J. Bone J. Surgery*, **75A**, pp. 694–699, 1993.

[51] Abdel-Rahman, E.M. & Hefzy, M.S., 3D dynamic behavior of the human knee joint under impact loading. *Med. Eng. Physics*, **20**, pp. 276–290, 1998.

[52] Rakotomanana, L.R., Contribution à la modélisation géométrique et thermodynamique d'une classe de milieux faiblement continus. *Arch. Rational Mech. Anal.*, **141**, pp. 199–236, 1998.

[53] Ramaniraka, N.A. & Rakotomanana, L.R., Models of continuum with microcrack distribution. *Mathematics and Mechanics of Solids*, pp. 301–336, 2000.

[54] Coleman, B.D. & Noll, W., The thermodynamics of elastic materials with heat conduction and viscosity. *Arch. Rational Mech. Anal.*, **13**, pp. 167–170, 1963.

CHAPTER 9

Tissue modeling and visualization using virtual reality

O. Rodríguez, R. Carmona, E. Coto & H. Navarro

Computer Graphics Lab, Universidad Central de Venezuela, Venezuela.

Abstract

Computer modeling and simulation of the human body and its behavior are very useful tools in situations where it is either too risky to perform a surgical procedure on a patient already suffering a traumatic situation, or too costly for *in vivo* experiments. Several non-invasive visualization techniques for medical data images have emerged in response to this need. Among them, virtual reality provides an ideal environment for training and simulation of surgical procedures.

In this chapter we will discuss relevant topics regarding the creation of a virtual reality system that allows the user to see and interactively manipulate 3D hard tissue models and other structures in order to improve surgical planning or determine a pathological condition. Several techniques of medical image segmentation and rendering are also discussed.

1 Introduction

Virtual reality might be seen like a highly sophisticated user 3D interface for a specific application, but the variety of topics involved in the process of its creation, makes of itself a field of study. We deal with a special case of medicine and bioengineering application regarding the use of medical images for the design and analysis of modeling tools and surgery planning and medical training.

Our goal is to provide the reader with the basic steps and techniques required for the creation of such an environment. Special emphasis is made in image segmentation, 3D visualization and navigation of virtual environments.

The chosen model to represent the Immersive Virtual Environment is a Workbench [1] interface for passive stereoscopic projection. The inputs are objects corresponding to surfaces or volumes of physical models, such as prosthesis or bones reconstructed from computer tomography (CT) data. The outputs are virtual objects that correspond to physical instantiations of information from the input objects projected on a flat surface.

In an ideal Virtual Reality System users have to be strongly convinced that they are actually performing a task, we call this realism. The user would interact with virtual objects as if they were real, i.e. feel real, handled properly and have the appropriate visual enhancement. On the other hand, virtual objects would respond to the appropriate actions demanded by the user or by the intrinsic behavior of the physical object. Virtual navigation techniques are necessary to achieve realism.

Most of the techniques discussed in this chapter can be applied on several medical image technologies, like magnetic resonance (MR), computed axial tomography scan (CAT), single photon emission computed tomography (SPECT) and ultrasound. The reader can find a brief description of these imaging technologies in [2].

We first discuss 3D data visualization methods that can be used to display medical image volume datasets in the workbench, and then we discuss image segmentation techniques to obtain the computer geometrical models of bones and implants that are used as input for the workbench. Next, virtual scene navigations methods are presented, that improves the realism of the simulations. We conclude the chapter, presenting a prototype of a workbench developed at the computer graphics lab (LCG).

2 3D data visualization

Volume dataset consists in 3D samples of scalar field $s(x, y, z)$, $x, y, z \in R$, arranged in a rectilinear grid. Each sample is called voxel (acronym of volume pixel). The dataset can be thought of as a set of 2D slices (fig. 1). Many techniques have been used to visualize 3D volume datasets. In most of the cases, they can be divided in two groups: volume rendering and surface rendering. In this section, we present aspects about capture and rendering techniques for volume datasets.

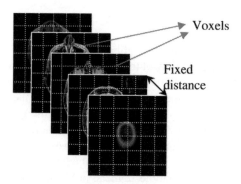

Figure 1: Volume dataset. Each voxel consists of one scalar, representing the numeric interpretation given by any device during sampling. The volume can be thought of as a set of slices, or parallel 2D images.

2.1 Volume rendering

Volume rendering is a close simulation of light propagation throughout a medium, which is represented by the volume. As light flows through the volume, it can be absorbed and emitted by the volume. Other types of interaction are also possible, but the complete optical model is simplified for visualization purposes [3]. Therefore, volume rendering algorithms produce an image by computing how much light reaches each pixel on an image plane (fig. 2).

The light emitted and absorbed by one voxel can be computed using a transfer-function. The transfer-function maps the scalar value s in a Red-Green-Blue (RGB) color with opacity A (fig. 3).

The volume rendering equation is showed in eqn (1). The exponential term represents the accumulated extinction along the viewing ray between the eye and the emission point sample $s(x(\lambda))$ [4].

$$C = \int_0^D c(s(x(\lambda))) \cdot e^{-\int_0^\lambda t(s(x(\lambda')))d\lambda} \, d\lambda. \tag{1}$$

In practice, often this integral is not computed. A numerical approximation is used, based on Riemann series in eqn (2).

$$C \approx \sum_{i=0}^n C_i \prod_{j=0}^{i-1} (1 - \alpha_j), \quad C_i = c_i * \alpha_i, \quad c_i = c(s(x(i*h))), \quad \alpha_i = t(s(x(i*h))). \tag{2}$$

Only samples every h units along the ray are considered (fig. 4).

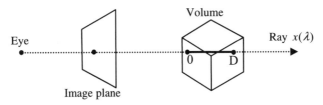

Figure 2: Volume rendering. For each pixel, one ray can be parameterized by $x(\lambda)$. The goal is to obtain the final color in the pixel, integrating reconstructed values for the parameterized segment in $[0,D]$.

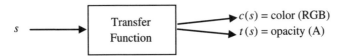

Figure 3: Transfer-function. Maps scalar values to RGBA.

The approximation can be computed in several ways. Ray Casting algorithms evaluate it from the nearest sample to the farthest, implementing directly eqn (2) as shown in eqn (3).

$$C = C_0 + C_1(1 - \alpha_0) + C_2(1 - \alpha_0)(1 - \alpha_1) + \cdots$$
$$+ C_n(1 - \alpha_0) \cdots (1 - \alpha_{n-1}). \tag{3}$$

This technique does not exploit cache performance because the volume is not accessed in storage order. But, early ray termination can be easily implemented by truncating eqn (2) when the pixel opacity reaches some threshold. In practice, this is satisfied by the following condition:

$$\prod_{j=0}^{i-1} (1 - \alpha_j) < 0.05. \tag{4}$$

Another approach used to accelerate the rendering speed is the Shear-warp factorization of the viewing transformation [3]. In this approach the viewing matrix is factorized in two matrices: shear and warping. Three copies of the volume are required, one for each axis. The copy more perpendicular to the viewing vector is selected for rendering. Slices are sheared using the shear transformation, such as they are viewport aligned. Sheared slices are projected into an intermediate image, traversing the volume and the image in storage order, improving cache performance. A warping is applied to the intermediate 2D image (fig. 5). Earlier implementations compute warping using 2D texture mapping [5, 6].

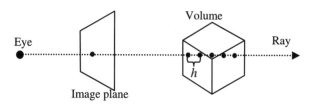

Figure 4: Samples used to approximate volume rendering equation.

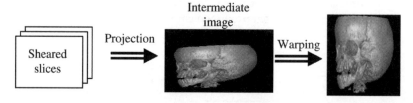

Figure 5: Shear-warp process.

2.2 Hardware accelerated volume rendering

Unfortunately, volume dataset cannot be directly displayed with current hardware graphics devices. Hardware requires a proxy geometry to be texturized with volume slices. This geometry is usually made out of quadrilateral polygons. They are rendered in back-to-front order (from the farthest to the nearest slice). Figure 6 shows the texture mapping process for one polygon, using texture coordinates, which are normalized in [0,1]. Texture coordinates are specified for each polygon vertex, and linearly interpolated for interior polygon points during rasterization, which is a phase of the graphics rendering pipeline where graphic primitives are reduced to fragments or pixels.

Volume composition is computed using the blending function provided by the hardware. Beginning with the farthest slice, a linear interpolation between the accumulated color S_{i+1} and voxel color c_i is computed using eqn (5).

$$
\begin{aligned}
S_0 &= C, \\
S_n &= \alpha_n c_n, \\
S_i &= \alpha_i c_i + (1 - \alpha_i) S_{i+1}, \quad \text{if } i < n.
\end{aligned}
\tag{5}
$$

Using OpenGL graphics library [7], supported by most current graphics hardware, this is equivalent to specifying the blending operation as the following:

glBlend(GL_SRC_ALPHA, GL_ONE_MINUS_SRC_ALPHA).

Finally, hardware oriented volume rendering can be divided in two techniques: object aligned polygons, which requires 2D texture mapping, and viewport aligned polygons, which requires 3D texture mapping. Recent works, improve these methods by pre-computing the integral in eqn (1) between any possible sample-pair, generating very high quality render. These techniques are described in the following sections.

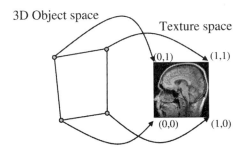

Figure 6: Texture mapping process. For each polygon vertex, texture coordinates are defined in texture space. Texture coordinates for internal polygon points are obtained by interpolation. Texture is re-sampled to get the associated voxel for a given point.

2.2.1 Object aligned polygons
This technique requires three volume copies [4]. Each volume copy is perpendicular to one axis in object space (fig. 7). For rendering, is selected the more perpendicular copy to the viewing vector *vv*. Polygons are texturized using the slices information (stack of 2D textures), and rendered in back-to-front order (i.e. from the farthest to the nearest slice). If the volume is too big, and all copies do not fit in texture memory, page faults could degrade the rendering speed considerably.

2.2.2 Viewport aligned polygons
In this case, polygons are parallel to the viewport, and texture coordinates are defined in 3D texture space (fig. 8) [8]. Intersections of one or more polygons with 3D textures can be computed by hardware using clamp, or even using clipping planes [7].

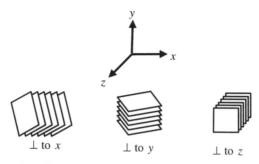

Figure 7: Three copies of the volume, one for each axis. Each volume copy consists in parallel slices of the volume, loaded into texture memory.

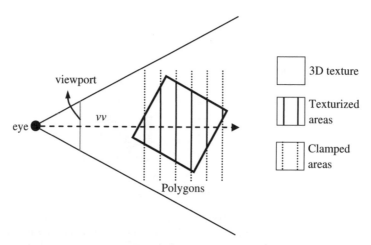

Figure 8: Volume rendering using 3D texture mapping (top view). Texturized polygons are parallel to the viewport.

Table 1: Comparison between hardware based volume rendering.

	Object aligned polygons	Viewport aligned polygons
Render Quality	Lower: increases artifacts in 45° angles	Higher
Distance between samples Perspective Projection	Varies per sample pair	Varies per sample pair
Distance between samples Parallel projection	Constant between samples in fixed angle, but varies for each angle	Constant for any angle and any samples pair
Hardware availability	More	Less
Sampling interpolation	Bi-linear	Tri-linear (better)
Speed	About three times faster	About three times slower
Volume copies	Three	One
Volume rotation	Rotates vertex polygon via model and view matrix	Rotates texture coordinates via texture matrix

Because polygons are parallel to the viewport, texture coordinates are rotated using a texture matrix in order to visualize the volume from any possible angle. In addition, it is also possible to implement volume scaling using a texture matrix.

Table 1 shows a brief comparison of volume rendering techniques between object aligned polygons and viewport aligned polygons.

2.2.3 Pre-integrated volume rendering

Pre-integrated volume rendering focuses in eqn (2); instead of composing point samples s_i, this technique composes pre-computed integral values between samples-pairs s_i, s_{i+1} [4]. The volume bounded by these slices is called a Slab. This technique considers slab by slab in the composition equation, instead of slice by slice as previous techniques. The integral between sample-pairs is based in eqn (1), and after some simplifications, we obtain

$$\alpha_i = 1 - e^{-\frac{\text{distance}}{s_{i+1} - s_i}(T(s_i) - T(s_{i+1}))} \quad \text{and} \quad c_i = \frac{\text{distance}}{s_{i+1} - s_i}\left(K^t(s_{i+1}) - K^t(s_i)\right), \quad (6)$$

where

$$T(s) = \int_0^s c(s)ds, \quad K^t(s) = \int_0^s t(s)c(s)ds. \quad (7)$$

Hardware implementations use multitexturing to map pairs of consecutive slices into a polygon. Values s_i and s_{i+1} from pairs of texture are used to index a 256×256

Red-Green-Blue-Alpha (RGBA) texture, where pre-integrated color and extinction are stored for every discrete sample-pair. It can be easily implemented using fragment program OpenGL extension [7].

2.3 Mixing surface and volume rendering

When we need to interact with volumes using 3D objects defined by surface polygons, or we want to put the volume and the iso-surface together for rendering, it is necessary to define a technique to mix both objects correctly; otherwise a visual confusion may appear (fig. 9(a)). Our implementation is based on Westermann [9] with 3D textures. Surface polygons and proxy geometry (quadrilateral shells) are intercalated during rendering, determining which polygons lie between pairs of consecutive shells p_i and p_{i+1} (fig. 9(b)). Hardware clipping planes are configured to remove polygon areas outside the volume limited by p_i and p_{i+1}. In order to improve search speed, surface polygons are depth-sorted before rendering.

2.4 Rendering large datasets

Large volume datasets are very common in medical data used in daily clinical routines as well as other applications. New technologies will improve the capabilities of newer acquisition devices and higher resolution scanner devices will provide larger and larger datasets. Unfortunately, current graphics cards cannot store large volume datasets in their texture memory. Moreover, most graphic hardware imposes power of two texture dimensions; consequently it is necessary to add padding voxels to the dataset, increasing even more the volume size, which is a limitation factor when large datasets need to be handled.

Bricking techniques are a well-known method to exploit cache coherence and have been proposed to avoid these rendering limitations [9]. The volume data is decomposed in bricks and sorted in *z-order*, which are rendered one by one independently, from the farthest to the nearest. Thus, a volume of any size can be rendered. Bandwidth limitations to transfer bricks into texture memory make interactive rendering impossible. Several improvements have been considered to deal with this problem. The first ideas were based on the decomposition of the original volume data in bricks using octrees to avoid storage and processing of empty areas [10, 11].

Multiresolution schemes have been considered by other authors. In those cases, the volume is downsampled to obtain several levels of details (LODs). Under some considerations, areas with higher (lower) priority are rendered with higher (lower) LOD.

LaMar *et al.* [12] used an octree to represent the volume hierarchy in LODs subdivided in bricks. They also define a new proxy geometry (spherical shells) to improve rendering quality. Additionally, Weiler *et al.* [13] reduced boundary artifacts at level transitions, considering consistent interpolation between consecutive levels. Boundary voxels of finer LODs are taken from next coarser LOD. This idea is applied to each pair of consecutive LODs, but not between pairs. Both works

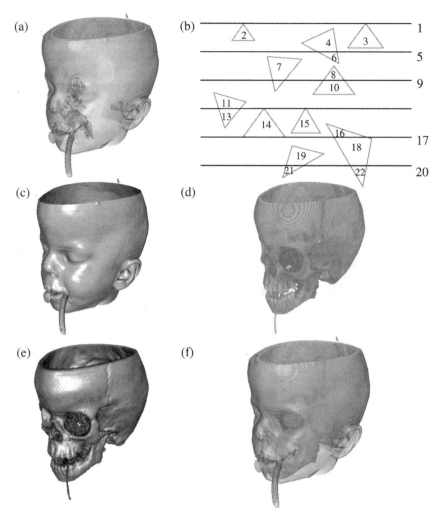

Figure 9: Mixing volume and surface rendering. (a) Transparent surface is displayed first with depth test. The result is a "visual-confusion". (b) Shells and surface polygons are depth-sorted. (c) Skin surface rendered with lighting. (d) Bones volume rendered without lighting. (e) Bones volume rendered with lighting. (f) Mixing surface (c) and volume (d).

consider an opacity correction factor for each LOD, taking into account the distance between slices. Boada *et al.* [14] also focused on the technique of LaMar, but they consider other issues to select bricks: level of importance (defined via ROI, or region of interest), homogeneity, and number of bricks. Li *et al.* [15] initially subdivided the source volume into subvolumes, looking for larger homogeneous areas. The motivation is that homogeneous areas must not be subdivided, because they require more polygons to render. For each subvolume, LODs are also generated. They select the LOD for each subvolume based on predicted rendering speed, maximum opacity, distance to the viewpoint, projected area and gaze distance, leading to low changes in rendering speed [14].

Guthe *et al.* [16] worked with loose wavelets compression, to reduce memory consumption, for huge datasets (i.e. the visible human). Least recently used (LRU) caching of uncompressed bricks is used. Plate *et al.* [17] focused on volume roaming using a lens with paging and prediction strategies. Prediction is based on the linear extrapolation of lens movement. Thus, future required bricks can be predicted and uploaded previously. They limited the number of uploaded bricks by frame, to avoid slowing down the rendering process, obtaining quite low resolution in some cases.

3 Medical image segmentation

Diagnostic imaging is an invaluable tool in medicine today. Computed tomography and other imaging modalities provide an effective means for non-invasively mapping the anatomy of a subject. These technologies are a critical component in diagnosis and treatment planning.

With the increasing size and number of medical images, the use of computers in facilitating their processing and analysis has become necessary. In particular, computer algorithms for the delineation, extraction or reconstruction of anatomical structures and other regions of interest are a key component in several tasks. These algorithms, called *image segmentation algorithms*, play a vital role in numerous biomedical imaging applications such as the study of anatomical structures [18], treatment planning [19] and computer integrated surgery [20].

Methods for performing segmentations vary widely depending on the specific application, image modality, and other factors. Furthermore, it depends also on the dimension of the desired segmentation, since image segmentation algorithms can be used to extract contours, surfaces or volumes. General image artifacts such as noise, partial volume effects, and motion can also have significant consequences on the performance of segmentation algorithms. In addition, each imaging modality has its own idiosyncrasies with which to contend. There is currently no single segmentation method that yields acceptable results for every medical image. There are more general methods that can be applied to a variety of data. However, methods that are specialized to particular applications can often achieve better performance by taking into account prior knowledge. Selection of an appropriate approach to a segmentation problem can therefore be a difficult dilemma.

The most common application of segmentation algorithms over medical images is contours extractions of tissue or anatomical structures. For contour extraction, Xu *et al.* [2] divided segmentation methods into eight categories: thresholding approaches, region growing approaches, classifiers, clustering approaches, Markov random field models, artificial neural networks, deformable models, and atlas-guided approaches. Although separated into several categories, multiple techniques are often used in conjunction for solving different segmentation problems.

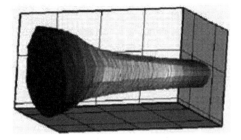

Figure 10: Coto *et al.* [19] used deformable models to reconstruct the surface of a knee for finite element analysis and knee arthoplasty simulation.

Each technique has its own advantages and disadvantages, and some of them are more widely used than others. However, not all of them can be extended to 3D space for surfaces and volumes extraction. It is possible to extract the surface of a bone using deformable models [19, 21] (fig. 10) but the intent to accomplish the same results using a simple thresholding technique will not succeed. However, Marching Cubes [22] is a thresholding-based technique that can successfully obtain the surface reconstruction of an anatomic structure. Artificial neural networks also have been used successfully to extract 3D representations of anatomical structures from medical images [23, 24]. A full description of competing methods is beyond the scope of this chapter and the readers are referred to references for additional details. The reader can find several surveys on image segmentation specifically for medical images in the literature [2, 25–27].

This section is focused on the segmentation of contours, surfaces and volumes from medical images using deformable models [28], since it is a technique that has been extensively studied and widely used in medical image segmentation, with promising results. The widely recognized potency of deformable models stems from their ability to segment, match, and track images of anatomic structures by exploiting (bottom-up) constraints derived from the image data together with (top-down) *a priori* knowledge about the location, size, and shape of these structures. Deformable models are capable of accommodating the often significant variability of biological structures over time and across different individuals. Furthermore, deformable models support highly intuitive interaction mechanisms that allow medical scientists and practitioners to bring their expertise to bear on the model-based image interpretation task when necessary.

Deformable models are curves or surfaces defined within an image domain that can move under the influence of internal forces, which are defined within the curve or surface itself, and external forces, which are computed from the image data. The internal forces are designed to keep the model smooth during deformation. The external forces are defined to move the model toward an object boundary or other desired features within an image. By constraining extracted boundaries to be smooth and incorporating other prior information regarding the object shape, deformable models offer robustness to both image noise and boundary gaps and allow integrating boundary elements into a coherent and consistent mathematical

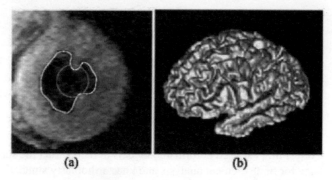

Figure 11: (a) Extraction of the inner wall of the left ventricle of a human heart from a 2D MRI image. (b) Reconstruction of the brain cortical surface from a 3D MRI image dataset.

description. Such a boundary description can then be readily used by subsequent applications. Moreover, since deformable models are implemented on the continuum, the resulting boundary representation can achieve subpixel accuracy, a highly desirable property for medical imaging applications. Figure 11 shows two examples of using deformable models to extract object boundaries from medical images. The result is a parametric curve in fig. 11(a) and a parametric surface in fig. 11(b).

We first introduce the most important variants and extensions of deformable models for contour extraction. Following we provide a review of the 3D extensions of this technique to obtain surfaces and volumes. However, because of its importance and wide application, we briefly discuss the Marching Cubes [22] technique in the surface reconstruction section.

3.1 Contour extraction

Deformable models owe its popularity in great part to the work of Kass *et al.* [29], where is proposed a parametric deformable model with an energy minimizing formulation that they called the active contour model or *snake*. The contour is said to be active because the minimization is performed continuously throughout the time, causing the contour to move dynamically and behave like a snake. Typically, users initialized a deformable model near the object of interest (fig. 12) and allowed it to deform into place. Users could then use the interactive capabilities of these models and manually fine-tune them. Since then, a great amount of research has been done regarding image segmentation using active model contours.

Amini, Weymonth and Jain [30] proposed a dynamic programming approach as a method to solve the minimization problem. Their work allows the introduction of hard constraints and moving the points of the snake within a discrete grid which does not require approximations. In addition, their strategy is numerically more stable and ensures the global optimality of the solution. However, the method is slow and has large memory requirements.

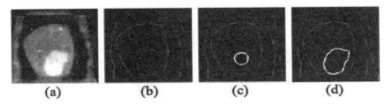

Figure 12: (a) CT image slice of left ventricle (b) Edge detected image. (c) Initial snake. (d) Snake deforms towards the boundary.

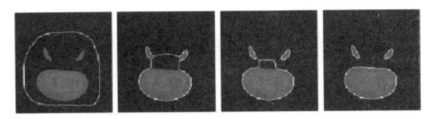

Figure 13: T-Snake shrinking and splitting on a human vertebra image slice.

Williams and Shah [31] presented a very stable and flexible greedy algorithm that allows hard constraints and is faster than the dynamic programming approach of Amini *et al.* [30] and the original strategy of Kass *et al.* [29]. However, the method is dependent of the initial snake since all the points are updated according to its previous neighbor.

Menet *et al.* [32] used a parametric spline to represent the contour, called B-Snake. This snake formulation allows local control, compact representation, and it also needs only a few parameters. Brigger [33] improves B-Snakes using a multiresolution approach.

Cohen [34] used an internal "inflation" force to expand a snake model past spurious edges towards the real edges of the structure, making the snake less sensitive to initial conditions. Cohen [34] also proposed changes in the image energy functional to make it more stable, along with optimal values for tension and rigidity coefficients.

Gunn and Nixon [35] developed a technique based on two snakes, called the dual snake technique. The user initializes an internal contour and an external contour, and then both contours are minimized and attracted to each other. This method gives the snake the ability to reject local minimums.

Lai and Chin [36], proposed a method for extraction of contours of any arbitrary shape, called g-snake. In addition, they proposed an efficient way to automatically initialize the snake using the generalized Hough Transform.

Terzopoulos and McInerney [21] developed a topology independent shape modeling scheme that allows a deformable contour to dynamically sense and change its topology, called T-Snake (fig. 13). Other researchers have also worked in the same direction [37, 38].

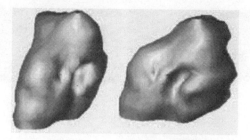

Figure 14: Two views of the reconstructed inside cavity of the left ventricle.

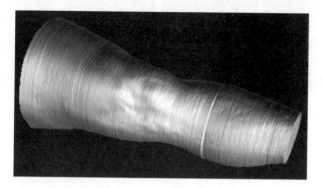

Figure 15: Reconstructed surface of a segment of the visible human right leg. This
          surface consists of 113,895 triangles and it was segmented from a set of
          650 images of 1748 × 966 pixels.

3.2 Surface extraction

Deformable models can also be used to segment surfaces of anatomical structures
from a CT or MRI image dataset. It is possible to segment a contour from an initial
image slice and once the user is satisfied with the result, the fitted contour model
may then be used as the initial boundary approximation for neighboring slices.
These models are then deformed into place and again propagated until all slices
have been processed. The resulting sequence of 2D contours can then be connected
to form a continuous 3D surface model. Cohen [34] already tried this approach
successfully (fig. 14).

   Coto *et al*. [39] also used this approach successfully for large number of images,
but using a T-Snake variant (fig. 15). This work also applies non-commercial 3D
meshers to obtain the tetrahedral mesh of the segmented structures.

   However, segmenting 3D image volumes slice by slice, either manually or by
applying 2D contour models, is a laborious process or requires a post-processing
step to connect the sequence of 2D contours into a continuous surface. Furthermore,
the resulting surface reconstruction can contain inconsistencies or show rings or
bands. The use of a true 3D deformable surface model on the other hand, can result

in a faster, more robust segmentation technique which ensures a globally smooth and coherent surface between image slices.

Kass *et al.* [40] first proposed the concept of deformable surfaces as an extension of their previous work on snakes. Many researchers have since explored the use of deformable surface models for segmenting structures in medical image volumes.

Terzopolous *et al.* [41] and Cohen *et al.* [42] used the finite element method (FEM) and physics-based techniques to implement elastically deformable models. These deformable surfaces are based on a thin-plate under tension surface spline, which controls and constrains the stretching and bending of the surface. The models are fitted to data dynamically by integrating Lagrangian equations of motion through time in order to adjust the deformational degrees of freedom. Furthermore, the FEM is used to represent the models as a continuous surface in the form of weighted sums of local polynomial basis functions. Pentland *et al.* [43] also developed physics-based models but used a reduced modal basis for the finite elements. Terzopoulos and McInerney [21] also extended the T-Snake model to 3D, with the name of T-Surfaces.

Miller *et al.* [44] created a deformable surface based on geometric restrictions with the name of Geometrically Deformable Models. This technique uses a collection of triangular faces which approximates a sphere. Each vertex on the sphere is deformed (moved) based on the local topology.

Thingvold [45] proposed a deformable surface with a B-Spline representation and Newton dynamics. Thingvold models elastic and plastic deformations on the surfaces, which makes possible the application of deformation forces over the surfaces that can be eliminated later. Currently, this is not possible with finite element surfaces.

Sakaue and Yamamoto [46] developed an Active Net model for the extraction of regions from images. The Active Net is a model of energy-minimizing net that is guided for image forces and internal constraints.

In a different approach, Szeliski *et al.* [47] used a dynamic, self-organizing oriented particle system to model surfaces of objects. Other notable works involving 3D deformable surface models and medical image applications can be found in [41, 48, 49].

3.2.1 Marching Cubes

The Marching Cubes technique [22] was introduced in 1987 to extract high quality meshes from volume datasets. Once given a threshold U corresponding to the surface to reconstruct, this algorithm traverses the entire volume voxel by voxel, determining how the voxel is cut by the surface. In this case, the voxel is thought of as a cube delimited by 8 volume samples. Every voxel can be either under or above the threshold. In other words, it is inside or outside the surface. Thus, we have $2^8 = 256$ possibilities. Lorensen and Cline [22] developed 15 patterns of surface-edge intersections, using complementary and rotational symmetry (fig. 16). However, there have been some ambiguities found in six configurations where there are at least two ways to triangulate a given voxel. This occurs when two *ambiguous*

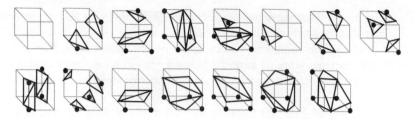

Figure 16: Patterns for Marching Cubes algorithm.

faces happen to be adjacent to each other. An ambiguous face has two diagonally opposite grid points marked (inside) and the other two diagonally opposite grid points unmarked (outside). If ambiguous patterns are not considered, they can lead to holes in the 3D surface. Some solutions have been presented to fix this problem [50–53]. Mainly, they use extra information (vertex average in ambiguous faces, neighborhood triangulation, bilinear interpolation in ambiguous faces and so on) to eliminate the ambiguity.

Other methods are based in triangulate tetrahedrons instead of cubes [54]. A tetrahedron has only 16 possible triangulations, which is reduced to 3 by symmetry. Even though the lookup table is small, the final mesh size increases considerably.

3.3 Volume extraction

Anatomic structures in the human body are either solid or thick-walled. To support the expanding role of medical images into tasks such as surgical planning and simulation, and functional modeling of structures such as bones, muscles, skin, or arterial blood flow, may require volumetric or solid deformable models rather than surface models. It also requires the ability to simulate the movement and interactions of these structures in response to forces, the ability to move, cut and fuse pieces of the model in a realistic fashion, and the ability to stimulate the simulated muscles of the model to predict the effect of the surgery. Recently, new investigations explore the use of volumetric or solid deformable models of the human face and head for computer graphics applications [55] and medical applications.

Radeva *et al.* [56] use B-Solids to find local deformations of the heart from MRI image datasets. A B-Solid is a 3D tensor product of three B-Splines that provides local control, compact representation and parametric smoothness. A B-Solid uses information on different slices, making the strategy robust and accurate (fig. 17).

Doi *et al.* [57] developed a physics-based approach using a 3D deformable mesh called 3D Active Grid, to automatically extract an arbitrary region from a 3D dataset. The 3D Active Grid is an extension of the Active Net, but the active grid is able to extract 3D regions using information inside and outside the object. Moreover, the generated geometry can be directly used in FEM, so the 3D Active Grid has many potential applications like virtual surgery simulations, anatomical structure modeling and so on.

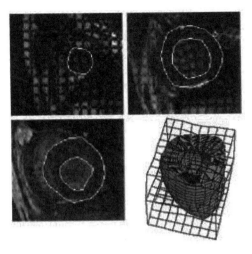

Figure 17: Heart contours and heart volumetric model located in a B-Solid.

Other notable works involving deformable solid models for medical image applications can be found in [58–60].

4 Scene navigation

One of the crucial aspects of a virtual environment is how the user navigates the scene. Usually, Virtual Environment Systems use non common visual displays to present the 3D computer generated world. The virtual environment presents a non-traditional interface paradigm, which requires the use of special devices, and novel ways to scroll the virtual world, in order to see every piece of information that is being displayed. There are several ways to do this, depending on the available hardware, the straight forward solution is to use a commodity mouse to navigate the scene. The problem with this approach, is that a mouse does not provide a natural mechanism for navigating a 3D scene, in fact, it was designed to navigate 2D scenes. A 3D mouse allows the user to move the virtual cursor spatially in three axes, and is able to give the 3D position of a point or object [61].

Another approach is to use a 3D position scanner, which provides the position of a sensor in 3D space. This sensor could, for example, be attached to a data glove or to a stylus, which are components that allow the user to navigate the scene using his hands. The objects which belong to a virtual surgery environment scene are predetermined, therefore, no scrolling of the data is required.

Another consideration to be taken during the interaction of the user and the virtual objects is the proper handling of the scene objects. The user will be moving objects in the virtual world like a bone, a surgery saw to cut a bone, or a prosthesis that will be implanted in a bone. Therefore, every time an object in the virtual world is moved by the user, we have to check if that object will collide with another object within the virtual world. In the case there is a collision of the two objects, depending on the type of objects participating in the collision, we have to perform the appropriate action. For example, the collision between a bone and a saw may result in the cutting of the bone, while the collision of a bone and a prosthesis may result in the placement of the prosthesis.

4.1 Collision detection methods

There are several methods for collision detection between different objects in a virtual world. The first thing to be considered is the type of rendered object we are handling. In the case of bones, virtual objects are rendered surfaces or volumes extracted from medical image data. Surgical instruments, such as the saw and drill, are usually modeled using surfaces designed using CAD/CAM software. Prosthetic objects are also modeled using this kind of software.

We only consider the case of having two active objects in the virtual environment at any time. One of these objects may be a bone, and the other a surgical instrument or prosthesis. After determining the types of objects that may coexist in our virtual world, we identify the types of collision that may occur.

If the bone is defined by a volume then we will have collisions between a volume and a surface. This type of collision is not easy to handle because the two representations (volume and surface) are very different. Volume rendering on real time was made possible recently, and collision detection involving volumes has not been thoroughly studied.

If the bone is defined by a surface, all the collisions will be between surfaces. This type of collision is the most studied in literature.

A well-known approach for collision detection between surfaces is to subdivide each object in a hierarchy of bounding volumes. The bounding volume can be a sphere, an axis aligned box, an oriented box, a cylinder, etc. [62–64].

The idea is to find a bounding volume that will contain the entire object. For example, if we are using bounding spheres, we will have to find a sphere containing all the triangles on the object (fig. 18).

After the initial bounding, the sphere is subdivided into two smaller spheres, and each triangle is classified to which sphere it belongs. In our example, we can identify two levels: level one sphere S1, and second level spheres S1.1 and S1.2.

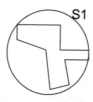

Figure 18: Bounding sphere for an object.

The same procedure is repeated until we reach very small spheres containing only one triangle. The advantage of using this scheme is that we do not have to test for collisions between every pair of triangles of the objects. Instead we have to test the bounding volumes (in this case spheres) to detect if there is a collision.

Figure 19 shows two objects each one with its bounding spheres.

In our example when intersecting the level one spheres, apparently there will be a collision, but checking the second level of bounding spheres (fig. 20) we find that there is no collision between the two objects.

Next, the spheres are organized using a hierarchy tree (fig. 21). The root of the tree is the bounding sphere of the object. This node has two children corresponding to the first subdivision of the object. A sphere corresponds to each child. This process continues until there is only one triangle in the sphere, or until the tree has some fixed size. If the object is too big, not always will it be possible to end the algorithm with a triangle in each sphere of the last level of subdivision. The corresponding tree will be too big and memory limitations will occur.

Depending on the virtual world we are working with, sometimes it is not necessary to check for collisions between triangles. If we are just walking on a building, it is possible that we do not need a high accuracy on the collisions, so it is not necessary to check collisions between triangles. On a surgical simulation environment we need to be very accurate, so it is necessary to detect collisions between triangles [65].

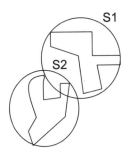

Figure 19: The bounding spheres of two intersecting objects.

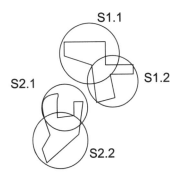

Figure 20: The second level bounding spheres of two objects.

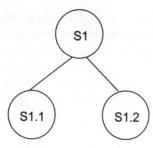

Figure 21: Sphere Tree.

The following example illustrates how expensive could be a detailed collision detection for triangles. Suppose we have a triangle A, with vertexes A1, A2, A3, and a triangle B, with vertexes B1, B2, B3. A lies on a plane P_A and B lies on a plane P_B. A and B collide if and only if any segment A1A2, A1A3 or A1A3 intersects with plane P_B, and any segment B1B2, B2B3, B1B3 intersects with plane P_A. To see if a segment V1V2 intersects with a plane P we have to evaluate V1 and V2 on P equation. If V1's and V2's evaluation on P signs differ, then the segment V1V2 intersects with the plane P. As we can see this is a very time-consuming task, so it is necessary to avoid them as much as possible.

5 A simple prototype of virtual reality workbench

When using projection systems to produce large displays, rear projection has the best quality images. Unfortunately this type of system employs a considerable floor space and ambient light may alter the projected images. As a consequence a big dark room is needed for rear projection. On the other hand for emulation of a medical surgery ambient, a flat surface is the ideal projection place for the images.

A workbench [1] (fig. 22) is a 3D interactive workspace where stereoscopic computer generated images are projected on a flat surface using a highly reflective mirror, shutter glasses, tracked gloves and stylus pen. A tracking system provides the user position to the system giving the appropriate viewpoint of the scene.

A PC-based graphics system can be constructed at a moderate cost and in a very simple to assemble way.

We can choose between active or passive stereoscopic projection. The first produces good quality image but requires highly sophisticated hardware for its implementation. In the case of passive stereoscopic projection a good cost-quality relationship can be achieved. Low-cost video projectors with high lumens capacity is a very important factor in the quality of the projected image. Also, glasses for this technique are very inexpensive compared to shutter liquid crystal display (LCD) glasses (fig. 23).

Polarized image projection for immersive systems requires two digital light processing (DLP) video projectors with a capacity of at least 1500 lumens, one for the

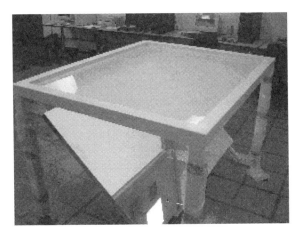

Figure 22: Workbench created at the Computer Graphics Lab.

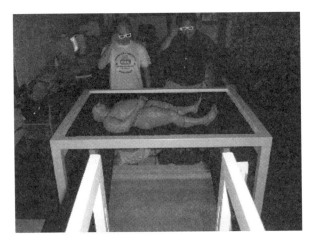

Figure 23: Passive stereoscopic projection is used.

image projected for the left eye and the other for the right eye. A pair of polarized filters and a display surface of a special material that preserves the polarization of the projected images is used in the projection bench.

A highly reflective mirror is used to project the image to the projection screen. The material of the projection screen display frame depends on the technology of the tracking system, but in most of the cases an isolator is used.

The system is PC-based with high standard graphics capabilities. Video card features for the system contemplates the use of graphic processor units (GPUs) with OpenGL hardware support with two video outputs.

5.1 Workbench's components

In this section we present a detailed description of the components of our first prototype of a virtual surgery room, entirely designed and constructed at the Computer Graphics Lab of the Central University of Venezuela. After the analysis and design of the prototype, one came to the evaluation and selection of the following necessary hardware devices for its construction.

The virtual surgery room environment is composed of a display platform, tracking devices, interface devices and the software system that makes possible the integration of all these components, displays the virtual environment and provides the feedback for the user actions.

As we mentioned before, the display platform is a workbench, having the following hardware components:

- Projection Screen: Diffusion screen with the property of preserving the polarization of the light.
- Mirror: A flat surface with a high index of reflection for a perfect reflection of the image.
- Projectors: Multimedia digital projectors featuring high illumination, high resolution images support and high refresh rates. An uphold for the projectors is also necessary, it must allow the adjustment of the position and orientation of the projectors.
- Projection frame: The support for the projection screen and the mirror. The material of the table can vary depending on the technology of the tracking device (wood, steel, etc.).
- Filters and lenses: Polarized filter for 3D projection.
- High performance PC, with a 3D graphics card: Since the same image must be displayed by both projectors, the graphic card must have 2 video outputs. We use a NVIDIA GeForce 4 Ti 4200 inside a Dell Precision Workstation.
- Polarized glasses.

Figure 24 shows how all the components are integrated to build up the virtual reality workbench.

The tracking device is an essential component in any virtual reality system. The more degrees of freedom the better, since one can have more information about the position and orientation of the objects. We use a Polhemus IsoTrack II which is an electromagnetic tracker with six degrees of freedom. The tracker provides the system with information about the position and orientation of the user head. This information is used to update the point of view, and to display the objects, so when the user moves he really feels like moving around the table. The tracker also provides information about the position and orientation of the pointing devices.

Pointing devices are also a typical input device component in virtual reality systems, and can vary from data gloves to 3D mouses and even infrared light emitters. We use a Polhemus Pen Stylus, connected to the PC though a RS-232 standard interface and also to the Isotrack II in order to track it. Using the Stylus

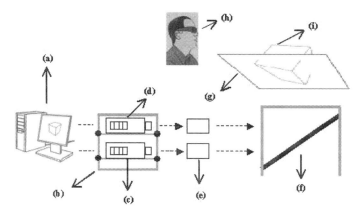

Figure 24: Components of VR System (a) PC with 3D graphic card with 2 outputs. (b) Support for video projectors. (c) Right Eye output. (d) Left Eye output. (e) Polarized filters. (f) High reflection mirror. (g) Projection screen. (h) User with polarized glasses. (i) 3D Object.

the user can select options, "touch" the displayed objects and perform several others functions using the system.

We developed a virtual reality engine that supports the applications developed for the virtual surgery room. The engine displays an initial virtual environment and then it takes information from the tracker and the stylus 15 times per second to update the virtual environment according to the user's input. The LCG staff has developed a few applications for the surgery room using the techniques described in previous section, like displaying the visible human using volume rendering techniques described earlier or displaying geometric models of bones or other structure, allowing the user to interact with the model using the stylus. We have also developed a friendly graphics user interface that is easy to use and learn.

In the future, our virtual reality system for surgery room will support more than one user and consuming processor applications, like FEM analysis will be running at real time. In order to address this new challenge we plan to migrate the entire system to a high-performance computer cluster, capable of performing huge amounts of computations in a few seconds.

References

[1] Kruger, W., Bohn, C., Fröhlich, B., Schüth, H., Strauss, W. & Wesche, G., The responsive workbench: a virtual work environment. *IEEE Computer*, **28(7)**, pp. 42–48, 1995.
[2] Xu, C., Pham, D.L. & Prince, J.L., Current methods in medical image segmentation. *Annual Review of Biomedical Engineering*, **2**, pp. 315–337, 2000.
[3] Lacroute, P. & Levoy, M., Fast volume rendering using a shear-warp factorization of the viewing transformation. *Proc. of ACM SIGGRAPH '94*,

eds. D. Schweitzer, A. Glassner & M. Keeler, ACM Press: New York, USA, pp. 451–458, 1994.

[4] Engels, K., Kraus, M. & Ertl, T., High quality pre-integrated volume rendering using hardware-accelerated pixel shading. *Proc. of ACM Siggraph/ Eurographics Workshop on Graphics Hardware 2001*, eds. G. Knittel & H. Pfister, ACM Press: New York, USA, pp. 9–16, 2001.

[5] Schulze, P., Niemeyer, L. & Lang U., The perspective shear-warp algorithm in a virtual environment. *Proc. of IEEE Visualization '01*, eds. M. Bailey, C. Hansen, H. Pfister & E. Swan, IEEE Computer Society Press: Washington DC, USA, pp. 207–214, 2001.

[6] Carmona, R., Shear-warp: una implementación eficiente. *Proc. of the XXVI Latinoamerican Conference on Informatics*, 2000.

[7] OpenGL, www.opengl.org.

[8] Wilson, O., van Gelder, A. & Wilhems, J., Direct volume rendering via 3D textures. Technical report UCSC-CRL-94-19, University of California, Santa Cruz, California, 1994.

[9] Westermann, R. & Ertl, T., Efficiently using graphics hardware in volume rendering applications. *Proc. of ACM SIGGRAPH '98*, eds. S. Cunningham, W. Bransford & M.F. Cohen, ACM Press: New York, USA, pp. 169–177, 1998.

[10] Srinivasan, R., Fang, S. & Huang, S., Volume rendering by template-based octree projection. *Proc. of the 8th Eurographics Workshop on Visualization in Scientific Computing*, eds. W. Lefer & M. Grave, Springer-Verlag, pp. 155–163, 1997.

[11] Tong, X., Wang, W., Tsang, W. & Tang, Z., Efficiently rendering large volume data using texture mapping hardware. *Proc. of the Joint Eurographics – IEEE TCCG Symposium on Visualization*, eds. E. Gröller & W. Ribarsky, Springer-Verlag: Vienna, Austria, pp. 121–134, 1999.

[12] LaMar, E., Hamann, B. & Joy, K., Multiresolution techniques for interactive texture-based volume visualization. *Proc. of IEEE Visualization '99*, eds. D. Ebert, M. Gross & B. Hamann, IEEE Computer Society Press: California, USA, pp. 355–362, 1999.

[13] Weiler, M., Westermann, R., Hansen, C., Zimmerman, K. & Ertl, T., Level-of-detail volume rendering via 3D texture. *Proc. of IEEE Volume Visualization and Graphics Symposium 2000*, eds. B. Lorensen, R. Crawfis & D. Cohen-Or, ACM Press: Utah, USA, pp. 7–13, 2000.

[14] Boada, I., Navazo, I. & Sopigno, R., A 3D texture-based octree volume visualization algorithm. *The Visual Computer*, **17(3)**, pp. 185–197, 2001.

[15] Li, X. & Shen, H., Time-critical multiresolution volume rendering using 3D texture mapping hardware. *Proc. of IEEE Volume Visualization and Graphics Symposium 2002*, eds. R. Crawfis, C. Jhonson & K. Mueller, IEEE Press: Massachusetts, USA, pp. 29–36, 2002.

[16] Guthe, S., Wand, M., Gonser, J. & Strasser, W., Interactive rendering of large volume data sets. *Proc. of the IEEE Visualization '02*, eds. R. Moorhead, M. Gross & K.I. Joy, ACM Press, pp. 53–60, 2002.

[17] Plate, J., Tirsana, M., Carmona, R. & Fröhlich, B., Octreemizer: a hierarchical approach for interactive roaming through very large volumes. *Proc. of the Symposium on Data Visualization 2002*, eds. D. Ebert, P. Brunet & I. Navazo, pp. 53–60, 2002.

[18] Worth, A.J., Makris, N., Caviness, V.S. & Kennedy, D.N., Neuroanatomical segmentation in MRI: technological objectives. *International Journal of Pattern Recognition and Artificial Intelligence*, **11**, pp. 1161–1187, 1997.

[19] Coto, E., Madero, A. & Rodriguez, O., A knee arthoplasty software tool for preoperative planning. *Proc. of the 1st International Congress on Computational Bioengineering*, eds. M. Doblare, H. Rodríguez & M. Cerrolaza, pp. 285–290, 2003.

[20] Grimson, W.E.L., Ettinger, G.J., Kapur, T., Leventon, M.E. & Wells, W.M., Utilizing segmented MRI data in image-guided surgery. *International Journal of Pattern Recognition and Artificial Intelligence*, **11**, pp. 1367–1397, 1997.

[21] Terzopoulos, D. & McInerney, T., *T-Snakes: Topology Adaptive Snakes*. Department of Computer Science, University of Toronto, 1999.

[22] Lorensen, W. & Cline, H., Marching Cubes: a high resolution 3D surface construction algorithm. *Proc. of the ACM SIGGRAPH '87*, ed. M.C. Stone, ACM Press: New York, USA, pp. 163–169, 1987.

[23] Busch, C. & Gross, M.H., Interactive neural network texture analysis and visualization for surface reconstruction in medical imaging, *Proc. of Eurographics '93*, eds. R.J. Hubbold & R. Juan, pp. 49–60, 1993.

[24] Reyes Aldasoro, C.C. & Algorri Guzmán, M.E., A combined algorithm for image segmentation using neural networks and 3D surface reconstruction using dynamics meshes. *Journal of the Mexican Society of Biomedical Engineering*, **21(3)**, pp. 73–81, 2000.

[25] Ayache, N., Cinquin, P., Cohen, I., Cohen, L., Leitner, F. & Monga, O., Segmentation of complex three dimensional medical objects: a challenge and a requirement for computer-assisted surgery planning and performance (Chapter 4). *Computer Integrated Surgery: Technology and Clinical Applications*, eds. R.H. Taylor, S. Lavallee, G.C. Burdea, & R. Mosges, MIT Press, pp. 59–74, 1996.

[26] Suetens, P., Bellon, E., Vandermeulen, D., Smet, M., Marchal, G., Nuyts, J. & Mortelmans, L., Image segmentation: methods and applications in diagnostic radiology and nuclear medicine. *European Journal of Radiology*, **17**, pp. 14–21, 1993.

[27] Terzopoulos, D. & McInerney, T., Deformable models in medical image analysis: a survey. *Medical Image Analysis*, **1**, pp. 91–108, 1996.

[28] Xu, C., Pham, D.L. & Prince, J.L., Image segmentation using deformable models (Chapter 3). *Handbook of Medical Imaging*, eds. M. Sonka & J.M. Fitzpatrick, SPIE Press, **2**, pp. 129–174, 2000.

[29] Kass, M., Witkin, A. & Terzopoulos, D., Snakes: active contour models. *International Journal of Computer Vision*, **1(4)**, pp. 321–331, 1987.

[30] Amini, A.A., Weymouth, T.E. & Jain, R.C., Using dynamic programming for solving variational problems in vision. *IEEE Transactions on Pattern Analysis and Machine Intelligence*, **12(9)**, pp. 855–867, 1990.

[31] Williams, D.J. & Shah, M., A fast algorithm for active contours and curvature estimation. *CVGIP: Image Understanding*, **55(1)**, pp. 14–26, 1992.

[32] Menet, S., Saint-Marc, P. & Medioni, G., B-Snakes: implementation and application to stereo. *Proc. of the Image Understanding Workshop*, pp. 720–726, 1990.

[33] Brigger, P., Hoeg, J. & Unser, M., B-Spline snakes: a flexible tool for parametric contour detection. *IEEE Transactions on Image Processing*, **9(9)**, pp. 1484–1496, 2000.

[34] Cohen, L.D., On active contour models and balloons. *Computer Vision, Graphics and Image Processing: Image Understanding*, **53(2)**, pp. 211–218, 1991.

[35] Gunn, R. & Nixon, M.S., A model based dual active contour. *Proc. of the British Machine Vision Conference '94*, ed. E. Hancock, BMVA Press: York, pp. 305–314, 1994.

[36] Lai, K. & Chin, R., Deformable contours: Modeling and extraction. *IEEE Transactions on Pattern Analysis and Machine Intelligence*, **17(11)**, pp. 1084–1090, 1995.

[37] Caselles, V., Catté, F., Coll, T., & Dibos, F. A geometric model for active contours. *Numerische Mathematik*, **66**, pp. 1–31, 1993.

[38] Leitner, F. & Cinquin, P., Complex topology 3-D objects segmentation. *Proc. of Model-Based Vision Development and Tools*, SPIE Proc. volume 1609, eds. R.M. Larson & H.N. Nasr, SPIE Press, pp. 16–26, 1992.

[39] Coto, E. & Rodríguez, O., T-Snakes y Triangulación de Delaunay como método de generación de mallados de estructuras anatómicas para la aplicación del Método de Elementos Finitos. *Simulación Numérica y Modelado Computacional*, Proc. of CIMENICS '04, eds. J. Rojo, M.J. Torres & M. Cerrolaza, pp. TC 11–18, 2004.

[40] Kass, M., Witkin, A. & Terzopoulos, D., Constraints on deformable models: recovering 3D shape and nonridgid motion. *Artificial Intelligence*, **36(1)**, pp. 91–123, 1987.

[41] McInerney, T. & Terzopoulos, D., A dynamic finite element surface model for segmentation and tracking in multidimensional medical images with application to cardiac 4D image analysis. *Computerized Medical Imaging and Graphics*, **19(1)**, pp. 69–83, 1995.

[42] Cohen, L. D. & Cohen. I., Finite-element methods for active contour models and balloons for 2D and 3D images. *IEEE Transactions on Pattern Analysis and Machine Intelligence*, **15(11)**, pp. 1131–1147, 1993.

[43] Pentland, A. & Sclaroff, S., Closed-form solutions for physically based shape modeling and recognition. *IEEE Transactions on Pattern Analysis and Machine Intelligence*, **13(7)**, pp. 715–729, 1991.

[44] Miller, J.V., Breen, D.E., Lorensen, W.E., O'Bara, R.M. & Wonzy, M.J., Geometrically deformed models: a method for extracting closed geometric models from volume data. *Computer Graphics*, **25(4)**, pp. 217–226, 1991.

[45] Thingvold, J., *Elastic and Plastics Surfaces for Modeling and Animation.* Dept. of Computer Science, The University of Utah, Salt Lake City, Utah, 1990.

[46] Sakaue, K. & Yamamoto, K., Active net model and its application to region extraction. *The Journal of the Institute of Television Engineering of Japan,* **45(10)**, pp. 1155–1163, 1991.

[47] Szeliski, R., Tonnesen, D. & Terzopoulos, D., Modeling surfaces of arbitrary topology with dynamic particles. *Proc. of Computer Vision and Pattern Recognition '93*, eds. G. Taubin & D.B. Coope, IEEE Press: New York, pp. 82–87, 1993.

[48] Delingette, H., Hebert, M. & Ikeuchi, K., Shape representation and image segmentation using deformable surfaces. *Image and Vision Computing*, **10(3)**, pp. 132–144, 1992.

[49] Sanderson, A.R., Shape recovery of volume data with deformable B-spline models. Ph.D. Thesis, Dept. of Computer Science, The University of Utah, Salt Lake City, Utah, 1996.

[50] Carmona, R. & Rodríguez, O., Cubos Marchantes: una implementación eficiente. *Proc. of the XXV Latinoamerican Conference on Informatics*, 1999.

[51] Mackerras, Paul., A fast parallel Marching-Cubes implementation on the Fujitsu AP1000. Technical Report TR-CS-92-10, The Australian National University, Department of Computer Science, 1992.

[52] Nielson, G. & Harmann, B., The asymptotic decider: resolving the ambiguity in Marching Cubes. *Proc. of IEEE Visualization '91*, eds. G.M. Nielson & L.J. Rosenblum, IEEE Press: Piscataway, NJ, pp. 83–91, 1991.

[53] Wilhelms, J. & van Gelder, A., Topological considerations in isosurface generation. *ACM Transactions on Graphics*, **13(4)**, pp. 337–375, 1994.

[54] Treece, G., Prager, R. & Gee, A., Regularized marching tetrahedra: improved iso-surface extraction. *Computer and Graphics*, **23(4)**, pp. 583–598, 1999.

[55] Lee, Y., Terzopoulos, D. & Waters, K., Realistic modeling for facial animation. *Proc. of ACM SIGGRAPH '95*, eds. I.V. Kerlow, C. Conn, A. Goodrich & R. Hennigar, ACM Press: California, USA, pp. 55–62, 1995.

[56] Radeva, P., Amini, A., Huang, J. & Marti, E., Deformable B-Solids and implicit snakes for localization and tracking of MRI-SPAMM data. *IEEE Proc. of Mathematical Methods in Biomedical Image Analysis*, ed. Mary E. Kavanaugh, IEEE Press: California, USA, pp. 192–201, 1996.

[57] Doi, A., Fujiwara, S., Matsuda, K. & Kameda, M., 3D Volume extraction and mesh generation using energy minimization techniques. *Proc. of 1st International Symposium on 3D Data Processing Visualization and Transmission (3DPVT '02)*, ed. Bob Werner, IEEE Press: California, USA, pp. 83–86, 2002.

[58] Delingette, H., Subsol, G., Cotin, S. & Pignon, J., Virtual reality and craniofacial surgery simulation. *Proc. of Visualization in Biomedical Computing 1994*, SPIE Proc. volume 2359, ed. Richard A. Robb, SPIE Press, pp. 607–618, 1994.

[59] Park, J., Metaxas, D. & Axel, L., Analysis of left ventricular wall motion based on volumetric deformable models and MRI-SPAMM. *Medical Image Analysis*, **1(1)**, pp. 53–71, 1996.

[60] Whitaker, R., Volumetric deformable models. *Proc. of Visualization in Biomedical Computing '94*, SPIE Proc. volume 2359, ed. Richard A. Robb, SPIE Press, pp. 122–134, 1994.

[61] Fröhlich, B. & Plate, J., The cubic mouse: a new device for three-dimensional input. *Proceedings Conference on Human Factors in Computing Systems 2000*, ed. M. Tremaine, ACM Press: The Hague, The Netherlands, pp. 526–531, 2000.

[62] Foley, J., Van Dam, A., Feiner, S. & Hughes, J., *Computer Graphics. Principles and practice, Second Edition in C*. Addison-Wesley Pub. Co., pp. 660–663, 1996.

[63] Gottschalk, S., Lin, M. & Manocha, D., OBB-Tree: A hierarchical structure for rapid interference detection. *Proc. of ACM SIGGRAPH '96*, ed. J. Fujii, ACM Press: New York, USA, pp. 171–180, 1996.

[64] Lin, M. & Gottschalk, S., Collision detection between geometric models: a survey. *Proceedings of the 8th IMA Conference on Mathematics of Surfaces*, ed. D. Hanscombe, Oxford University Press, pp. 37–56, 1998.

[65] Kaiser, K., 3D Collision detection. *Game Programming Gems*, ed. Mark DeLoura, Charles River Media Inc., pp. 390–402, 2000.

CHAPTER 10

Biomechanics and the cyber-infrastructure: delivering the bone and other models to the surgeon

T. Impelluso and C. Negus

Department of Mechanical Engineering, San Diego State University, CA, USA.

Abstract

While recent research into hard tissue modeling has trended toward examination of cellular and microscopic effects, this chapter presents the case for a cyber-infrastructure suitable for models which bridge the length scale gap from the continuum down to the microscopic. The emerging technologies of the cyber-infrastructure have made it feasible to deliver models into the surgical ward to assist in surgical planning. Models which blend the computational facility of macroscopic models with advances at and below the cellular level offer the most promise for this endeavor. This chapter begins with a summary and classification of salient macroscopic bone models. The authors then present a novel 3D macroscopic model inspired by current cellular understanding of remodeling which predicts internal and architectural remodeling given a dynamic stimulus. A brief excursion into muscle mechanics modeling is followed by a presentation of the terminology of the proposed cyber-infrastructure. The authors then present a description of the type of software architecture that will be needed to deliver the power of biomechanical bone models into the surgical ward. The same architecture can be used not only to assist in surgical planning, but also to bridge the length scale gap between the various ontological levels of bone modeling.

1 Introduction

The algorithms of computational mechanics have advanced the field of biomechanics. For example, the finite element method (FEM) is widely used to study material deformation of human skin or bone, the multi-body dynamics method (MDM) is used to study the motion of linked bodies such as the skeletal system, and computational fluid dynamics methods (CFDMs) are used to study blood flow. Commercial computational mechanics programs have gained wider use due largely to the emergence of powerful graphical interfaces. It is a fairly easy task to take a graphics file of a human bone, mesh it (in the parlance of finite element applications), and conduct an analysis to study the deformation of bone material under applied loads.

Is it possible, however, that large-scale commercial packages have the potential to hinder further growth of the field of biomechanics? After all, the aforementioned methods – FEM, MDM, CFDM – were developed by engineers to aid in the analysis of artificial structures as opposed to analysis of human tissue that might suggest supplementing the algorithms with a suite of other modules such as optimization, fluid flow, etc. Is the field in danger of becoming dulled by the use of these software packages, answering only those questions which are easily framed within the limitations of the graphical interface?

It is the contention of these authors that biomechanicians have arrived at a plateau in the computational evolution of the field. Commercial software tools too often dictate the boundaries of inquiry. This is particularly the case in biomechanics research for clinical applications where commercial codes are most likely to be used. Such commercial codes actually hinder the full integration of biomechanical models and their delivery into the surgical ward. For above all else, biomechanical theories face their ultimate test, not in the laboratory, but in the clinic.

This chapter advocates a view that computers and computer programs serve academicians, rather than the other way around. This chapter shows how we can push new boundaries in biomechanics by taking the time to appreciate the advances that our colleagues in the field of computer science have achieved. Some of these advances are described in terms of a new "cyber-infrastructure" for biomechanics. Cyber-infrastructure (CI), a term coined by the National Science Foundation (NSF) Computer and Information Science and Engineering Directorate, broadly defines the large-scale integration of hardware, high-performance communications networks, data repositories, and other advanced computing technologies for the purpose of dramatically increasing the scope and facilitating deployment of scientific research. It is the hope of the authors that this chapter provides a vision for a CI for biomechanics into which the achievements of other authors in the text can be fully appreciated. It is also the hope of these authors that readers will review these other chapters in light of this proposed shift in computational biomechanics.

The CI proposed is presented in the context of bone and muscle mechanics research. Consequently, much of the chapter consists of a review of theories pertaining to these. Section 2 is a review of continuum bone remodeling mechanics, for the sake of revealing how a new computational paradigm could enhance future algorithmic design. This section ends with a description of a novel bone remodeling code (Section 2.5) that not only incorporates some current biological understanding of remodeling, but draws inspiration from growth in the CI. Section 3 is a parallel (albeit shorter) excursion into soft tissue mechanics. Section 4 provides a few necessary definitions pertaining to the cyber-infrastructure. Section 5 presents a new biomechanical software architecture which could couple bone and muscles mechanics, among others. Finally, Section 6 presents issues regarding the delivery of biomechanical models into the surgical ward. The chapter closes with a call for action: now is the time for researchers in biomechanics to avail themselves of advances in the CI.

2 Bone remodeling algorithms

Models of mechanical adaptation of bone are often classified as being either phenomenological or mechanistic [1]. Hart [2] later proposed a third category: global optimization models. In this chapter, optimization models will be grouped under the "phenomenological" heading since they seek to satisfy some observed global goal, such as minimizing global bone mass, without regard to the actual remodeling mechanism occurring in the bone. Phenomenological models treat the adaptation mechanism as a "black box" aiming simply to simulate cause (mechanical loading) and effect (changes in morphology) without regard to the biological mechanisms at work [3]. Models in the mechanistic class (see e.g., [2, 4, 5] or [6, 7]) seek to predict morphology changes by leveraging knowledge (or at least a postulate) of the underlying biology driving the adaptation process. The mechanistic approach "offers the promise of not only extending the descriptive and predictive capabilities of phenomenological models, but may offer insights into manipulation of the bone response, and development of pharmacological therapeutic agents" [3].

Is such a clean distinction between approaches still necessary? There has been, in the last decade, a perceptible shift of effort to models incorporating cellular-level effects which has, in the process, shed light on such phenomena as fluid drag on the pericellular matrix surrounding osteocytic processes. This shift corresponds to a broader preference for "*mechanobiology*" over "*biomechanics*" [8]. These authors believe that emerging models can be built on a continuum scaffold (e.g., the finite element method applied at the organ level) and enhanced by cellular-level theories whose effects are averaged over a continuum length scale. As discussed in the excellent summary by Hart [2], phenomenological models can be direct beneficiaries of insights provided by mechanistic research, the result of which is to decrease the length scale of the phenomenological "black box". Further, what makes the resulting computational models particularly exciting is not only the synthesis of these two types of models, but also their potential to fully exploit the CI described later in this chapter. This CI is not simply jargon for "parallel processing" or "computational efficiency" (though it will employ both) but implies that an extensible computer architecture exists which accommodates new theoretical model-modules as they emerge.

This section seeks to survey bone remodeling algorithms and the continuum-level theories on which they are based. Emphasis has been placed on an algorithmic presentation of the internal and architectural remodeling theories in order to elucidate their computational characteristics. They are divided into three categories based primarily on the origin of their underlying theories, though this is a coarse simplification of the interconnected spectrum of algorithms found in the literature. The first class are those based on Cowin's theory of adaptive elasticity; the second class use Carter's concept of a daily stress stimulus; the final section describes recent illustrative models which do not neatly fit into either previous class. Before these models are described in detail, some preliminary definitions are needed.

2.1 Continuum-level remodeling iterative equations

Algorithms based on continuum theories tend to follow the same outline [9]. First, an *initial state* is defined in which initial conditions, material properties, and initial stresses are specified. Next, a *solution* phase iterates among four classes of equations, illustrated in fig. 1 and described here:

1. **Stimulus definition.** Bone material properties at a point must change in response to some mechanical signal such as principal stress, strain, strain-energy density, or rate of one of these. This remodeling signal is called the stimulus.
2. **Remodeling correlation.** A well defined rule which describes changes in the independent variables as a function of the stimulus is needed.
   (a) If some measure of bone porosity is chosen as the independent remodeling variable (such as bulk density ρ, or volume fraction v) then the model describes *internal adaptation*. Changes in cortical bone (which is essentially isotropic), are often predicted using internal adaptation models.
   (b) If, in addition to porosity, some variable describing orientation of the structural matrix is taken as independent (such as through a fabric tensor, H, Section 2.2.2) or principal material direction θ_I (Section 2.4.2.4) then the model describes *architectural adaptation*. Changes in trabecular bone (which

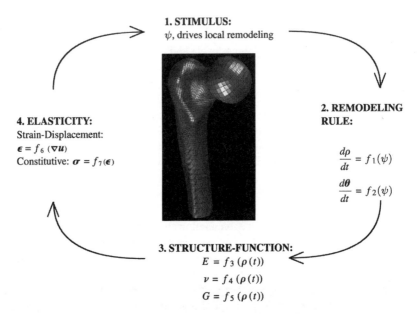

1. STIMULUS:
ψ, drives local remodeling

2. REMODELING RULE:

$$\frac{d\rho}{dt} = f_1(\psi)$$

$$\frac{d\theta}{dt} = f_2(\psi)$$

3. STRUCTURE-FUNCTION:
$$E = f_3(\rho(t))$$
$$v = f_4(\rho(t))$$
$$G = f_5(\rho(t))$$

4. ELASTICITY:
Strain-Displacement:
$\epsilon = f_6(\nabla u)$
Constitutive: $\sigma = f_7(\epsilon)$

Figure 1: Remodeling iterative equations.

is essentially orthotropic in the continuum), are often predicted using architectural adaptation models.

(c) *Surface remodeling* describes changes in the exterior geometry of bone. For the sake of clarity of presentation, most models in this section will focus on internal and architectural remodeling.

3. **Structure-function relationships.** The engineering constants known as Young's modulus E, shear modulus G, and Poisson's Ratio ν all describe bone function, and must be dependent on the bone structure variable(s), which is found from the above remodeling rule. These bone-function variables are often calculated using empirical relationships.

4. **Elasticity equations.** A new stress and strain will result from a change in stiffness magnitude, and in the case of architectural remodeling, orientation. These are calculated from the equations of elasticity.

The last phase is a new *equilibrium* configuration, met after a specified number of iterations or after some convergence criteria is met.

While all of the algorithms below iterate among the four equations in some manner, only some attach meaningful physical significance to configurations at intermediate iterations. While some algorithms simply seek to determine a new equilibrium morphology that results from a change in loading, others intend to predict the time-evolution of the remodeling process. The former will classified as "*remodeling equilibrium*" while the latter will be called "*time-evolving*" algorithms.

2.2 Cowin's adaptive elasticity

The first comprehensive theory that mathematically correlated mechanical stimulus in cortical bone to changes in bone structure appeared in the now widely cited papers by Cowin and co-workers [10–14]. Their objective was to create a thermo-mechanical model of bone as a porous, elastic solid and to model the adaptation processes (mass deposition or resorbtion resulting in changes in porosity) as being stimulated by strain. The theory was later supplemented to include architectural adaptation and time-evolution.

2.2.1 Internal adaptation: cortical bone remodeling

Cowin and Hegedus [10] start with the assumption that bone is biphasic: a structural matrix perfused with fluid. Next, they develop field equations for the conservation laws of mass, momentum, and energy as well as an entropy inequality. These were written with respect to a temporally changing bulk density $\rho(t)$, defined in terms of the bone volume fraction, v and the average density of the bone matrix, γ:

$$\rho(t) = \gamma v(t). \tag{1}$$

At this point, a constitutive equation for stress is developed from the balance laws, constitutive assumptions, and thermodynamic constraints. If remodeling is assumed isothermal, then the two variables driving remodeling, defined by Cowin as the net rate of mass addition c, and the specific free energy Ψ, are simply functions of the reference, unstrained volume fraction v_0, and the deformation gradient F,

$$c = c(v_0, F), \quad \Psi = \Psi(v_0, F). \tag{2}$$

Changes in value of c and Ψ result in changes in the density and elastic constants (and hence overall stiffness) of the bone material.

These general assumptions allowed for the complete definition of a boundary value problem in the sequel [11]. Here, the theory is specialized for the case of small strains.

For this case the strain tensor at a point in the continuum bone material is,

$$\epsilon = \frac{1}{2}\left[\nabla u + (\nabla u)^{\mathrm{T}}\right], \tag{3}$$

where u is the displacement vector. The following update equation for bone structure (change in volume fraction, $e = v - v_0$) is obtained:

$$\dot{e} = \frac{de}{dt} = a(e) + A_{ij}(e)\epsilon_{ij} + \frac{1}{2}B_{ijkl}\epsilon_{ij}\epsilon_{kl}, \tag{4}$$

where A_{ij} and B_{ijkl} are remodeling tensors which must be determined experimentally.

The net surface remodeling expressed in terms of the normal velocity of a particle on the surface of a bone is [14]:

$$\frac{dX}{dt} = C_{ij}\left[\epsilon_{ij} - \epsilon_{ij}^0\right], \tag{5}$$

where dX/dt is the velocity of a particle of surface bone, C_{ij} is a tensor element to be determined experimentally, and $\epsilon_{ij} - \epsilon_{ij}^0$ is the difference between the local strain and the strain at *remodeling equilibrium* – the strain at which no net remodeling occurs.

The above theory was first implemented in simulations in the work of Cowin and Firoozbakhsh [15, 16]. In an attempt to develop an update algorithm for density and surface velocity, Hart [17, 18] used finite element techniques to determine the remodeling constants A, B, and C in eqns (4) and (5) though ultimately concluded these were difficult to reliably estimate. This difficulty was later alleviated by assumptions Cowin would make in his "approximate noninteracting microstructure theory" [19] described in the following section.

2.2.2 Architectural adaptation: trabecular bone remodeling
In 1986, Cowin formalized the trabecular bone alignment observations of Wolff [20] through his introduction of the second rank *fabric tensor* [21]. The fabric tensor is a "quantitative stereological measure of the microstructural arrangement of trabeculae and pores in the cancellous bone tissue" [21]. The measure Cowin uses to define the components of the second rank tensor is the *mean intercept length*.

"The mean intercept length is the average distance between two bone/marrow interfaces measured along a line" [21]. To characterize the anisotropy of bone in three dimensions, the mean intercept length is characterized by ellipsoids and must be represented mathematically by a second rank tensor. This tensor is defined by Harrigan and Mann [22] as $\mathbf{M}$. Cowin defines the fabric tensor, $\mathbf{H}$ in terms of the mean intercept length tensor:

$$\mathbf{H} = \mathbf{M}^{-1/2}. \tag{6}$$

(Note that the square root of $\mathbf{M}$ exists since it is positive definite and symmetric.)

In 1992, Cowin published a comprehensive theory for trabecular bone adaptation that included evolution equations for bulk density and fabric which were based on his previous works [19]. Total strain (ϵ) was separated into dilatational ($tr(\epsilon)\mathbf{1}$) and deviatoric ($\hat{\epsilon}$) components:

$$\epsilon = \hat{\epsilon} + tr(\epsilon)\mathbf{1},$$

$$\epsilon_{ij} = \hat{\epsilon}_{ij} + \epsilon_{ij}\delta_{ij}. \tag{7}$$

The earlier update eqn (4) for bulk density was simplified by dropping higher order strain terms and assuming a dependence only on the dilatational portion (the trace) of the strain tensor:

$$\dot{e} = (f_1 + f_2 e)\left[tr(\epsilon) - tr(\epsilon_0)\right]. \tag{8}$$

The salient assumption that led to this theory was that evolution of two measures of microstructure, bulk density ρ, and fabric $\boldsymbol{H}$, were independent of each other. If a normalized fabric tensor $\mathbf{K}$ is defined as

$$\mathbf{K} = \mathbf{H} - \frac{1}{3}\mathbf{1}, \tag{9}$$

then this assumption states,

$$\frac{d\mathbf{K}}{dt} = \frac{d\mathbf{K}(\mathbf{K}, \hat{\epsilon})}{dt} \tag{10}$$

and

$$\frac{d\rho}{dt} = \frac{d\rho(\rho, \epsilon)}{dt}. \tag{11}$$

The lack of functional dependence (or physical *noninteraction*) of these two microstructure measures led to the theory being called *approximate noninteracting microstructure theory*. Specific forms for eqns (10) and (11) are given in Algorithm 1.

2.2.2.1 Two-dimensional application   An idealized 2D numerical implementation of this theory is given in [21]. This example assumes transverse isotropy, so that when written with respect to its principal directions the normalized fabric tensor is,

$$\mathbf{K} = \begin{bmatrix} K_1 & 0 & 0 \\ 0 & K_2 & 0 \\ 0 & 0 & -K_1 - K_2 \end{bmatrix}. \tag{12}$$

The equilibrium solution is found using Algorithm 1.

2.2.2.2 Three-dimensional application Fritton, in her 1994 Ph.D. dissertation, extended Cowin's 2D model to 3D and incorporated it into a finite element program, RFEM3D [25]. In order to integrate Cowin's constitutive equation with the existing finite element program, the constitutive equation in Algorithm 1 is recast into the linear matrix equation

$$\sigma_{ij} = C_{ijkl}\epsilon_{kl} \quad \text{or} \quad \{\sigma\} = [D]\{\epsilon\}. \tag{13}$$

Fritton's 3D work ([25]) is outlined in Algorithm 2.

The remodeling rate constants used in the above theory were chosen so that the model would reach equilibrium in approximately 160 days to agree with clinical observations.

2.3 The Stanford models

A series of models from researchers at Stanford University were based on a fundamentally different approach than adaptive elasticity. They are collectively called the "Stanford Models" in this work, though perhaps that is misleading as there now exist many permutations by researchers around the world. One distinguishing characteristic of the Stanford class of models is the use of a daily stimulus, ψ which incorporates effects of multiple load cases. A few highlights of this approach follow.

2.3.1 Internal adaptation
In 1986, Fyhrie and Carter, two researchers at the VA rehabilitation R&D Center in Palo Alto, CA, developed an adaptive theory which predicted internal adaptation, as quantified by the bulk density [26]. The theory could also predict equilibrium trabecular orientation at each step, though architecture was not an independent variable and was not related to stiffness through a structure-function relationship.

The early Stanford model did not employ the open system, thermomechanical, matrix-fluid model of Cowin. Fyhrie and Carter assumed bone is a self-optimizing material which seeks to maximize structural integrity while minimizing bone mass (or volume fraction). "To measure the degree to which the bone meets these conflicting goals we postulate a remodeling objective function, $\tilde{Q}(\rho, \theta, \sigma)$, which measures the optimality of the bone under a given load, where $\tilde{Q}$ is a positive function of the apparent density, ρ and orientation θ of the anisotropic material axes with respect to the principal directions of the given static stress state θ" [26]. While this sounds like a global remodeling criteria, it is actually enforceable at every local point throughout the bone.

1. **Initial State**
   (a) Stress, $\boldsymbol{\sigma}_0$.
   (b) Strain, $\boldsymbol{\epsilon}_0$.
   (c) Fabric, $\boldsymbol{H}_0$ and volume fraction, ν_0.
2. **Remodeling** (Time-evolving)
   (a) New stress state, $\boldsymbol{\sigma}^*$.
      Applied at some angle, τ to a reference axis and is assumed constant for $0 < t < \infty$.
   (b) Constitutive equation:
      Given $\boldsymbol{\sigma}^*$, use a form derived using representation theorems (For a proof, see [23]) to solve for strains, $\boldsymbol{\epsilon}$:

$$\boldsymbol{\sigma} = (g_1 + g_2 e) tr(\boldsymbol{\epsilon})\mathbf{1} + (g_3 + g_4 e)\boldsymbol{\epsilon} + \cdots$$
$$g_5 (\mathbf{KE} + \mathbf{EK}) + g_6 [\mathbf{1} tr(\mathbf{KE}) + tr(\mathbf{E})\mathbf{K}].$$

   (c) Stimulus.
      The difference from a reference strain at remodeling equilibrium, $\boldsymbol{\epsilon} - \boldsymbol{\epsilon}_0$.
   (d) Remodeling rules.
      Internal:

$$\frac{de}{dt} = (f_1 + f_2 e)\left(tr\,\boldsymbol{\epsilon} - tr\,\boldsymbol{\epsilon}^0\right).$$

      Architectural: (For the deviatoric portion of the normalized fabric tensor)

$$\boldsymbol{K}^{(i)} = \boldsymbol{K}^{(i-1)} = \Delta\boldsymbol{K} \text{ from the equation}$$

$$\frac{d\mathbf{K}}{dt} = h_1\left(\hat{\boldsymbol{\epsilon}}^{(i)} - \hat{\boldsymbol{\epsilon}}_0\right) + h_2\left[\mathbf{1} tr(\mathbf{K})\left(\hat{\boldsymbol{\epsilon}}^{(i)} - \hat{\boldsymbol{\epsilon}}_0\right)\cdots\right.$$
$$\left. - \frac{3}{2}\left(\mathbf{K}\left(\hat{\boldsymbol{\epsilon}}^{(i)} - \hat{\boldsymbol{\epsilon}}_0\right) + \left(\hat{\boldsymbol{\epsilon}}^{(i)} - \hat{\boldsymbol{\epsilon}}_0\right)\mathbf{K}\right)\right].$$

   (e) Structure-function relations.
      Empirical structure-function relationships from Turner *et al.* (1990) [24] are manifested in constants g_1 through g_6 in the constitutive equation.
3. **Equilibrium**
   (a) Reached when the angles between the principal axes of $\boldsymbol{\sigma}^*$ and the principal axes of fabric and strain reach zero.

Algorithm 1: Cowin 2D, time-evolving, architecture remodeling.

1. **Initial State**
   (a) Fabric(normalized), K and volume fraction, e_0.
   (b) Elasticity tensor, D_0 .
       This is calculated using K_0 and e_0.
   (c) Strain, ϵ_0.
       Calculated from a FE analysis for the initial load case.
   (d) Stress, σ_0.
       Calculated using constitutive relation $\{\sigma\} = [D]\{\epsilon\}$.
2. **Remodeling** (Time-evolving, for each iteration, i).
   (a) Apply new load condition, $f^{(i)}$.
   (b) New strain field, $\epsilon^{(i)}$.
       Resulting from the new ith load.
   (c) Fabric remodeling rule:

   $$K^{(i)} = K^{(i-1)} = \Delta K \text{ from the equation}$$

   $$\frac{d\mathbf{K}}{dt} = h_1\left(\hat{\epsilon}^{(i)} - \hat{\epsilon}_0\right) + h_2\left[\mathbf{1}tr\left(\mathbf{K}\right)\left(\hat{\epsilon}^{(i)} - \hat{\epsilon}_0\right)\cdots\right.$$
   $$\left. - \frac{3}{2}\left(\mathbf{K}\left(\hat{\epsilon}^{(i)} - \hat{\epsilon}_0\right) + \left(\hat{\epsilon}^{(i)} - \hat{\epsilon}_0\right)\mathbf{K}\right)\right].$$

   (d) Volume fraction remodeling rule:

   $$e^{(i)} = e^{(i-1)} + \Delta e \text{ from the equation}$$

   $$\frac{de}{dt} = (f_1 + f_2 e)\left[tr(\epsilon^{(i)}) - tr(\epsilon_0)\right].$$

   (e) Structure-function relation.
       $$D^{(i)} = f\left(K^{(i)}, e^{(i)}\right).$$
   (f) Constitutive equation (linear elastic):
       $$\{\sigma^{(i)}\} = \left[D^{(i)}\right]\{\epsilon^{(i)}\}.$$
   (g) Repeat.
       Return to step 2b if convergence criteria is not met.
3. **Equilibrium**
   (a) Reached when new strain $\epsilon^{(i)}$ reaches equilibrium strain, ϵ_0.

Algorithm 2: Fritton 3D, time-evolving, architecture remodeling.

Fyhrie and Carter worked two cases: one where strain energy density is optimized and one where the remodeling objective is failure stress. Carter and co-workers [27, 28] later enhanced this theory by including the effects of multiple loading conditions experienced *in vivo* thus allowing daily stress history to manifest itself (see Section 2.3.1.1). "The strain energy density principle assumes that the bone has the goal of optimizing its stiffness using the least material for a given stress" [26] (see Section 2.3.1.2). The ultimate strength principle "assumes that the bone has the goal of optimizing its strength using the least material for a given load" [26] (see Section 2.3.1.3).

These optimization criteria were integrated into a 3D FE model of the proximal femur. A static distributed load was applied to the femoral head. Two stress fields, the von Mises and the strain-energy stress, were plotted. The stress fields for a 2D slice of the model were compared qualitatively with density patterns found in a 2D X-ray slice of the femur.

2.3.1.1 Addition of multiple load cases   The "given stress" described above should not be a result of a single, static load, Carter and co-workers later suggested, but instead be a manifestation of multiple loads of varying intensity over some characteristic time period [27]. When strain energy density is optimized for this resultant stress, the bone is in equilibrium: there is no net change in bone mass or structure. The goal, then, became a constitutive relation between equilibrium bone morphology and an "effective stress" which encompasses the effects of multiple loading.

To this end, Carter and co-workers propose there is a certain daily stimulus, ψ which is necessary to maintain bone mass [27]. Should ψ fall below its equilibrium value at some site within a bone, there will be a local loss of mass. A higher stimulus than needed (at a point) will result in local bone deposition.

2.3.1.2 Stimulus based on strain energy optimization   In the case of strain energy optimization, the form for the stimulus they developed for a model with nlc ("number of load cases per day") load cases was:

$$\psi \propto \sum_{j=1}^{nlc} n_j (U_{bj})^k, \qquad (14)$$

where subscript j indicates load case, U_{bj} is the strain energy density in the bone tissue (described further below), n_j is the number of cycles of the jth load case, and k is a constant. Note that implicit in the above equation is the assumption that the order that the loads are applied is not important in remodeling. This assumption seems reasonable based on the large disparity in time scales of load application and remodeling. Also note that while the number of cycles per load affects the stimulus, the frequency of those cycles do not.

Trabecular bone is a structure made up of struts of mineralized tissue and pockets of marrow. As a result, continuum variables attempting to describe this structure are often defined as "apparent" values. As in the adaptive elasticity theory described in Section 2.2.1, volume fraction v can be described in terms of bulk density ρ and bone matrix density γ.

$$v = \frac{\rho}{\gamma}. \qquad (15)$$

Since,

$$U = \frac{U_b}{v} = U_b \frac{\rho}{\gamma}$$

eqn (14) can now be written in terms of continuum level strain energy density, U:

$$\psi \propto \frac{1}{\rho^k} \sum_{j=1}^{nlc} n_i U_j^k. \tag{16}$$

Because the prediction of equilibrium morphology is desired, ψ is held constant and the equilibrium value of apparent density relates to U through:

$$\rho \propto \left[\sum_{j=1}^{nlc} n_j U_j^k \right]^{1/k}. \tag{17}$$

To write apparent density in terms of some scalar effective stress induced by each load case, Carter and co-workers [27] introduce the energy stress, $\bar{\sigma}_{energy}$ where:

$$\bar{\sigma}_{energy} = \sqrt{2 E_{ave} U}. \tag{18}$$

E_{ave} is the average of the elastic moduli. (Energy stress is derived from the definition for strain energy density in linear elasticity: $U = \frac{1}{2}\sigma^T S \sigma$, S = compliance matrix.) A constitutive equation relating the apparent density and a scalar effective stress is now possible:

$$\rho \propto \left[\sum_{j=1}^{nlc} n_j \bar{\sigma}_{energy\,j}^m \right]^{1/2m}, \tag{19}$$

where $m = 2k$.

2.3.1.3 Stimulus based on failure stress optimization   In the case of optimizing ultimate stress, the daily stimulus is defined by Carter *et al.* [27] in terms of a scalar effective stress (such as the von Mises) for the jth load case, $\bar{\sigma}_j$:

$$\psi \propto \sum_{j=1}^{nlc} n_j \left(\frac{\bar{\sigma}_j}{\bar{\sigma}_{ult}} \right)^m, \tag{20}$$

where $\bar{\sigma}_{ult}$ is the effective (continuum) ultimate stress which Carter and Hayes [29] noted to be approximately linear to ρ^2. A constitutive relation between effective stress and apparent density can now be written for the strength principle:

$$\rho \propto \left[\sum_{j=1}^{nlc} n_j \bar{\sigma}_j^m \right]^{1/2m}, \tag{21}$$

which is the same form as that derived from the strain energy principle (eqn (19)).

2.3.1.4 2D, remodeling equilibrium applications   In their 2D models [28, 30] (described below), Carter and co-workers assumed isotropy in each element which left stiffness to be described by a single constant, the elastic modulus E. The isotropy assumption was only applicable on an elemental level: the modulus was allowed to vary from element to element. While they did not model architectural adaptation, they did provide a technique for *predicting* the orientation of the equilibrium trabecular structure.

Once bulk density for each element is calculated from one of the two optimization approaches above, the magnitude of the elastic modulus for that element, E was calculated using the empirical structure-function [29]:

$$E = 3790\rho^3. \tag{22}$$

As just mentioned, the orientation of the elastic modulus is not changed in this iterative scheme. Because the elasticity tensor has been reduced to a single scalar modulus, E, this is an *isotropic* remodeling formulation. Instead, the model surmises the final principal material direction (and hence, trabecular orientation) based on a superposed normal stress, σ_n^*, which is calculated for a desired location in the bone as follows:

$$\sigma_n^* = \left[\sum_{j=1}^{nlc} \left(\frac{n_j}{n_t} \right) |\sigma_{nj}|^m \right]^{1/m}, \tag{23}$$

where nlc is the number of load cases, n_j is the number of cycles in the jth load case, n_t is the total number of cycles, σ_{nj} is the normal stress (which is a function of angle, θ) for the jth load case, and m is a weighting constant. When σ_n^* is plotted as a function of angle for a desired location, an ellipse is generated. Carter proposes the major trabecular direction to coincide with the major axis of this effective normal stress ellipse.

A schedule of three load cases (l_j, $j = 1, 3$) corresponding to number of cycles n_j was used to represent bone stresses induced by activities during an "average day" The first load case was generated from a survey of the literature [31, 32]. The other two load cases "were constructed solely on the basis of what we believed to be reasonable conditions in the extremes of normal activities" [30]. The 2D internal remodeling algorithm is summarized in Algorithm 3.

Carter also proposed that the adaptive theory he first put forth with Fyhrie [26] was actually extensible to all phases of bone growth and adaptation, not just adult remodeling [33]. In this expanded theory, the stress history plays a crucial role in regulating *gene expression*. In this view, genetic influences and mechanical stress history are not competing influences on bone morphology. Rather, stress history regulates genetic expression. Carter adapts the optimization theory for developing bones undergoing *in utero* and neonatal ossification [34], for adult bones in maintenance, and bones in a degenerative state due to fracture or disease. In each case, multiple loads are used to develop an expression for stimulus appropriate to

1. **Initial State**
   (a) Strain, ϵ_0.
   (b) Stress, σ_0.
   (c) Material properties, homogeneous.
       $E = 1000\text{MPa}$, $\nu = 0.2$ in each element.
2. **Remodeling** (For each iteration, i)
   (a) For each load, l_j, $j = 1, nlc$
       (All of the calculations below are understood to be "per element".)
       i. Elasticity Equations: Strain, $\epsilon_j^{(i)}$ Calculated using FEA. Constitutive equations (linear elastic):

       $$\sigma_j^{(i)} = C_j^{(i)} \epsilon_j^{(i)}.$$

       ii. Strain energy density (SED).
       $$U_j^{(i)} = \tfrac{1}{2} \sigma_j^{(i)} \epsilon_j^{(i)} \sigma_j^{(i)\mathrm{T}}$$
       iii. Energy stress.
       $$\bar{\sigma}_j^{(i)} = \sqrt{2E_j^{(i)} U_j^{(i)}}$$
   (b) Stimulus.

   $$\psi^{(i)} = \left[\sum_{j=1}^{nlc} n_j \left(\bar{\sigma}_j^{(i)} \right)^M \right]^{(1/2M)}.$$

   (c) Remodeling rule.
       $\rho^{(i)} = K\psi^{(i)}$
   (d) Structure-function relationship.
       $E^{(i)} = 3790\rho^{(i)}$.
3. **Equilibrium**
   (a) If left to run indefinitely, each element would tend to the pathological state of complete density saturation or resorption. After 7 iterations, however, density distributions appeared reasonable.

Algorithm 3: Carter 2D, remodeling equilibrium, internal remodeling.

the stage of bone growth and the theory is implemented in a 2D finite element model.

2.3.1.5 2D, Time evolving applications In the previous works by Carter, no attempt was made at introducing a time scale. Only the homeostatic bone architecture was desired. In 1990, Beaupré and co-workers supplemented Carter's adaptive

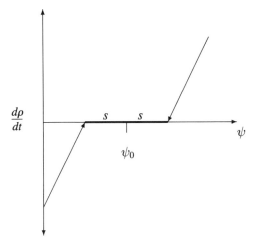

Figure 2: Piecewise linear remodeling rule with "lazy-zone" of half-width s.

optimization theory to include calculation of the remodeling rate (both internal and surface) [35]. Their goal was the definition of the initial value problem governing the remodeling process:

$$\frac{d\rho}{dt} = f(\psi_b),$$

$$\rho(t = 0) = \rho_0, \tag{24}$$

$$\psi(t = 0) = \psi_0.$$

The remodeling rule was written as a function of tissue-level (e.g., in an individual trabecular strut) stimulus, ψ_b. Here the subscript emphasizes that it is felt in the bone matrix. It is assumed that a location in a bone will cease net remodeling when the stimulus at that point equals the value of some "attractor state" stimulus, $\psi_{b_{AS}}$, shown in fig. 2 as actually being a range of stimuli of width $2s$. Until that attractor state is reached, the error can be measured by the difference,

$$e = \psi_b - \psi_{b_{AS}}, \tag{25}$$

where the subscript "b" distinguishes the measure from some continuum-level apparent values. This error driven remodeling technique has also been success-fully employed by others (see e.g., [31, 36]). While Cowin [37] and others have suggested a non-linear form for 24, Beaupré used an idealized piecewise linear function (illustrated in fig. 2) for the density remodeling rule [38]:

$$\frac{d\rho}{dt} = \begin{cases} c(\psi_b - \psi_{b_{AS}} + c \cdot s & \psi_b - \psi_{b_{AS}} \leq -s \\ 0 & -s \leq \psi_b - \psi_{b_{AS}} \geq s \\ c(\psi_b - \psi_{b_{AS}}) - c \cdot s & \psi_b - \psi_{b_{AS}} \geq s. \end{cases} \tag{26}$$

Here, c is an empirical constant, and s describes the half-width of a "lazy zone" [39]. Similarly, the elastic modulus, E was calculated using a piecewise structure-function relation [40]:

$$E = \begin{cases} k_1 \rho^{2.5} & \rho \leq 1.2\,\mathrm{g/cm^3} \\ k_2 \rho^{3.3} & 1.2\,\mathrm{g/cm^3} \leq \rho \leq 1.92\,\mathrm{g/cm^3} \\ 1.45\,\mathrm{MPa} & \rho = 1.92\,\mathrm{g/cm^3} \end{cases} \tag{27}$$

for constants k_1 and k_2 and a saturation density equal to that of cortical bone, $1.92\,\mathrm{g/cm^3}$.

In the companion paper [38], the time evolving model was implemented in a 2D finite element model. The computational algorithm used by Beaupré is summarized in Algorithm 4.

2.3.2 2D Architectural adaptation

Though the time-dependent model of Beaupré was capable of updating the elastic modulus for each element at each iteration, it ultimately remained an isotropic model. The predicted modulus in each element was a scalar, not an anisotropic tensor.

Jacobs et al. [41, 42] added adaptation of the anisotropic stiffness tensor, C to the time-evolving model of Beaupré. The tensor was decomposed into an isotropic and anisotropic portion:

$$\dot{C} = \dot{C}_{iso} + \dot{C}_{aniso}. \tag{28}$$

Perturbations of the isotropic and anisotropic tensors were based on calculations involving the principal stresses. In this way, principal material directions influence calculation of principal stresses at each iteration. This 2D model is described in further detail in Algorithm 5.

2.3.3 3D Architectural adaptation

A more recent implementation of the Stanford model is described in Wirtz et al. [43] and is based on the work of Pandorf et al. [44]. Working from cadaveric human femurs, they created a 3D CAD model from 2D serial CT scans. This model was then coarsely auto-meshed with hex elements using an image processing system. Density was assigned based on the intensity of the CT scan at that point. Other material values such as moduli, Poisson's ratio, and ultimate strength were calculated from the density using empirical relations determined from a comprehensive search of available anisotropic bone data [45]. Destructive serial sectioning was necessary to determine principal material orientation, which were assigned to each element. This data was used as the initial configuration in a 3D FE remodeling algorithm. The model was converted to a tetrahedral-element mesh, and Beaupré's time-evolution of density remodeling algorithm was implemented. Evolution of principal material directions for each element was governed by a continuum damage mechanics model used by Jacobs et al. [46] described in Section 2.4.1.

1. **Initial state**
   (a) Strain, ϵ_0.
   (b) Stress, σ_0.
   (c) Material properties, homogeneous.
       $E = 500\,\text{MPa}$, $\nu = 0.2$ in each element.
2. **Remodeling** (For each iteration, i)
   For each load, l_j, $j = 1$, nlc (number of load cases)
   (All of the calculations below are understood to be "per element".)
   (a) Elasticity equations:
       Strain, $\epsilon_j^{(i)}$ Calculated using FEA
       Constitutive equations (linear elastic):

$$\sigma_j^{(i)} = C_j^{(i)} \epsilon_j^{(i)}.$$

   (b) Energy stress:
       i. Strain energy density (SED).

$$U_j^{(i)} = \tfrac{1}{2} \sigma_j^{(i)} \epsilon_j^{(i)} \sigma_j^{(i)\,\mathrm{T}}$$

       ii. Continuum-level energy stress.

$$\bar{\sigma}_j^{(i)} = \sqrt{2E_j^{(i)} U_j^{(i)}}$$

       iii. Tissue-level energy stress.

$$\bar{\sigma}_{b_j}^{(i)} = \left(\frac{\rho_c}{\rho^{(i)}} \right)^2 \bar{\sigma}_j^{(i)}$$

       where ρ_c is the density of cortical bone.
   (c) Stimulus.

$$\psi_b^{(i)} = \left[\sum_{j=1}^{nlc} n_j \left(\bar{\sigma}_{b_j}^{(i)} \right)^M \right]^{(1/M)}$$

   (d) Remodeling rule (Internal):
       Piecewise-linear (eqn (26)).
   (e) Structure-function relationship.
       Piecewise-linear (eqn (27)).
3. **Equilibrium**
   (a) The analysis terminated when the element with the largest change in density from one iteration to the next was less than $0.02\,\text{g/cm}^3$.

Algorithm 4: Beaupré 2D, time-evolving, internal adaptation.

2.4 Other models

A number of recent computational remodeling algorithms, while sometimes borrowing ideas from Cowin and or the Stanford models, are not easily classified in

1. **Initial state**
   (a) Strain, ϵ_0.
   (b) Stress, σ_0.
   (c) Material properties, homogeneous.
   $E = 500$ MPa.
2. **Remodeling** (Time-evolving, for each iteration i)
   For each load, l_j, $j = 1, nlc$ ($nlc = 3$)
   (All of the calculations below are understood to be "per element".)
   (a) Elasticity equations:
   Strain, $\epsilon_j^{(i)}$ Calculated using FEA

   Constitutive equations (linear elastic): $\sigma_j^{(i)} = C^{(i)} \epsilon_j^{(i)}$
   (b) Stimulus. (Calculated per load case.)
   Average principal stress:

   $$\sigma_{\text{ave}}^{(i)} = \frac{\sigma_I^{(i)} + \sigma_{II}^{(i)} + \sigma_{III}^{(i)}}{3}.$$

   (c) Remodeling rule.
   Internal: Beaupré's piecewise for bulk density eqn (26) with $\psi^{(i)} = \sigma^{(i)}$.
   Architectural: Imbedded in the structure-function relation below.
   (d) Structure-function relation:
   Different rules are used for $\dot{C}_{\text{iso}}$ and $\dot{C}_{\text{aniso}}$ as follows:
      i. For $\dot{C}_{\text{iso}}^{(i)}$:
        Use Beaupré's structure-function relationship for the isotropic model, eqn (27) to calculate modulus $\dot{E}$.
        $\dot{C}_{\text{iso}}^{(i)} = f\left(\dot{E}^{(i)}\right)$.
      ii. For $\dot{C}_{\text{aniso}}^{(i)}$ Use the following logical criteria:
        If $\sigma_I^{(i)}$ or $\sigma_{II}^{(i)} > \sigma_{\text{ave}}^{(i)}$ scale the corresponding principal stiffness in that direction by some factor $\gamma > 1$.
        If $\sigma_I^{(i)}$ or $\sigma_{II}^{(i)} < \sigma_{\text{ave}}^{(i)}$ reduce the corresponding principal stiffness in that direction by some factor $\gamma < 1$.
3. **Equilibrium**
   (a) The algorithm was allowed to run for 300 days (or 100 repetitions of the 3-day loading schedule).

Algorithm 5: Jacobs 2D, time-evolving, architecture remodeling.

either category. Some, for example, have tried to leverage the substantial increases in computer processing speed to create massive meshes of the actual trabecular structure. This section summarizes a few of these innovative approaches.

2.4.1 Global criterion models

Another adaptive anisotropic model by Jacobs *et al.* [46] was inspired by the principles of continuum damage mechanics (CDM). In CDM theory, the elasticity tensor is a modifiable tensor, operated on by a scalar *damage parameter, d*. In Jacobs application of CDM to bone remodeling, a global optimization criterion is ultimately reduced to a local anisotropic remodeling criteria by satisfying mathematical requirements at every point in the global domain. (In particular, Jacobs *et al.* determined the optimum value for bone adaptation "effectiveness" defined as "the difference between the power associated with the applied external loads and the resulting rate-of-change in the total internal energy" [46].) Since the anisotropic characteristics of the stiffness tensor are predicted, this is an architectural adaptation model. The model used multiple load cases (as with Beaupré) but unlike previous work, density and anisotropy changes were calculated for each load case in succession. (Beaupré's algorithm superposed the stresses induced by all of the different load cases and *then* adapted bone apparent density.) Jacobs applied his model to a 2D slice of the proximal femur. It is summarized in Algorithm 6.

Jacobs ran the above algorithm for five alternating load conditions over a period of 300 days.

Bagge [47] used a similar optimization criteria as Jacobs: maximize stiffness thereby minimizing strain energy density. A time-evolving remodeling algorithm used a series of ten load cases, applied in successive time steps. A method employing Lagrange multipliers was used to determine a remodeling rule for volume fraction v. Density and anisotropic moduli were calculated using a structure-function relation for v. (Bagge used correlations for material properties which were found from a micro-finite element analysis of an idealized "unit" of trabecular structure [47, 48].) Reorientation of principal material directions was accomplished by performing a weighted average of the stiffness tensor C calculated for each element in a finite element analysis and determining the principal material directions of the average stress at each element. The remodeling rate was limited to a maximum value based on experimental observations. Finally, the model incorporated a "loading memory" (also used by Levenston *et al.* [49]) which helped model the time lag between application of a loading stimulus and manifestation in bone morphology.

2.4.2 Local criterion models

2.4.2.1 Local continuum damage mechanics model   Doblaré and García 50–52] noted that while the global Jacobs model [46] predicted trabecular material directions well, the ratio of principal to transverse magnitudes was excessive. They set out to again use CDM to derive a more realistic (and, they note, thermodynamically consistent) prediction of anisotropic material properties. Where Jacobs developed update equations for apparent density ρ and the elasticity tensor C, Doblaré and García chose ρ and a *damage tensor D* as the internal variables which

1. **Initial State**
   (a) Strain, ϵ_0.
   (b) Stress, σ_0.
   (c) Material properties, homogeneous.
       Density $\rho_0 = 0.5 \text{ g/cm}^3$, $E = 356 \text{ MPa}$, $\nu = 0.2$
2. **Remodeling** (Time-evolving, for each iteration i).
   For each load, l_j, $j = 1$, nlc
   (All of the calculations below are understood to be "per element".)
   (a) Elasticity equations:
       Strain, $\epsilon_j^{(i)}$
       Calculated using FEA Constitutive equations (linear elastic),

$$\sigma_j^{(i)} = C_j^{(i)} \epsilon_j^{(i)}.$$

   (b) Stimulus.
       Calculated per load case so $\psi_j^{(i)} = \bar{\sigma}_j^{(i)}$, where $\bar{\sigma}$ is the energy stress given by eqn (18).
   (c) Remodeling rule.
       Use Beaupré's remodeling rule for apparent density eqn (26).
   (d) Structure-function relation:
       Two possibilities depending on whether $\dot{\rho}$ is positive or negative. In both cases, $\dot{C}_j^{(i)} = f\left(\dot{\rho}_j^{(i)}, \rho_j^{(i)}, \bar{\sigma}_j^{(i)}, \epsilon_j^{(i)}\right)$.
3. **Equilibrium**
   (a) Algorithm allowed to run for 300 days. If it was allowed to run longer, the model predicted unphysiological material properties.

Algorithm 6: Jacobs Second, 2D, time-evolving, architecture.

would describe bone microstructure. The damage tensor is actually closely related to Cowin's fabric tensor [21]:

$$D = 1 - H^2.\tag{29}$$

The tensor is not a measure of material damage (such as from microcracking), but instead describes the porosity and orientation of the structure. The stimulus derived in the model is based on strain. The resulting remodeling law resulted in predictions of anisotropy magnitude and orientation which were in good qualitative agreement with *in vivo* measurements, but was very complex mathematically. Examples involving the proximal femur with intramedullar and extramedular fixations were conducted using a user-defined material subroutine in a commercial finite element package.

2.4.2.2 Strain energy based adaptive elasticity   In an approach that had similarities to both adaptive elasticity and aspects of the Stanford Model, Huiskes *et al.* [53] used strain energy density (SED) error, $((U - U_n)$ where U_n is the local homeostatic equilibrium SED) to drive both internal and external surface remodeling. Elastic modulus was updated using a piece-wise defined criteria similar to Carter's:

$$\frac{dE}{dt} = \begin{cases} c(U - (1+s)U_n) & U > (1+s)U_n \\ 0 & (1-s)U_n \le U \le (1+s)U_n \\ c(U - (1-s)U_n) & U < (1-s)U_n. \end{cases} \tag{30}$$

The model was implemented in a commercial 2D finite element model of the femur with plane strain four node quadrilateral elements. The SED was calculated at each integration point and then averaged to give a single value within each element. Thus, remodeling was driven by a local criterion. Ad hoc logical precautions prevented devolution into unreal situations. An expansion of this model was done by Weinans *et al.* [54] to include a time-evolving expression for density distribution.

2.4.2.3 Minimization of spatial strain gradients   Turner and co-workers [55] proposed that trabecular bone remodels in a manner that tends to keep continuum (apparent) level strains uniform, thus minimizing spatial strain gradients. This acts to eliminate large pressure gradients which could lead to failure. This results in an update equation for Young's modulus which was similar in form to that of Cowin [10]:

$$\frac{\Delta E}{E} = B_1 \left(\frac{|\epsilon_1| + |\epsilon_2|}{2} - 3500\,\mu\text{strain} \right), \tag{31}$$

where $3500\,\mu$strain was selected as a "target strain" for remodeling, as opposed to the use of a "lazy-zone" as in other models.

The theory was tested in a 2D model of the femur using commercial finite element software. It was found that this approach was more successful at minimizing strain gradients than the SED model used by Huiskes and others.

2.4.2.4 Principal stress based, anisotropic remodeling   While the Jacobs CDM model was derived from a global optimization criterion which led to a local remodeling rule, Impelluso's model [56, 57] for material property prediction was based from the start on a local criterion: that the principal directions θ_C of the orthotropic material tensor C, at any given point, align themselves with the principal directions θ_σ of stress, σ. This criterion, very much in keeping with Wolff's law of trabecular realignment (see the micrograph in fig. 3 for an illustration of trabecular trajectories), was tested in two dimensions using a simple static loading scheme. While previous researchers calculated bone bulk density for each element from the scalar stimulus, Impelluso implemented theories from cellular solids [58] to correlate the apparent strain calculated in each element with the density. Total bone mass was also constrained from iteration to iteration.

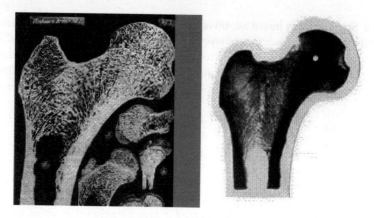

Figure 3: Micrograph of femoral head.

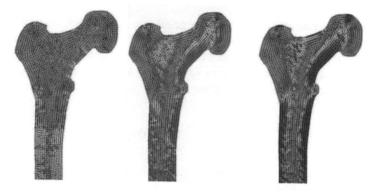

Figure 4: Density evolution in 2D Impelluso model. Dark gray = 2200 kg/m^3, light gray = 50 kg/m^3.

Impelluso also added a safeguard to prevent pathologically high strains from occurring during iteration. Because a linear elastic constitutive law was used in the finite element algorithm, the results are only valid for small strains. Density evolution results are shown in fig. 4. In the early iterations, when bone density was low (in keeping with clinical experience of bone atrophy which accompanies fixation), normal loading conditions could result in large deformations. To prevent this, load magnitude was low in early iterations and increased to typical daily values as density was added to a global "pool" of available bone mass. The Impelluso model is summarized in Algorithm 7.

Miller *et al.* [59], like Impelluso, used the local principal stress criterion and incorporated it into the definition of stimulus derived by Carter. Where Carter's model was written in terms of an "effective stress" based on strain energy density,

1. **Initial State**
    (a) Strain, ϵ_0.
    (b) Stress, σ_0.
    (c) Material properties, random.
2. **Remodeling** (Time-evolving, for each iteration i).
    (All calculations below are understood to take place "per element".)
    (a) Apply a static load.
    (b) Elasticity equations:
        Strain, $\epsilon^{(i)}$ Calculated using FEA
        Constitutive equation (linear elastic),

    $$\sigma^{(i)} = C^{(i)}\epsilon^{(i)}.$$

    (c) Remodeling rule.
        Internal: $\rho^{(i)} = f\left(\epsilon^{(i)}\right)$.
        Architectural: $\theta_C^{(i)} = \theta_\epsilon^{(i)}$.
    (d) Structure-function relation.
        $E_{1,2} = f(\rho^{(i)})$
        Fill the elasticity tensor $C^{(i)}$ using $\theta_C^{(i)}$ and $E_{1,2}$.
3. **Equilibrium**
    (a) Reached when the element with the maximum change in density is within a preset tolerance.

Algorithm 7: Impelluso 2D, remodeling equilibrium, architecture adaptation.

Miller's was written in terms of principal stress as follows:

$$\psi_{k(i)} = \frac{1}{E_{k(i)}}\left(\sum_j n_j \sigma_{k(i,j)}^m\right)^{1/m}, \tag{32}$$

$$i = 1\dots \text{ number of elements,}$$
$$j = 1\dots \text{ number of load cases,}$$
$$k = 1,2\text{: principal, transverse direction,}$$
$$E = \text{Young's Modulus,}$$

where m is the usual weighting constant found in Carter's model (a value of $m = 4$ was used by Jacobs). The stimulus was used with the remodeling rate equations of Beaupré [35]:

$$\frac{dE_{k(i)}}{dt} = \begin{cases} c\left[\psi_{k(i)} - \psi_0(1+s)\right] & \psi_{k(i)} \geq \psi_0(1+s) \\ 0 & \psi_0(1-s) \leq \psi_{k(i)} \geq \psi_0(1+s) \\ c\left[\psi_{k(i)} - \psi_0(1-s)\right] & \psi_{k(i)} \leq \psi_0(1-s). \end{cases} \tag{33}$$

2.4.3 Trabecular level and below

Recent applications of finite element analysis to bone remodeling have attempted to simulate morphological changes that occur to individual trabeculae. Adachi and co-workers [60] modeled a 5 mm cube of cancellous bone obtained from a canine femur using micro-CT scans (μCT) to map individual voxels to finite elements. Each voxel was 20 μm, resulting in a model with approximately 2.3 million elements. The stimulus for remodeling was chosen to be "nonuniformity" in stress which exists at a point in an individual trabeculae. This stimulus was used with a remodeling rate equation to either add or remove individual voxels to the surfaces of the trabeculae. Tsubota *et al.* [61, 62] attempted to use this technique to predict remodeling in a two-dimensional representation of a femur with a somewhat arbitrary initial trabecular morphology. The initial trabecular structure, containing about 0.67 million elements, was obtained not by μCT scans, but by randomly generating a pattern of circular trabeculae whose characteristic dimensions were consistent with values of the fabric tensor published by Cowin [63]. While the model demonstrated trabecular reorientation toward principal stresses surprisingly well, the trabecular density at an apparent level was not realistic.

2.5 A new algorithm of bone remodeling

How can emerging models of functional adaptation better exploit both advances in mechanistic models and the CI? Suggested in this section is one approach currently being researched by the authors. This bone remodeling algorithm hopes to avail itself of the CI potential through:

- a parallelized, explicit FE code capable of fast solution to large scale problems via remote supercomputer
- extensibility which allows for seamless integration with MD and CFD codes (e.g., to couple with muscle motion, or blood flow) or modules incorporating osteon-level activity as they emerge.

To this end, the algorithm is designed to use a dynamic, rate-type remodeling stimulus. It is proposed that this parallel, dynamic FE algorithm not only opens the door for solution to large-scale problems, but is very much in keeping with current understanding of remodeling mechanisms which have found that dynamic loads are crucial to maintenance of bone mass. (See, e.g., [64–66]. Turner has a nice summary of dynamically induced remodeling at the continuum level [67]. For a sampling of cellular-level research on dynamically induced drag on osteocytic processes and the pericellular matrix, see [68–70].)

2.5.1 Hypoelastic dynamic functional adaptation

Current research by the authors hopes to incorporate the need for dynamic loads as a remodeling stimulus in a model which will be extensible as understanding of remodeling grows. A 3D model femur from the Standardized Femur Project [71] was meshed with approximately 50,000, 8-noded hexahedral elements. A dynamic load is applied to the femoral head and greater trochanter corresponding to observed magnitudes, rates, and directions. The model is fixed at mid-diaphysis. The rate of deformation tensor D will be calculated per element and used as the stimulus to a piecewise linear remodeling rule. To account for potentially significant cumulative elemental rotations, a (path-dependent) hypoelastic constitutive law will be used with the Jaumann stress rate. The model is summarized here.

2.5.1.1 Finite element implementation
- The finite element semidiscretization equation (spatially discrete, temporally continuous) is derived by writing the equation of virtual work for small velocities:

$$[m]\{\ddot{d}\} = \{p\} = \{r_{\text{ext}}\},\qquad(34)$$

$$\{p\} = \int_{V_e} [B]^T \{\sigma\}dV,\qquad(35)$$

where $[m]$ is the elemental mass matrix $\{\ddot{d}\}$ is the vector of nodal acceleration, $\{p\}$ is the vector of internal loads, $\{r_{\text{ext}}\}$ is the vector of external loads, $[B]$ is the strain-displacement matrix, and $\{\sigma\}$ is the stress vector resulting from the hypoelastic constitutive equation.

2.5.1.2 Remodeling algorithm
- Constitutive law: The current stress state is found using a path-dependent hypoelastic constitutive law: $\dot{\sigma} = C(K, \rho)D + W\sigma + \sigma W^T$. Objectivity is achieved by accounting for spin terms W, which arise as an element rotates. The current objective stress rate is numerically integrated to get the current stress $\{p\}_t$,

$$\int [B]^T \left\{ ([C(\theta_{\hat{\epsilon},\rho})]\{D\} + [W]^T\{\sigma\} + \cdots \right.$$
$$\left. \sigma^T \left[W^T\right]\right)_{t-\frac{\Delta t}{2}} \Delta t + \{\sigma\}_{t-\Delta t} \right\}.\qquad(36)$$

- Stimulus, ψ: A function of the rate of deformation, D. For small deformation gradients F, D is very nearly equal to the rate of strain: $D = F^{-T}\dot{\epsilon}F^{-1}$. The rate of deformation tensor is the symmetric part of the velocity gradient, $D = (1/2)\left((\partial v/\partial x) + (\partial v/\partial x)^T\right)$.
- Remodeling rules:
  - Internal: Piecewise linear with lazy zone.
  - Architectural: Principal material directions of orthotropy align with the principal directions (θ) of the continuum deviatoric strain, $\hat{\epsilon} = \epsilon - \frac{1}{3}tr(\epsilon)\mathbf{1}$. This is accomplished through multiplication by a transformation matrix, $[T]$:

$$[C]^{(i+1)} = [T(\theta_{\hat{\epsilon}})][C]^{(i)}[T(\theta_{\hat{\epsilon}})]^T.\qquad(37)$$

- Structure-Function Relation: from Yang *et al.* [72]:

$$E_1 = 1240E_t\phi^{1.80}, \qquad E_2 = 885E_t\phi^{1.89}, \qquad E_3 = 528.8E_t\phi^{1.92},$$
$$2G_{23} = 533.3E_t\phi^{1.92}, \quad 2G_{13} = 633.3E_t\phi^{1.97}, \quad 2G_{12} = 972.6E_t\phi^{1.98},$$
$$v_{23} = 0.256\phi^{-0.09}, \qquad v_{13} = 0.316\phi^{-0.19}, \qquad v_{12} = 0.176\phi^{-0.25},$$
$$v_{32} = 0.153\phi^{-0.05}, \qquad v_{31} = 0.135\phi^{-0.07}, \qquad v_{21} = 0.125\phi^{-0.16}.$$

3 Using FE to create a virtual muscle

While this text concerns itself with hard tissue, this section focuses on ways to exploit the CI to advance biomechanics. To this end, a brief excursion into muscle mechanics is presented, not as an end in itself, but to demonstrate the possibility of integrating the bone and muscle.

A muscle bundle consists of groups of muscle fibers. Fibers, in turn, are composed of groups of myofibrils as seen on the left in fig. 5. A unit of the myofibril is indicated in the figure as a myofilament. A myofilament, in its turn, consists of two molecular structures: myosin and actin. In addition, myofibrils are surrounded by the sarcoplasmic reticulum. Upon innervation, the sarcoplasmic reticulum releases calcium. Calcium serves as a chemical inducement to drive the "heads" on the myosin complex to act as a "zipper" and pull – on both ends – along the actin

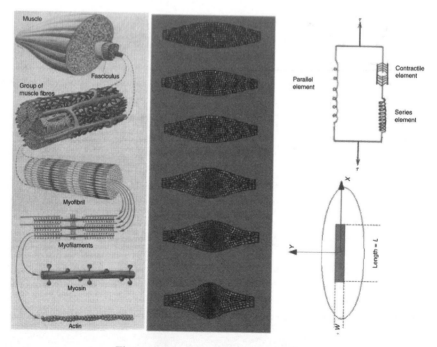

Figure 5: Models of muscle actuation.

molecule. This "zippering", "pulling" or "ratcheting" is what causes the muscle to contract and bulge.

A 1D mechanical model, Hill's model (upper right in fig. 5), has been actively used in biomechanical research. Hill's model represents an active muscle as composed of three elements. Two elements are arranged in series: a contractile element, which at rest is freely extensible (zero tension), but when activated is capable of shortening; and an elastic element arranged in series with the contractile element. To account for the elasticity of the muscle at rest, a third "parallel elastic element" is added.

The Hill type muscle model, used for nonlinear length-tension properties to calculate dynamic power output, remains the primary investigative tool in musculoskeletal biomechanics [73, 74]. While modifications for subtle "tuning" have been created [75], the model remains nearly the same as originally described by Hill in 1938 [76]. The model has been used for a variety of projects involving reptilian, amphibian, arthropoda, icthian, avian and human locomotion. However, the primary use for the model involves human loco-motor strategies for walking, running, jumping and cycling. This new muscle mechanics algorithm will extend the reach of these biomechanical models by creating a new model that exploits the tools of the emerging CI.

This model of active 2D muscle mechanics is essentially an inversion of the FE method. Consider the schematic shown in the bottom right of fig. 5. The external ellipse-like boundary represents the external boundary of a FE mesh of a 2D muscle bundle. The shaded box in the center of the ellipse on the right of fig. 5 can be considered a zone of influence. A strain is applied to all FE elements within this zone of influence. From the strain and elastic properties, the stress in each element can be computed. The resulting forces on each node can be computed from the stresses. Finally, these nodal forces are actually applied and the final FE analysis is conducted. Results are seen in the center of fig. 5. (It is important to state that compatibility is not violated, as this algorithm does NOT apply the strains, but only the approximate forces that "could" induce such strains.)

Naturally, there are many issues to address. Should the applied strain be ramped down non-linearly or linearly? Or should it be constant over the zone of influence? How wide should the zone be (in the figure, there is only one large zone)? How long should the zone be? How many zones should there be (if they are very small, there could be hundreds within a muscle)? Where should they be? Should enervation occur through a frequency or amplitude based impulse? These are some of the many questions that invite the participation of physiologists. It may be possible that this new paradigm of inverting the FE method could open the door to the creation of new empirical equations and new parametric constants which could ultimately be related to physiological parameters in much the same way that the parameters in Hill's model have been used in the past thirty to forty years. A critical question would be how such a 3D active muscle mesh would be "loaded" onto a bone (say, the femur) and how it would effect human gait, remodeling, and fracture fixation. Thus, while this approach can generate a muscle to be used in bone loading cases, it also invites research into new approaches to muscle modeling itself.

4 An overview of the CI

As mentioned in Section 2, much of the current research in bone mechanics has been away from the macroscopic bone models summarized in this chapter toward more mechanistic (that is, cellular-level and below) ones. It was also suggested that this distinction is no longer necessary; that an integrated approach can exploit knowledge gained at and below the cellular level with the clinical utility and computational attractiveness of macroscopic models.

Ultimately, if these models are to be deployed in the clinic to enhance surgical planning, models will have to be guided by microscopic understanding, but the predictions will be at the macroscopic level. For example, a surgeon may have to decide on a proper course of action, dictated by the peculiarities for a particular patient, such as where to place fixation plates. The patient may have, for example, a lytic lesion, or perhaps due to a misarticulation between the hip and femoral head, a pathological distribution of density or trabecular architecture. In these cases, predicted macroscopic response to surgical intervention will be necessary.

To extend the scenario, suppose that after intervention, it was advantageous to study remodeling during a normal gait. A model in which a muscle bundle could be used as an actuator to move the femur and tibia would be very useful. In this way, bone models can be integrated with muscle models to more fully exploit macroscopic approaches. The model could be extended again to include an embedded femoral artery in the muscle. This would require, in addition to the FE and MD codes, a CFD code for blood flow.

All these cases require macroscopic models to be readily accessible by the clinician and also require a computational platform on which they can be integrated and delivered to the surgical ward. The remainder of this chapter addresses these issues. It commences with some preliminary definitions from computer science.

4.1 Computer science definitions

These selected definitions reveal some of the CI techniques and characteristics that will be used to construct a new CI.

4.1.1 Application programming interface (API)
An API is a collection of software functions and structures that are made available to a programmer. This collection of code, often referred to as a library, facilitates software development by collecting a group of commonly used and related functionality together into a reusable form. Use of API's free a programmer from the tedium of redeveloping common code functionality.

4.1.2 Sockets
A socket is the standard underlying software API for computer network communications. Sockets operate with four basic steps whose functionality can best be described by a "telephone" metaphor. First, a telephone jack is installed in the wall.

This is akin to creating the socket with the socket call. Next, a phone is attached to the phone jack in order that calls can be made. This is akin to the socket bind function. Third, the telephone company is notified that the phone is ready to receive calls and a phone number is associated with the jack. This is akin to the socket listen function. Finally, since the phone is ready and waiting for calls it can receive: answering the call is akin to the socket accept function. Note that the socket API is very low level, and there are numerous communications packages layered on top of the socket API, making for easier network communications, such as the message passing interface (MPI) or parallel virtual machine (PVM).

4.1.3 Fork

A fork is a fairly advanced UNIX system API. In the most basic terms, a fork is a mechanism whereby a program creates another running copy of itself. This copy is, in every sense, identical to the original. Both copies continue execution from the point of the fork, and would, under normal circumstances, perform the exact same functions up until their termination. Using fork technology processes are able to determine which running version is the original, and which is the copy.

4.1.4 Exec

When a program makes an exec call, another advanced UNIX system API, it stops what it was doing and begins running the functionality defined within the exec call. The new exec functionality can be completely unrelated to the functionality that was being performed. An exec call can execute any program that it has available. Used in conjunction with a fork, this can be a very powerful mechanism allowing one program to run any other program, while maintaining the integrity of peripheral computer resources and devices. A fork is accomplished as follows. First, program "A" forks itself, creating an identical running copy: program "Ac". Next, both "A" and "Ac" must identify if they are the original or the copy. The original program "A" continues as before, but the copy program execs an instance of a new program "B" in its same memory space. The result is an instance of program "A" and a new instance of program "B" both of which are actively running.

4.1.5 Process

In the parlance of computer science, a program is the series of instructions that are stored (either in memory or on the hard drive) while a process is the actual instance of that program when it runs. One program can have many processes, but each process will only be running one program at a time. Consider the example where a program is running: at startup, that program will have one process. If the program were to fork/exec itself, then it would now have two different processes. If each of these were to fork/exec itself, then the program would have four different processes, and so on. There is a special type of process, called a Daemon, which is unique in that it does not belong to any user, and is instead associated only with the operating system.

4.1.6 Client/server model

The client/server model is a functional model for process management that is very common in computer programming. In this model, there is a single server process whose function is to provide a defined service. Typically a server is structured so that it runs indefinitely on a certain machine (as a daemon), waiting for requests for that service from clients. The clients are other processes, often on other machines, which communicate with the server, generally, through a socket, and request functionality. The client/server model is powerful because it allows for a single process (the server) to perform a specialized action on demand over and over again.

4.1.7 Shared memory

Use of shared memory enables a common block of memory to be accessed and modified by many different processes. This is a convenient tool for allowing different processes to communicate with one another in a regulated manner. For instance, if one process needed to know the result of a computation that was being carried out by another process, the result could be stored in common shared memory. Of course complications would arise if two or more processes wanted to write to the same block of memory at roughly the same time or if a process wanted a result before it was ready.

4.1.8 Semaphores

Semaphores regulate access to certain resources such as shared memory. A semaphore works by restricting access to certain sections of code that deal with critical resources. Before a process can enter a critical section (update shared memory), it checks the semaphore. If the semaphore is raised, the process must wait. If the semaphore is not raised then the process raises the semaphore and enters the shared memory arena. Once it completes its work, the process lowers the semaphore, freeing the critical resource for use by another process. Semaphores must be carefully managed to avoid causing processes to stall by waiting for a resource that is never freed.

5 An implementation of a CI for biomechanics

A macroscopic biomechanical analysis of human organs or organ systems requires the coupling of the core algorithms of mechanical engineering: FE for tissue deformation analyses, MD for motion analyses, and CFD for blood flow analyses. Further, more accurate models can be created that include coupled molecular dynamics, cell physics, physiological models and so on. A coupled model as ambitious as this would require a new biomechanical CI platform.

For now, consider the multi-phase model described in Section 4: arterial blood supply to a muscle-actuated femur during gait. This will require the couple algorithms of finite element analysis (for arterial deformation and muscle deformation), multi-body dynamics (for femur/tibia motion) and fluid dynamics (for blood flow). In standard MD analysis, linkages are presumed rigid. The motion of rigid linkage systems can be analyzed using traditional explicit integration methods. Multi-body dynamics analyses provide the time-varying position of the links and the joint contact forces between them. If the links are deformable however, an analysis must also be conducted to solve for their deformation. Thus, after an iteration of the MD method to obtain contact forces and the updated position of the links an FE analysis can be conducted to obtain the new deformed geometry. If updated bone properties were desired, a remodeling scheme from Section 2 could also be implemented here. With this new deformed geometry, the configuration of the system is updated in shared memory before proceeding to the next iteration of the MD method. Since either process can alter the state of the linkage system (FE deforms the links and MD moves them), it is critical to use ensure that only one process at a time is updating the data. Semaphores are used to ensure such data integrity.

5.1 A new architecture

Consider the solution scenario as indicated in fig. 6. Upon receipt of a request from a client ("help me solve a coupled problem such as blood flow in an artery embedded in a muscle/bone linkage system"), the server **forks/execs** (Sections 4.1.3 and 4.1.4) a process scheduler. The scheduler parses the incoming data frame, interprets the request and takes the necessary actions. The scheduler creates a *shared memory arena* (Section 4.1.7) which is an active region of memory accessible by other concurrent processes. Information pertinent to the FE and MD *processes* (Section 4.1.5) (mesh connectivity, boundary conditions, material properties, geometric properties, joints, and link inertial parameters) is stored in appropriate segments of the shared memory. Then the scheduler instantiates the necessary *semaphores* (Section 4.1.8)

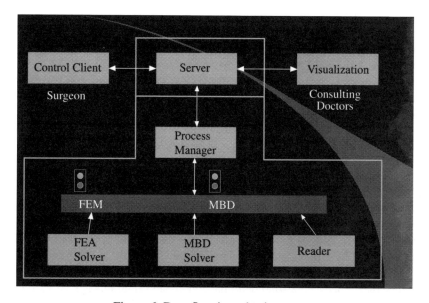

Figure 6: Data flow in a physics server.

which enable processes to self-regulate their access to the shared memory. The scheduler then **forks/execs** secondary physics-based child processes and schedules them to fulfill the client request: FE process (deformation and possible remodeling), MD process (motion), and CFD process (blood flow). Each physics-based child process immediately attaches to the shared memory arena. Processing then commences.

The shared memory arena describes the state of the object. First, the FE process raises the semaphore and locks the memory to prevent another process from altering the data while it conducts its incremental analysis. The FE process then establishes state equilibrium by replacing the data in the shared memory arena with new data resulting from its *deformation analysis* (updates node geometry of links, etc.) and then lowers the semaphore. Next the MD process raises the semaphore, locks the memory, establishes dynamic equilibrium, deposits an updated configuration of the data resulting from its dynamic analysis, and lowers the semaphore. The scenario iterates with each process taking its turn. This approach avoids the mathematical complexities of coupled physical analyses while the use of semaphores, as lightweight processes, does not degrade optimization. While there do exist traditional means to couple the algorithms of applied mechanics, this platform reveals a new use and extension of the CI for biomechanics.

The authors now elaborate on this architecture by including contact algorithms and providing further detail. In order to simplify the computational theater, it is assumed that the linkage system is driven by prescribed joint motion with respect to time. In addition, a fluid is contained in an elastic tube that is embedded in a deforming solid. The MD process commences processing the FE process blocks on a read of the contact forces from the MD process. Upon delivery of the forces, the FE establishes state equilibrium by modifying its data resulting from its deformation analysis (updates node geometry of links, etc.). This will occur on each FE target mesh. Next the CONTACT receives data from each mesh and assesses contact criteria. If contact occurs, contact resisting forces are applied. The FE process computes the new geometry according to the new contact forces, and lowers the semaphore. The CONTACT repeats: updates contact forces, and delivers back the status. The above processes between FE and CONTACT processes will be iterated until the CONTACT process accepts the tolerance set *a priori* for the contact. As the last step of each time increment, the MD awakens, updates the reaction forces required for the prescribed motion based on the revised contact forces, and lowers the semaphore.

If the CFD analyses in the deformable tube are requested for prescribed wall position and pressure variation at the upstream boundary, CFD process is invoked at each time step. In this scenario the second contact event is invoked between the vessel wall and fluid, in addition to the first contact event between the rigid linkage and the deformable body. The new contact event is independent from the first event. Each time, both the FE and CFD processes will be invoked. Then the second CONTACT process assures the continuity between the wall deformation and the fluid velocity at the interior wall. This process is also iterative as discussed for the contact between a solid deformable body and rigid linkage. At each time step, each contact process must be iterated until a pre-set tolerance is met.

5.2 A new network protocol

The Standard for the Exchange of Earthquake Data (SEED) is an international standard format for the exchange of digital seismological data. SEED was designed for use by the earthquake research community, primarily for the exchange between institutions of unprocessed Earth motion data. The SEED database defined the protocols by which seismic data was transferred over the net; in so doing, it enabled researchers to develop hardware and software tools to facilitate seismic research and analysis. A second aspect of this work is to research the proper design of an analogous protocol for biomechanics data sharing.

For the sake of computational efficiency, data frame structures for *transmission* and data process structures for *analysis* should be identical as this would facilitate memory acquisition for processing and communication. The type of process (FE or MD for example) will be in the header file of the first data frame along with other pertinent information.

The data frames (fig. 7) will be designed to include all pertinent information including (in an order that will be the subject of research): material properties, geometric properties, boundary conditions, numerical methods constants, target architecture, and backup architecture. Naturally, the spawned processes will communicate with each other and this communication will adhere to rigorous data frame designs. Researching data frame formats for the transmission of physics-based simulations is a critical task if one hopes to deliver the power of mechanics to real-time simulators.

Two final points must be made. First, a well developed CI and data transmission protocol will allow researchers to place their algorithms on the web for access. This will hopefully foster the movement from pure research to development and use in the clinic. Second, this CI would serve as the conduit by which macroscopic models can be used to bridge the length scale gaps to the micro level. Nothing prevents one from deploying cellular-level model algorithms as codes spawned by a server. Proper data frame design would inform the macroscopic processes that, before continuing to the next iteration, they should wait for data from

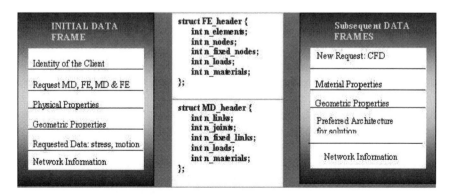

Figure 7: Data frames to support network architecture.

gap-bridging processes. In these ways, the CI would simultaneously enhance model sophistication and clinical practicality; two goals traditionally at odds.

6 A call to action

In January of 2003, the National Science Foundation (NSF) Advisory Committee on Environmental Research and Education in the United States published a report [77] that identified CI as a suite of tools and research essential to the study of engineering systems. In response to the January report, the NSF hosted a June workshop to provide preliminary input to the Directorate for Engineering in considering how to best make investments – 1 billion dollars (US) per year on engineering alone, as advocated by the Atkins report – that support the creation and use of new CI capabilities to support engineering research and education over the next decade.

This chapter has introduced a new view of applied mechanics and the CI. The definitions and efforts described here will hopefully spur new research endeavors by practitioners of applied bio and computational mechanics. The authors offer a final scenario as a motivation.

A surgeon must prepare for a medical procedure: the placement of a stent in an artery near the heart valve. The surgeon would like to prepare for the intervention by first conducting a simulation. Clearly, the following algorithms are needed: fluid mechanics (for the blood flow), finite element methods (for modeling the deformation of the artery, perhaps shell models for the layered musculature of the heart itself), and perhaps, MD (to model the interaction of the valve mechanism and papillary muscles). These programs must orchestrate their analysis, be fast, and deliver their results to an appropriate visualization tool. In addition, the surgeon might also have the need and option of choosing a host of constitutive models for viscous blood flow, heart valve and papillary muscle properties.

This scenario suggests a need for creating a new type of computational platform. The purpose of such a platform would be to integrate the extant computational algorithms of mechanics and deliver their power to engineers, surgeons and animators in a fundamentally new way. The scenarios also suggest the need to properly define data transmission protocols between such a physics platform and the visualization tools. These two efforts – platform construction and data frame design – are an intrinsic part of the CI's use in applied mechanics and is far more intricate than simple data mining, data retrieval and inspection that many are proposing.

This new platform represents an opportunity to take a new approach to a diverse array of problems facing engineers whose solutions are limited in scope, cumbersome or impossible with traditional software approaches. These problems include: flexible multi-bodies, solid-fluid interaction, coupled heat and deformation analyses, process parallelization for applied mechanical problems, and a wide array of numerical convergence and stability issues. An intellectual investment now in this research at the intersection of applied mechanics and computer science will allow for a dramatic increase in the scope and facility of biomechanics research in the future.

Acknowledgments

The authors wish to thank the US Defense Advanced Research Projects Agency (DARPA) and the US National Science Foundation whose funding made our research possible.

References

[1] Hart, R.T. & Fritton, S.P., Introduction to finite element based simulation of functional adaptation of cancellous bone. *Forma*, **12**, pp. 277–299, 1997.

[2] Hart, R.T., Bone modeling and remodeling: Theories and computation. *Bone Mechanics Handbook, 2nd Edition*, ed. S.C. Cowin, CRC Press: Boca Raton, FL, Chapter 31, 2001.

[3] Cowin, S.C., A review and critique of a bone tissue adaptation model. *Eng. Trans.*, **51(2–3)**, pp. 113–193, 2003.

[4] Hart, R.T. & Davy, D.T., Theories of bone modeling and remodeling. *Bone Mechanics*, ed. S.C. Cowin, CRC Press: Boca Raton, FL, pp. 253–277, 1989.

[5] Oden, Z.M., Hart, R.T., Forwood, M.R. & Burr, D.B., A priori prediction of functional adaptation in canine radii using a cell based mechanistic approach. *Trans. 41st Orthopaedic Research Society*, Orlando, FL, p. 296, 1995.

[6] Mullender, M.G., Huiskes, R. & Weinans, H., A physiological approach to the simulation of bone remodeling as a self-organizational control process. *J. Biomechanics*, **27(11)**, pp. 1389–1394, 1994.

[7] Mullender, M.G. & Huiskes, R., Proposal for the regulatory mechanism of Wolff's law. *J. Orthopaedic Res.*, **13(4)**, pp. 503–512, 1995.

[8] van der Meulen, M.C.H. & Huiskes, R., Why mechanobiology?: A survey article. *J. Biomechanics*, **35(4)**, pp. 401–414, 2002.

[9] Hollister, S.J., Computational modeling of biological tissues, notes from BME/ME 506, 1996. University of Michigan, www.engin.umich.edu/class/bme506/.

[10] Cowin, S.C. & Hegedus, D.H., Bone remodeling i: theory of adaptive elasticity. *J. Elasticity*, **6**, pp. 313–326, 1976.

[11] Hegedus, D.H. & Cowin, S.C., Bone remodeling ii: small strain adaptive elasticity. *J. Elasticity*, **6**, pp. 337–352, 1976.

[12] Cowin, S.C. & Nachlinger, R.R., Bone remodeling iii: uniqueness and stability in adaptive elasticity. *J. Elasticity*, **8**, pp. 285–295, 1978.

[13] Cowin, S.C., Continuum models of the adaptation of bone to stress. *Mechanical Properties of Bone*, ed. S.C. Cowin, American Society of Mechanical Engineers: New York, NY, pp. 193–210, 1981.

[14] Cowin, S.C. & Buskirk, W.C.V., Internal remodeling induced by a medullary pin. *J. Biomechanics*, **11(5)**, pp. 269–275, 1978.

[15] Cowin, S.C. & Firoozbakhsh, K., Bone remodeling of diaphyseal surfaces under constant load: theoretical predictions. *J. Biomechanics*, **7(6)**, pp. 471–484, 1981.

[16] Firoozbakhsh, K. & Cowin, S.C., Devolution of inhomogeneties in bone structure – predictions of adaptive elasticity theory. *J. Biomechanical Eng.*, **102(4)**, pp. 287–293, 1980.

[17] Hart, R.T., *Quantitative response of bone to mechanical stress.* Ph.D. thesis, Case Western Reserve University, Cleveland, OH, 1983.

[18] Hart, R.T., Davy, D.R. & Heiple, K.G., A computational method for stress analysis of adaptive elastic materials with a view toward applications in straininduced bone remodeling. *J. Biomechanical Eng.*, **106**, pp. 342–350, 1984.

[19] Cowin, S.C., Sadegh, A.M. & Luo, G.M., An evolutionary Wolff's law for trabecular architecture. *J. Biomechanical Eng.*, **114**, pp. 129–136, 1992.

[20] Wolff, J., *Das Gesetz Transformation der Knocken.* Hirschwald Verlag: Berlin, 1892.

[21] Cowin, S.C., Wolff's law of trabecular architecture at remodeling equilibrium. *J. Biomechanics*, **108**, pp. 83–86, 1986.

[22] Harrigan, T. & Mann, R.W., Characterization of microstructural anisotropy in orthotropic materials using a second rank tensor. *J. Material Science*, **19**, pp. 761–767, 1984.

[23] Gurtin, M.E., *An Introduction to Continuum Mechanics.* Academic Press: New York, 1981.

[24] Turner, C.H., Cowin, S.C., Rho, J.Y., Ashman, R.B. & Rice, J.C., The fabric dependence of the orthotropic elastic constants of cancellous bone. *J. Biomechanics*, **32(6)**, pp. 549–561, 1990.

[25] Fritton, S.P., *Computational simulation of trabecular bone adaptation.* Ph.D. thesis, Tulane University, New Orleans, LA, 1994.

[26] Fyhrie, D.P. & Carter, D.R., A unifying principle relating stress to trabecular bone morphology. *J. Orthopaedic Res.*, **4**, pp. 304–317, 1986.

[27] Carter, D.R., Fyhrie, D.P. & Whalen, R.T., Trabecular bone density and loading history: regulation of connective tissue biology by mechanical energy. *J. Biomechanics*, **20(8)**, pp. 785–794, 1987.

[28] Carter, D.R., Orr, T.E., Fyhrie, D.P., Whalen, R.T. & Schurman, D.J., Mechanical stress and skeletal morphogenesis, maintenance, and degeneration. *Trans. 33rd Orthopaedic Research Society*, San Francisco, CA, p. 462, 1987.

[29] Carter, D.R. & Hayes, W.C., The behavior of bone as a two-phase porous structure. *J. Bone and Joint Surgery*, **59-A(7)**, pp. 954–962, 1977.

[30] Carter, D.R., Orr, T.E. & Fyhrie, D.P., Relationships between loading history and femoral cancellous bone architecture. *J. Biomechanics*, **22(3)**, pp. 231–244, 1989.

[31] Pauwels, F., *Biomechanics of the Locomotor Apparatus: contributions on the functional anatomy of the locomotor apparatus.* Springer-Verlag: New York, 1980.

[32] Rybicki, E.F., Simonen, F.A. & Weiss, E.B., On the mathematical analysis of stress in the human femur. *J. Biomechanics*, **5**, pp. 203–215, 1972.

[33] Carter, D.R., Mechanical loading history and skeletal biology. *J. Biomechanics*, **20(11)**, pp. 1095–1109, 1987.

[34] Carter, D.R., Orr, T.E., Fyhrie, D.P. & Schurman, D.J., Influences of mechanical stress on prenatal and postnatal skeletal development. *Clinical Orthopaedics and Related Research*, **219**, pp. 237–250, 1987.

[35] Beaupré, G.S., Orr, T.E. & Carter, D.R., An approach for time-dependent bone modeling and remodeling – theoretical development. *J. Orthopaedic Res.*, **8**, pp. 651–661, 1990.

[36] Kummer, B., Computer simulation of the adaptation of bone to mechanical stress. *Proc. of the San Diego Biomedical Symposium*, San Diego, CA, volume 10, pp. 5–12, 1971.

[37] Cowin, S.C., Bone remodeling of diaphyseal surface by torsional loads: theoretical predictions. *J. Biomechanics*, **20**, pp. 1111–1120, 1987.

[38] Beaupré, G.S., Orr, T.E. & Carter, D.R., An approach for time-dependent bone modeling and remodeling – application: A preliminary remodeling simulation. *J. Orthopaedic Res.*, **8**, pp. 662–670, 1990.

[39] Carter, D.R., Mechanical loading histories and cortical bone remodeling. *Calcified Tissue International*, **36**, pp. S19–S24, 1984.

[40] Gibson, L.J., The mechanical behavior of cancellous bone. *J. Biomechanics*, **18**, pp. 317–328, 1985.

[41] Jacobs, C.R., Simo, J.C., Beaupré, G.S. & Carter, D.R., Anisotropic adaptive bone remodeling simulation based on principal stress magnitudes. *Trans. 41st Orthopaedic Research Society*, Orlando, FL, p. 178, 1995.

[42] Jacobs, C.R., Simo, J.C., Beaupré, G.S. & Carter, D.R., A principal stress-based approach to the simulation of anisotropic bone adaptation to mechanical loading. *Comput. Methods Biomech. Biomed. Eng.*, pp. 85–94, 1996.

[43] Wirtz, D.C., Pandorf, T., Portheine, F., Radermacher, K., Schiffers, N., Prescher, A., Weichert, D. & Niethard, F.U., Concept and development of an orthotropic fe model of the proximal femur. *J. Biomechanics*, **36**, pp. 289–293, 2003.

[44] Pandorf, T., Haddi, A., Wirtz, D.C., Lammerding, J., Forst, R. & Weichert, D., Numerical simulation of adaptive bone remodeling. *J. Theoretical and Applied Mechanics*, **37(3)**, pp. 639–658, 1999. Published by: The Polish Society of Theoretical and Applied Mechanics.

[45] Wirtz, D.C., Pandorf, T., Portheine, F., Radermacher, K., Schiffers, N., Prescher, A., Weichert, D. & Forst, R., Critical evaluation of known bone material properties to realize anisotropic fe-simulation of the proximal femur. *J. Biomechanics*, **33**, pp. 1325–1330, 2000.

[46] Jacobs, C.R., Simo, J.C., Beaupré, G.S. & Carter, D.R., Adaptive bone remodeling incorporating simultaneous density and anisotropy considerations. *J. Biomechanics*, **30(6)**, pp. 603–613, 1997.

[47] Bagge, M., A model of bone adaptation as an optimization process. *J. Biomechanics*, **33**, pp. 1349–1357, 2000.

[48] Pedersen, P., On bone mechanics, modeling and optimization. *Meccanica*, **37**, pp. 335–342, 2002.

[49] Levenston, M.E., Beaupré, G.S., Carter, D.R. & Jacobs, C.R., A fading memory of recent loading enhances short-term bone adaptation simulations. *Bone*

Structure and Remodeling, eds. A. Odgaard & H. Weinans, World Scientific Publishing Company, Inc.: Singapore, pp. 201–212, 1994.

[50] Doblaré, M. & García, J.M., Application of an anisotropic bone-remodeling model based on a damagerepair theory to the analysis of the proximal femur before and after total hip replacement. *J. Biomechanics*, **34**, pp. 1157–1170, 2001.

[51] Doblaré, M. & García, J.M., Anisotropic bone remodeling model based on a continuum damage-repair theory. *J. Biomechanics*, **35**, pp. 1–17, 2002.

[52] Doblaré, M. García, J.M. & Cegoñino, J., Development of an internal bone remodeling theory and applications to some problems in orthopaedic biomechanics. *Meccanica*, **37**, pp. 365–374, 2002.

[53] Huiskes, R., Weinans, H., Grootenboer, H.J., Dalstra, M., Fudala, B. & Sloof, T.J., Adaptive bone-remodeling theory applied to prosthetic-design analysis. *J. Biomechanics*, **20(11,12)**, pp. 1135–1150, 1987.

[54] Weinans, H., Huiskes, R. & Grootenboer, H.J., The behavior of adaptive boneremodeling simulation models. *J. Biomechanics*, **25(12)**, pp. 1425–1441, 1992.

[55] Turner, C.H., Anne, V. & Pidaparti, R.M.V., A uniform strain criterion for trabecular bone adaptation: do continuum-level strain gradients drive adaptation? *J. Biomechanics*, **30(6)**, pp. 555–563, 1997.

[56] Impelluso, T.J., A density distributing locally orthotropic 2-d femur remodeling algorithm. *International Society of Bioengineers*, Schlieren, Switzerland, 2001.

[57] Impelluso, T.J., Locally orthotropic femur remodeling. *American Society of Biomechanics*, La Jolla, CA, 2001.

[58] Gibson, L.J. & Ashby, M.F., *Cellular Solids: Structure and Properties.* Cambridge Solid State Science Series, 1988.

[59] Miller, Z., Fuchs, M.B. & Arcan, M., Trabecular bone adaptation with an orthotropic material model. *J. Biomechanics*, **35**, pp. 247–256, 2002.

[60] Adachi, T., Tsubota, K., Tomita, Y. & Hollister, S.J., Trabecular surface remodeling simulation for cancellous bone using microstructural voxel finite element models. *J. Biomechanical Eng.*, **123**, pp. 403–409, 2001.

[61] Tsubota, K., Adachi, T. & Tomita, Y., Functional adaptation of cancellous bone in human proximal femur predicted by trabecular surface remodeling simulation toward uniform stress state. *J. Biomechanics*, **35**, pp. 1541–1551, 2002.

[62] Tsubota, K., Adachi, T. & Tomita, Y., Cancellous bone adaptation in proximal femur predicted by trabecular surface remodeling simulation. *BED-50 ASME Bioengineering Conference*, pp. 299–300, 2001.

[63] Cowin, S.C., The relationship between the elasticity tensor and the fabric tensor. *Mechanics of Materials*, **4**, pp. 137–147, 1985.

[64] Lanyon, L.E. & Rubin, C.T., Static versus dynamic loads as an influence on bone remodeling. *J. Biomechanics*, **17**, pp. 897–906, 1984.

[65] Rubin, C.T. & Lanyon, L.E., Regulation of bone formation by applied dynamic loads. *J. Bone and Joint Surgery (Am)*, **66**, pp. 397–402, 1984.

[66] O'Connor, J.A., Lanyon, L.E. & MacFie, H., The influence of strain rate on adaptive bone remodeling. *J. Biomechanics*, **15**, pp. 767–781, 1982.

[67] Turner, C.H., Three rules for bone adaptation to mechanical stimuli. *Bone*, **23(5)**, pp. 399–407, 1998.

[68] Weinbaum, S., Cowin, S.C. & Zeng, Y., A model for the excitation of osteocytes by mechanical loading-induced bone fluid shear stresses on osteocytic processes. *J. Biomechanics*, **27(3)**, pp. 339–360, 1994.

[69] You, L. & Cowin, S., A model for strain amplification in the actin cytoskeleton of osteocytes due to fluid drag on pericellular matrix. *J. Biomechanics*, **34**, pp. 1375–1386, 2001.

[70] You, L., Cowin, S.C., Schaffer, M.B. & Weinbaum, S., Fluid now induced strain amplification in bone cells. *Trans. 47th Orthopaedic Research Society*, San Francisco, CA, p. 563, 2001.

[71] The standardized femur program home page, Int. Soc. of Biomechanics. www.cineca.it/hosted/LTM-IOR/back2net/standfem/standfem.html.

[72] Yang, G., Kabel, J., van Rietbergen, B., Odgaard, A. & Huiskes, R., The anisotropic hooke's law for cancellous bone and wood. *J. Elasticity*, **53**, pp. 125–146, 1999.

[73] Wagner, H. & Blickhan, R., Stabilizing function of antagonistic neuromusculoskeletal systems: an analytical investigation. *Biol. Cybern.*, **89(1)**, pp. 71–79, 2003.

[74] Lloyd, D.G. & Besier, T.F., An EMG-driven musculoskeletal model to estimate muscle forces and knee joint moments in vivo. *J. Biomechanics*, **36(6)**, pp. 765–776, 2003.

[75] Manal, K. & Buchanan, T.S., A one parameter neural activation to muscle activation model: estimating isometric joint moments from electromyograms. *J. Biomechanics*, **36(8)**, pp. 1197–1202, 2003.

[76] Fung, Y.C., *Biomechanics: Mechanical Properties of Living Tissues, 2nd Ed.* Springer-Verlag, 1993.

[77] Atkins, D., Revolutionizing science and engineering through cyberinfrastructure. Technical report, National Science Foundation, 2003.

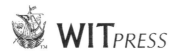

WITPRESS

Modelling in Medicine and Biology VI

Editors: *M. URSINO, University of Bologna, Italy,* **C.A. BREBBIA***, Wessex Institute of Technology, UK,* **G. PONTRELLI***, C.N.R., Istituto per le Applicazioni del Calcolo, Rome, Italy and* **E. MAGOSSO***, University of Bologna, Italy*

Featuring contributions from the Sixth International Conference on Modelling in Medicine and Biology, this volume covers a broad spectrum of topics including the application of computers to simulate biomedical phenomena. It will be of interest both to medical and physical scientists and engineers and to professionals working in medical enterprises actively involved in this field.

Areas highlighted include: Simulation of Physiological Processes; Computational Fluid Dynamics in Biomedicine; Orthopaedics and Bone Mechanics; Simulations in Surgery; Design and Simulation of Artificial Organs; Computers and Expert Systems in Medicine; Advanced Technology in Dentistry; Gait and Motion Analysis; Cardiovascular System; Virtual Reality in Medicine; Biomechanics; and Neural Systems.

Series: Advances in Bioengineering, Vol 2
ISBN: 1-84564-024-1 2005 apx 500pp apx £175.00/US$280.00/€262.50

WIT*Press*
Ashurst Lodge, Ashurst, Southampton, SO40 7AA, UK.
Tel: 44 (0) 238 029 3223
Fax: 44 (0) 238 029 2853
E-Mail: witpress@witpress.com

Wall-Fluid Interactions in Physiological Flows

Editors: *M.W. COLLINS, London South Bank University, UK,* **G. PONTRELLI***, C.N.R., Istituto per le Applicazioni del Calcolo, Rome, Italy and* **M.A. ATHERTON***, London South Bank University, UK*

All fluid flow problems in the human body involve interaction with the vessel wall. This volume presents a number of studies where primarily mathematical modelling has been applied to a variety of medical wall-fluid interaction problems. The medical applications discussed are highly varied, while some key clinical areas are also addressed. Unusually, a number of important medical challenges involving fluid flow are considered in combination with the relevant solid mechanics.

For the researcher this book offers new scope for developing and demonstrating a mastery of the scientific principles involved.

Partial Contents: Numerical Simulation of Arterial Pulse Propagation Using One-Dimensional Models; Modelling the Reopening of Liquid-Lined Lung Airways; A Finite-Volume Model of the Guldner 'Frogger' - A Training Device for Skeletal Muscle in Cardiac Assist Use Both in Training Mode and Coupled to a Ventricular Assist Device; Geometric Constraints in the Feto-Placental Circulation - Umbilical Cord Coiling and Ductus Venosus Dilation; Numerical Modelling of Blood Flow in a Stented Artery.

Series: Advances in Computational Bioengineering, Vol 6
ISBN: 1-85312-899-6 2004 204pp £75.00/US$120.00/€112.50

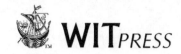

Human Respiration

Anatomy and Physiology, Mathematical Modelling, Numerical Simulation and Applications

Editor: V. KULISH, Nanyang Technological University, Singapore

Books on human respiration are usually written either only by physicians or engineers. The product of close collaboration between both, this volume presents the latest developments and major challenges in the area of biomedical engineering concerned with studies of the human respiratory system.

The contributors cover the anatomy and physiology of human respiration, some of the newest macro- and microscopic models of the respiratory system, numerical simulation and computer visualisation of gas transport phenomena, and applications of these models to medical diagnostics, treatment and safety.

Series: Advances in Bioengineering, Vol 3
ISBN: 1-85312-944-5 2005 apx 350pp
apx £115.00/US$184.00/€172.50

Simulations in Biomedicine V

Editors: Z.M. ARNEZ, University Medical Centre Ljubljana, Slovenia, C.A. BREBBIA, Wessex Institute of Technology, UK, F. SOLINA, University of Ljubljana, Slovenia and V. STANKOVSKI, University Medical Centre Ljubljana, Slovenia

This book contains papers presented at the Fifth International Conference on Computer Simulations in Biomedicine. These are divided under headings such as: Simulation of Physiological Processes; Artificial Limbs & Joints - Orthopaedics & Biomechanics; Data Acquisition & Computer Vision - Analysis & Diagnostics; Applications of Artificial Intelligence in Medicine; and Virtual & Intelligent Environments.

Series: Advances in Computational Bioengineering, Vol 7
ISBN: 1-85312-965-8 2003 544pp
£179.00/US$269.00/€268.50

Vascular Grafts

Experiment and Modelling

Editor: A. TURA, LADSEB-CNR, Italy

An extensive summary of all the haemodynamic, geometric, and mechanical elements which can influence the success or failure of graft implantations. The contributions come from a variety of research units with international reputations and this allows the reader to compare alternative approaches to similar problems.

Series: Advances in Fluid Mechanics, Vol 34
ISBN: 1-85312-900-3 2003 440pp
£138.00/US$213.00/€207.00